Digital Transformation of the Health Sector in Africa

A Framework for Inclusive, Scalable and Sustainable Health Systems Digitalization

Lishan Adam

First published in the United States in 2026

ISBN: 978-1-972592-02-1 Paperback

ISBN: 978-1-972592-03-8 Hardback

Table of Contents

List of Tables

List of Figures

PREFACE

Africa stands at this precise moment in history at an inflection point that may not recur. The convergence of factors is extraordinary: the fastest-growing population; a mobile connectivity revolution that has leapfrogged the infrastructure constraints of the twentieth century; a generation of digitally fluent health workers; a hard-earned post-pandemic confidence that African institutions can move with speed and purpose when the stakes demand it; and — crucially — a growing political recognition that dependence on external systems and financing is not a foundation. It is a vulnerability.

At the same time, the continent bears wounds that no technology can ignore. Thirteen health workers per 10,000 people and 420 million people who live more than an hour's travel from a hospital. Health systems where out-of-pocket payments still push millions into poverty each year. A quadruple burden of disease that no single platform can address.

This book was written to highlight the link between digital technologies and health, beginning with the COVID-19 pandemic and extending through the disruptions in global health funding in 2025—particularly the abrupt withdrawal of bilateral aid that supported fragile digital health systems across the continent. The purpose was to vividly demonstrate this connection to inspire decision-makers, civil society groups, academia, and medical informatics students.

The literature on digital health in Africa has grown substantially over the past decade. Much of it is excellent. Yet it has tended toward one of two modes: the granular case study — illuminating but difficult to generalize — or the sweeping framework — comprehensive but disconnected from implementation realities. This book fills the gap by outlining a comprehensive architecture for digital health in developing-country contexts, particularly in Africa.

The Digital Health Technology Stack introduced in Chapter 4 is, to my knowledge, the most coherent and practical organizing model for African digital health published to date. It does not claim that technology alone determines outcomes. Its five foundation layers — infrastructure, identity, interoperability, data, and applications — are inseparable from the seven cross-cutting enablers that determine whether those foundations ever become functional health systems: workforce, research, ecosystem, strategy, governance, regional cooperation, and financing. The insight that the enabling environment consistently defeats technology is not new. What is new is the rigor with which this book maps the relationship between the two and the clarity with which it shows that investing in one without the other is, in effect, investing in failure.

The most politically important argument in this book is also the quietest. It runs through every chapter like a thread: digital health, without deliberate and structural commitment to equity, will not reduce Africa's health disparities. It will reorganize them. A health information system that systematically undercounts the rural poor produces bad data. Bad data produces bad decisions. Bad decisions produce bad outcomes. Equity is not a value added to the technical agenda. It is a precondition for the technical agenda to mean anything at all.

The same logic applies to the book's treatment of African-led solutions. This is not nationalism dressed as policy. The claim that DHIS2, deployed across 47 African countries; OpenMRS, running in thousands of facilities across the continent; the Community Health Toolkit; and the dozens of platforms built by African innovators have outperformed imported alternatives in resource-constrained settings is empirical. Solutions built for African realities — intermittent power, low bandwidth, mobile-first workflows, and the continent's specific epidemiological and linguistic contexts — perform better in those settings.

I also realize that books about technology and the future face a particular problem: the future arrives before they are finished. By the time you read this, some of what the book describes has already shifted. The AI governance landscape, the continental interoperability frameworks, and the financing architecture — all are in motion. The aim of this book is to provide a framework — a way of thinking about digital health transformation that will remain useful long after specific statistics have been superseded. The questions the book poses — who bears the cost, who governs the data, who holds the intellectual property, who decides what equity means in practice — are not questions with answers that expire. They are the permanent questions.

I have seen enough digital health strategies come and go to learn to be cautious about any single volume's capacity to change practice. But I have also seen, over a long career, how the absence of a shared language impedes collective action — how much time is lost to arguments over definitions, to reinventing existing frameworks, and to failing to learn from what neighboring countries have tried and found wanting. This book offers that shared language. I believe it will become a standard reference for everyone working to build the health systems that Africa's people deserve. Read it with urgency. Argue with it where you disagree. Use it to build something that will still be standing — and improving people's lives.

Lishan Adam

PART 1

Context of Digital Transformation in the Health Sector in Africa

Chapter 1: Introduction

This opening chapter sets out the book's purpose, scope, and analytical foundations. It explains why digital health transformation has become the defining imperative for African health systems in the post-COVID-19 era. It presents eight core arguments that guide the analysis, defines key concepts in the African context, describes the research methodology, and outlines the book's structure. The chapter provides the conceptual roadmap for the detailed analysis that follows.

1.1 Purpose and Scope

The digital transformation of the health sector is a crucial goal for achieving universal health coverage and improving population health outcomes in the twenty-first century. This shift is especially urgent—and more difficult—to implement in Africa, where healthcare systems face persistent infrastructure gaps, workforce shortages, and resource limitations, all while managing a dual burden of communicable and non-communicable diseases (World Health Organization, 2021). The COVID-19 pandemic, which spread across the continent starting in early 2020, served as both a catalyst and a testing ground for digital health innovation, accelerating the adoption of technologies that had previously faced resistance and exposing significant gaps in digital readiness (Nachega et al., 2021).

This book explores the state of digital health transformation in Africa in the post-COVID-19 era—a period marked by unprecedented momentum for change, heightened awareness of health system vulnerabilities, and a growing recognition that digital technologies are not merely optional enhancements but vital infrastructure for building resilient, responsive, and equitable healthcare. The purpose of this work is threefold:

- First, to provide a comprehensive assessment of where African countries currently stand in their digital health development;

- Second, to analyze the core building blocks, policy frameworks, and implementation challenges that influence the success or failure of digital health initiatives; and

- Third, to present evidence-based strategies and practical recommendations to accelerate digital health transformation throughout the continent.

The scope encompasses all African Union Member States, recognizing both the diversity of contexts and the shared challenges that unify the continent's health systems. The analysis covers multiple aspects of digital health transformation, including clinical care delivery, public health surveillance, health system management, medical education, pharmaceutical supply chains, and health research (Wamala & Augustine, 2022). It spans the full spectrum of digital health technologies—from basic health information systems and mobile health apps to emerging artificial intelligence and machine learning capabilities that promise to transform diagnostics, treatment planning, and epidemic preparedness (Budd et al., 2020).

This volume targets a diverse audience: policymakers and government officials responsible for health and information technology strategies; healthcare administrators and clinical leaders implementing digital solutions; technology entrepreneurs and private sector innovators developing health technologies; development partners and donors supporting health systems strengthening; academic researchers studying digital health implementation; and students preparing for careers at the intersection of health and technology. While the book maintains analytical rigor and draws on extensive research evidence, it is written to be accessible to readers without specialized technical backgrounds, using clear language and concrete examples to clarify complex concepts.

1.2 Imperatives for Digital Transformation in the Health Sector

The COVID-19 pandemic underscored the importance of timely data, coordination, and adaptable service delivery in managing public health emergencies. Many African health systems faced challenges, including delayed reporting, limited testing capacity, and fragmented information flows. At the same time, the pandemic showed that digital solutions are feasible even in resource-limited settings when political will and urgency are present. Beyond emergency response, digital transformation is essential for addressing long-term health issues: managing the growing burden of non-communicable diseases, improving maternal and child health outcomes, strengthening pharmaceutical supply chains, and reaching remote and underserved populations. Digital tools improve efficiency, transparency, and accountability, leading to more effective use of limited resources (World Bank, 2022).

Importantly, digital health aligns with broader development goals. Investments in connectivity, data systems, and digital skills not only improve health outcomes but also boost economic growth, innovation, and government capacity. In this way, digital health transformation serves as both a sector-specific priority and a cross-sector enabler of development. The African Union's Agenda 2063, the Sustainable Development Goals, and the WHO Global Strategy on Digital Health 2020–2025 all recognize digital health as a key driver of broader development objectives (WHO, 2021).

1.3 Definition of Digital Health Transformation

Digital health uses information and communication technologies to improve health outcomes, enhance healthcare delivery, strengthen health systems, and empower patients and communities (WHO, 2021). This broad definition encompasses several related terms that have evolved over time: eHealth (electronic health), mHealth (mobile health), telehealth and telemedicine, health information systems, health informatics, and health technology. Although there are subtle distinctions among these terms, this book uses "digital health" as a general term for all applications of digital technologies to health challenges, consistent with WHO's current perspective.

Figure 1.1. presents the digital health technology spectrum in Africa: current adoption levels (bars) compared with transformative potential (line). Foundational technologies, such as health information systems and mHealth, have the highest current adoption. In contrast, emerging technologies, including AI, IoMT, blockchain, and genomics, have low adoption but very high transformative potential.

Figure 1.1. Digital Health Technology Spectrum in Africa: Current Adoption Vs. Transformative Potential

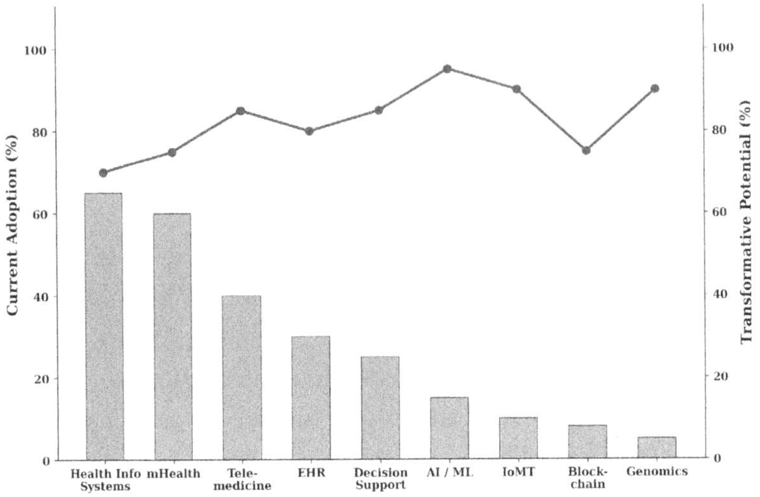

Sources: WHO (2021), Budd et al. (2020), Esteva et al. (2019).

Digital transformation is broader than technology adoption alone. While **digitization** refers to converting analog information into digital form (such as scanning paper records), **digitalization** involves using digital technologies to alter processes or business models. D**igital transformation** requires a fundamental rethinking of how organizations create value, deliver services, and engage stakeholders in the digital age (Vial, 2019). In healthcare, digital transformation means more than implementing electronic health records or telemedicine platforms; it involves reimagining how healthcare is organized, delivered, and financed—using digital technologies as the foundation (Kraus et al., 2021).

These key concepts and definitions, with source attributions, are used throughout this book. The definitions provide the terminological foundation for the analysis in subsequent chapters.

Table 1.1. Key Concepts and Definitions

Term	Definition
Digital Health	The use of information and communication technologies to improve health outcomes, enhance healthcare delivery, strengthen health systems, and empower patients and communities.
Digitization	Converting analog information into digital format (e.g., scanning paper records).
Digitalization	Using digital technologies to change existing processes or create new business models.
Digital Transformation	A fundamental rethinking of how organizations create value and deliver services using digital technologies.
eHealth	The use of electronic means to deliver health information, resources, and services.
mHealth	The use of mobile and wireless technologies for health objectives.
Telemedicine	Delivery of healthcare services at a distance using telecommunications technology.
Health Information System (HIS)	A system designed to manage health data, including collection, storage, management, and transmission.
Electronic Health Record (EHR)	A digital version of a patient's medical history maintained over time.
Interoperability	The ability of different information systems, devices, and applications to access, exchange, and use data in a coordinated manner.
Health Data Governance	The framework for managing the availability, usability, integrity, and security of health data.
Leapfrogging	Skipping intermediate developmental stages to adopt advanced technologies directly.

Source: Author's Elaboration

In the African context, digital health transformation has several distinct features:

- First, it often involves **leapfrogging**—skipping intermediate developmental stages to adopt advanced technologies, as the continent did by bypassing landline infrastructure to embrace mobile telephony (James, 2009). Countries with minimal legacy health information systems may be better positioned to implement modern, interoperable systems than those burdened by decades-old infrastructure.

- Second, transformation occurs in **resource-scarce** environments, requiring solutions that function with intermittent connectivity, limited electricity, and minimal technical support—constraints that foster innovation in low-cost, durable, and user-friendly technologies (Katurura & Cilliers, 2018).

- Third, African digital health transformation is marked by **innovation at the margins**, with many breakthrough solutions emerging from African entrepreneurs and organizations rather than being imported from high-income countries (Foster & Heeks, 2013).

1.4 Core Arguments and Key Messages

This book presents eight key arguments that challenge conventional beliefs about digital health in resource-limited settings and offer a realistic yet hopeful outlook for Africa's digital health future. These arguments guide the analysis throughout the book and are revisited with supporting evidence in later chapters.

Digital Health as Infrastructure—the main argument of this book is that digital health should be seen as essential health system infrastructure rather than just a set of applications or short-term projects. Just as health systems rely on physical facilities, trained staff, and essential medicines, they also depend on information systems, data, data standards, connectivity, and analytics capabilities to operate effectively. This perspective has significant implications for financing, governance, and institutional design: infrastructure requires ongoing investment, long-term maintenance, and dedicated institutional ownership—none of which are typical of the project-based, donor-funded approach that has dominated digital health in Africa for decades (WHO, 2021; Scott et al., 2017).

The COVID-19 inflection point—the pandemic marked a critical moment in Africa's digital health progress. Although digital health initiatives had existed on the continent for many years, progress was slow, fragmented, and often unsustainable (Mehl & Labrique, 2014). The pandemic compelled rapid change out of necessity: countries that had spent years debating telemedicine rules rapidly rolled out virtual care platforms; governments that had previously resisted electronic health records suddenly prioritized digital patient tracking; and healthcare workers who had avoided using technology became proficient with digital tools. Countries swiftly adopted digital solutions for monitoring, contact tracing, telemedicine, supply chain management, and vaccine certification (Whitelaw et al., 2020). However, many of these efforts were implemented under emergency conditions, raising questions about their long-term sustainability, compatibility, and integration into national health systems—topics this book explores in depth.

Figure 1.2 COVID-19 as a Catalyst: Digital Health Adoption in Africa, Before and After the Pandemic.

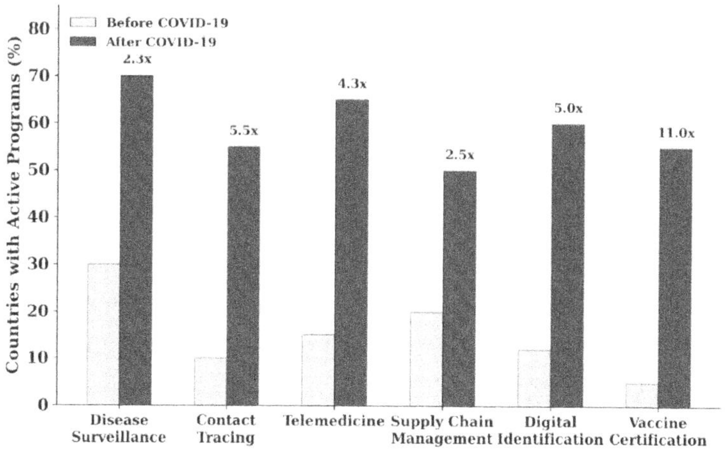

Source: WHO Africa (2022), Nachenga et al. (2021), Whitelaw et al. (2020)

The catalytic effect of COVID-19 on digital health adoption across six domains in Africa, as measured by the proportion of countries with active programs before and after the pandemic, indicates the scale of acceleration, with telemedicine and digital identification showing the most dramatic growth.

African-led solutions and contextual adaptation— the history of international development, including digital health initiatives, is marked by well-meaning efforts that failed because they overlooked local contexts, underestimated implementation challenges, or created dependencies on external expertise and funding (Aanestad & Jensen, 2011). Successful digital health transformation in Africa requires solutions tailored to environments with unreliable electricity and Internet access, built on open-source technologies that prevent vendor lock-in, integrated with existing clinical workflows rather than disrupting them, and owned and maintained by African institutions and professionals. Africa's digital health future depends not on importing technologies developed elsewhere but on adapting to local contexts, fostering local innovation, and developing African-led solutions that leverage the continent's unique strengths—including its mobile-first digital culture, its vibrant technology entrepreneurship ecosystem, and its proven capacity for leapfrog innovation (Katurura & Cilliers, 2018; Foster & Heeks, 2013).

The Systems Challenge—the most common reason digital health initiatives fail is not technical shortcomings but inadequate attention to the enabling conditions that determine whether technologies are adopted, sustained, and expanded (Greenhalgh et al., 2017). As the technology stack model developed in Chapter 4 demonstrates, the architecture of digital health comprises five foundational layers—physical infrastructure and connectivity, digital identity and registries, interoperability and data exchange, data management and analytics, and applications and services. Yet these technical foundations alone are not enough. Seven cross-cutting enablers influence whether investments in the foundation layers succeed or fail: digital health strategy; governance, policy, and standards; digital health skills and workforce; research and development priorities; the healthTech ecosystem; regional cooperation; and financing and sustainability.

This distinction between foundations and enablers offers a key insight: there are usually more enablers than foundations, and it is generally the enablers—not the technology—that determine outcomes. A country might invest heavily in connectivity infrastructure and implement advanced electronic health record systems yet still fall short of meaningful digital health transformation because it lacks a coherent national strategy to coordinate investments, governance frameworks to protect data and build public trust, a skilled workforce to implement and sustain systems, a research ecosystem to generate local evidence, a private healthtech sector to develop and adapt solutions, or sustainable funding to maintain systems beyond initial deployment. The history of digital health in Africa is filled with examples of technically sound systems that failed because one or more of these enablers were absent (Scott et al., 2017; Kivuti-Bitok et al., 2024).

The implication for policymakers is clear: digital health transformation requires investments in enablers that are just as deliberate and substantial as those in foundational elements. Achieving successful transformation requires simultaneous progress across all twelve aspects of the stack—comprising five foundations and seven enablers—rather than completing one before starting another. The World Health Organization's assessment indicates that the largest gaps between importance and readiness are in the cross-cutting enablers—especially governance, workforce, and financing—highlighting that the enabling environment, not just the technical infrastructure, determines success.

Regional Collaboration—many African countries are too small and face resource constraints that prevent them from developing comprehensive digital health ecosystems independently, negotiating favorable terms with technology vendors, or supporting specialized training institutions (Fritz et al., 2015). Regional approaches enable shared infrastructure, joint procurement, cross-border exchange of patient data, collaborative research networks, and economies of scale in capacity building. Institutions such as the Africa Center for Disease Control and Prevention (Africa CDC), the African Union Commission, and Regional Economic Communities provide platforms for coordinated strategies and shared resources (Adepoju et al., 2017).

Equity and inclusion—achieving health equity in the digital age requires deliberate strategies to ensure digital technologies do not widen existing disparities. Digital health can improve access for underserved rural communities, connect remote facilities with specialists, and empower patients through information and self-management tools (Bashshur et al., 2020). However, without careful attention to equity—across urban–rural, gender, income, education, and age groups—digital health risks creating a two-tier healthcare system that benefits the already privileged while leaving the most vulnerable even further behind (Nouri et al., 2020).

Figure 1.3 illustrates a multi-dimensional digital divide in African healthcare, highlighting disparities across urban–rural and gender dimensions for six indicators. The largest gaps are in health-specific digital applications (telemedicine, health apps), where access is limited for rural and female populations.

Figure 1.3 The Digital Divide in African Healthcare: Urban-Rural and Gender Dimensions

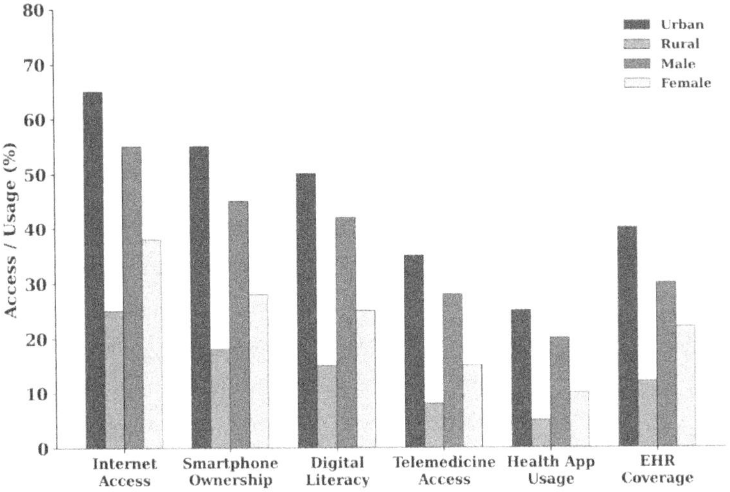

Source: GSMA (2023), ITU (2022), Nouri et al. (2020)

1.5 Methodology and Research Approach

This book synthesizes evidence from diverse sources and methodological approaches to provide a comprehensive, rigorous, and practical analysis of digital health transformation in Africa. The research combines systematic literature reviews, case studies, and expert consultations. It also draws on the authors' extensive implementation experience across African contexts.

Literature Review and Evidence Synthesis

A comprehensive review of published and grey literature supports this work. Academic databases—including PubMed, Web of Science, Scopus, and Google Scholar—were systematically searched for peer-reviewed articles on digital health in Africa published between 2010 and 2025, with a particular focus on post-2019 publications addressing the impacts of COVID-19. The academic literature was complemented by grey literature from international organizations such as the WHO, and other agencies like ITU, UNICEF, the Inter-American Development Bank, the African Development Bank, and the World Bank, as well as bilateral development agencies, foundations, and research institutions. Reports from the Health Information Systems Programme (HISP), the Digital Square initiative, and country-specific assessments conducted by WHO provided valuable insights into implementation, which are often missing from academic publications (Honeyman et al., 2020; Labrique et al., 2018).

The evidence synthesis recognizes that digital health research draws on multiple disciplines—ranging from randomized controlled trials assessing health outcomes to qualitative studies examining implementation processes, to design science focused on developing and testing information systems (Paré et al., 2015). When high-quality evidence was available, systematic reviews and meta-analyses were prioritized. When evidence was limited or contradictory, implementation experiences and expert opinions informed the analysis, and gaps were clearly identified (Aranda-Jan et al., 2014).

Throughout the book, case studies illustrate key concepts, document implementation experiences, and draw lessons. Cases were selected to reflect geographic diversity across all African regions, variation in country income levels and health system maturity, a range of digital health interventions, and a range of outcomes, including notable successes and instructive failures. International cases were deliberately selected to illustrate best practices and failures in the Global South, as well as in countries that delivered digital health in the Global North. The case study approach aligns with established methods in information systems research and implementation science, recognizing that understanding how and why interventions work (or fail) in specific contexts is as important as knowing whether they work on average (Yin, 2017; Greenhalgh et al., 2017).

Analytical Framework

The book employs an integrated analytical framework drawing on multiple theoretical perspectives: health systems thinking, which emphasizes the links between digital health and other parts of the health system (Marchal et al., 2014); implementation science frameworks, which guide the analysis of adoption, fidelity, and sustainability (Proctor et al., 2011); information systems success models, which inform assessments of technology design and organizational impacts (DeLone & McLean, 2016); and political economy analysis, which illuminates how power dynamics, incentives, and governance structures influence digital health outcomes (Sheikh et al., 2014).

Limitations and Caveats

Several limitations must be acknowledged. The evidence base for digital health in Africa is limited for many interventions and outcomes, and publication bias toward successful interventions and English-speaking countries likely skews the available literature. Rapid technological change means that some content may quickly become outdated, particularly regarding specific technologies and solutions. Africa's diversity means that generalizations necessarily oversimplify: what works in one setting may not work in another. The author's perspectives reflect specific experiences and professional networks, which may not encompass all viewpoints. These limitations have been addressed through rigorous methodology, an extensive literature review, diverse case study selection, and cautious interpretation of the evidence (Aranda-Jan et al., 2014).

Table 1.2. Research Method

Method	Description
Systematic Literature Review	Comprehensive searches of PubMed, Scopus, Web of Science, Google Scholar for peer-reviewed articles (2010–2025), complemented by grey literature from WHO, ITU, World Bank, and other organizations.
Case Study Analysis	In-depth examination of digital health implementations across African regions, selected for geographic diversity, income variation, and intervention type.
Expert Consultation	Engagement with digital health practitioners, policymakers, technology developers, and academic researchers across the continent.
Comparative Analysis	Cross-country and cross-regional comparison of digital health strategies, policies, and outcomes using standardized frameworks.
Analytical Frameworks	Integration of health systems thinking, implementation science, information systems success models, and political economy analysis.

1.6 Structure and Organization

The book is divided into four parts, each with a specific analytical purpose, that collectively provide a comprehensive overview of Africa's digital health transformation—from background and current conditions to essential requirements and future strategic directions.

- Part 1: Setting the Scene lays the foundation by exploring Africa's health sector landscape, available digital technologies for transformation, and essential cross-cutting issues such as equity, privacy, and sustainability.
- Part 2: Discusses the foundations of Digital Health. Chapters 7 through 10 cover the five foundational layers: infrastructure and connectivity (Chapter 7), digital identity and registries (Chapter 8),

interoperability and health information exchange (Chapter 9), and data management, quality, and analytics (Chapter 10).

- Part 3 covers the enablers of digital health. Chapters 11 through 17 address the seven cross-cutting enablers: digital health skills and workforce (Chapter 11), research and development priorities (Chapter 12), the healthtech ecosystem and private-sector engagement (Chapter 13), national health strategies (Chapter 14), governance policies and standards (Chapter 15), regional cooperation (Chapter 16), and financing and sustainability (Chapter 17). This structure reflects a central argument of the book: that enabling conditions are at least as important as technical foundations, and that investment in enablers must accompany investment in infrastructure.

- Part 4: Strategic Pathways (Chapter 18) synthesizes lessons, recommends priority interventions and implementation roadmaps, clarifies stakeholder roles, and concludes with a call to action for all invested in Africa's digital health future.

1.7 Conclusion

This introductory chapter has established both the urgency and the analytical framework for understanding digital health transformation in Africa. The continent stands at a pivotal juncture: the convergence of post-pandemic momentum, expanding mobile connectivity, a growing cadre of African technology innovators, and increasing political commitment to digital governance creates conditions for transformative change that are unlikely to recur in the near term.

The chapter advances several foundational propositions that will be examined in depth throughout the remainder of this book. Chief among them is the argument that digital health must be reconceived as essential infrastructure—requiring the same sustained investment, institutional stewardship, and strategic planning that governments apply to physical health facilities and human resources for health. The prevailing project-based, donor-dependent model has produced fragmented systems, duplicated efforts, and unsustainable interventions. A paradigm shift toward infrastructure thinking is a prerequisite for meaningful progress.

Equally important is recognizing that technology alone does not determine outcomes. The distinction between foundational layers and cross-cutting enablers—and the fact that enablers outnumber foundations—underscores a consistent pattern in the history of digital health on the continent: technically competent systems often fail when governance, workforce capacity, financing mechanisms, or strategic coordination are lacking. Policymakers and implementers who invest disproportionately in technology acquisition while neglecting the enabling environment are likely to repeat the failures of the past two decades.

The COVID-19 pandemic demonstrated what is possible when urgency overrides institutional resistance. The two- to fourfold acceleration in digital health adoption across multiple domains—documented in the evidence above—confirms that African health systems can adapt quickly. The real question is no longer whether digital transformation is possible, but whether the necessary political will, institutional structures, and financial support are in place to sustain and expand it.

The multi-dimensional digital divide identified in this chapter presents both a moral imperative and a practical constraint. If digital health transformation proceeds without deliberate equity strategies, it risks reinforcing the disparities it purports to address—concentrating benefits among urban, educated, male, and economically advantaged populations while leaving the most health-vulnerable communities further marginalized. Equity must be embedded in design, deployment, and evaluation from the outset, not treated as an afterthought.

Finally, the methodological approach outlined here—combining a systematic literature review, case study analysis, expert consultation, and multi-framework analysis—reflects the subject's complexity. Digital health transformation sits at the intersection of technology, health systems, governance, economics, and social equity. No single disciplinary lens is sufficient. The integrated framework adopted in this book aims to provide a comprehensive yet grounded analysis that the moment demands.

The chapters that follow build on these foundations, moving from broad contextual analysis to a detailed examination of each foundational layer and cross-cutting enabler, and then to strategic recommendations tailored to different country contexts and regional realities. The goal throughout is to equip readers—whether policymakers, practitioners, researchers, or students—with both the conceptual understanding and the practical guidance needed to advance Africa's digital health transformation.

References

Aanestad, M., & Jensen, T. B. (2011). Building nation-wide information infrastructures in healthcare through modular implementation strategies. Journal of Strategic Information Systems, 20(2), 161–176. https://doi.org/10.1016/j.jsis.2011.03.006

Adepoju, I. O., Albersen, B. J., De Brouwere, V., van Roosmalen, J., & Zweekhorst, M. (2017). mHealth for clinical decision-making in sub-Saharan Africa: A scoping review. JMIR mHealth and uHealth, 5(3), e38. https://doi.org/10.2196/mhealth.7185

Aranda-Jan, C. B., Mohutsiwa-Dibe, N., & Loukanova, S. (2014). Systematic review on what works, what does not work and why of the implementation of mobile health (mHealth) projects in Africa. BMC Public Health, 14, 188. https://doi.org/10.1186/1471-2458-14-188

Bashshur, R. L., Doarn, C. R., Frenk, J. M., Kvedar, J. C., Shannon, G. W., & Woolliscroft, J. O. (2020). Beyond the COVID pandemic, telemedicine, and health care. Telemedicine and e-Health, 26(11), 1310–1313. https://doi.org/10.1089/tmj.2020.29288.rb

Benson, T., & Grieve, G. (2016). Principles of health interoperability: SNOMED CT, HL7 and FHIR (3rd ed.). Springer. https://doi.org/10.1007/978-3-319-30370-3

Budd, J., Miller, B. S., Manning, E. M., et al. (2020). Digital technologies in the public-health response to COVID-19. Nature Medicine, 26(8), 1183–1192. https://doi.org/10.1038/s41591-020-1011-4

DeLone, W. H., & McLean, E. R. (2016). Information systems success measurement. Foundations and Trends in Information Systems, 2(1), 1–116. https://doi.org/10.1561/2900000005

Esteva, A., Robicquet, A., Ramsundar, B., et al. (2019). A guide to deep learning in healthcare. Nature Medicine, 25(1), 24–29. https://doi.org/10.1038/s41591-018-0316-z

Floridi, L., Cowls, J., Beltrametti, M., et al. (2018). AI4People—An ethical framework for a good AI society. Minds and Machines, 28(4), 689–707. https://doi.org/10.1007/s11023-018-9482-5

Foster, C., & Heeks, R. (2013). Conceptualising inclusive innovation. European Journal of Development Research, 25(3), 333–355. https://doi.org/10.1057/ejdr.2013.7

Fritz, F., Tilahun, B., & Dugas, M. (2015). Success criteria for electronic medical record implementations in low-resource settings: A systematic review. Journal of the American Medical Informatics Association, 22(2), 479–488. https://doi.org/10.1093/jamia/ocu038

Greenhalgh, T., Wherton, J., Papoutsi, C., et al. (2017). Beyond adoption: A new framework for theorizing and evaluating nonadoption, abandonment, and challenges to the scale-up, spread, and sustainability of health and care technologies. Journal of Medical Internet Research, 19(11), e367. https://doi.org/10.2196/jmir.8775

Greenhalgh, T., Koh, G. C. H., & Car, J. (2020). COVID-19: A remote assessment in primary care. BMJ, 368, m1182. https://doi.org/10.1136/bmj.m1182

Honeyman, M., Maguire, D., Evans, H., & Davies, A. (2020). Digital technology and health inequalities: A scoping review. Public Health Wales NHS Trust.

James, J. (2009). Leapfrogging in mobile telephony: A measure for comparing country performance. Technological Forecasting and Social Change, 76(7), 991–998. https://doi.org/10.1016/j.techfore.2009.04.002

Katurura, M. C., & Cilliers, L. (2018). Electronic health record system in the public health care sector of South Africa: A systematic literature review. African Journal of Primary Health Care & Family Medicine, 10(1), e1–e8. https://doi.org/10.4102/phcfm.v10i1.1746

Kivuti-Bitok, L. W., Leshan, L., & Osero, J. (2024). Digital health innovations in Kenya: Opportunities and challenges. BMC Health Services Research, 24(1), 45. https://doi.org/10.1186/s12913-024-10512-x

Kraus, S., Schiavone, F., Pluzhnikova, A., & Invernizzi, A. C. (2021). Digital transformation in healthcare: Analyzing the current state-of-research. Journal of Business Research, 123, 557–567. https://doi.org/10.1016/j.jbusres.2020.10.030

Labrique, A. B., Wadhwani, C., Williams, K. A., et al. (2018). Best practices in scaling digital health in low and middle-income countries. Globalization and Health, 14(1), 103. https://doi.org/10.1186/s12992-018-0424-z

Marchal, B., Dedzo, M., & Kegels, G. (2014). A realist evaluation of the management of a well-performing regional hospital in Ghana. BMC Health Services Research, 10, 24. https://doi.org/10.1186/1472-6963-10-24

Mehl, G., & Labrique, A. (2014). Prioritizing integrated mHealth strategies for universal health coverage. Science, 345(6202), 1284–1287. https://doi.org/10.1126/science.1258926

Nachega, J. B., Atteh, R., Ihekweazu, C., et al. (2021). Contact tracing and the COVID-19 response in Africa: Best practices, key challenges, and lessons learned. American Journal of Tropical Medicine and Hygiene, 104(4), 1179–1187. https://doi.org/10.4269/ajtmh.20-1513

Nouri, S., Khoong, E. C., Lyles, C. R., & Karliner, L. (2020). Addressing equity in telemedicine for chronic disease management during the COVID-19 pandemic. NEJM Catalyst Innovations in Care Delivery, 1(3). https://doi.org/10.1056/CAT.20.0123

Paré, G., Tate, M., Johnstone, D., & Kitsiou, S. (2015). Contextualizing the twin concepts of systematicity and transparency in information systems literature reviews. European Journal of Information Systems, 25(6), 493–508. https://doi.org/10.1057/ejis.2016.10

Proctor, E., Silmere, H., Raghavan, R., et al. (2011). Outcomes for implementation research. Administration and Policy in Mental Health, 38(2), 65–76. https://doi.org/10.1007/s10488-010-0319-7

Reich, M. R., Harris, J., Ikegami, N., et al. (2016). Moving towards universal health coverage: Lessons from 11 country studies. The Lancet, 387(10020), 811–816. https://doi.org/10.1016/S0140-6736(15)60002-2

Rosenbaum, S. (2010). Data governance and stewardship. Health Services Research, 45(5 Pt 2), 1442–1455. https://doi.org/10.1111/j.1475-6773.2010.01140.x

Scott, R. E., Mars, M., & Scalvini, S. (2017). The role of digital technologies in strengthening health systems. Journal of Telemedicine and Telecare, 23(10), 877–878. https://doi.org/10.1177/1357633X17735858

Sheikh, K., Schneider, H., Agyepong, I. A., Lehmann, U., & Gilson, L. (2016). Boundary-spanning: Reflections on the practices and principles of Global

Health. BMJ Global Health, 1(1), e000058. https://doi.org/10.1136/bmjgh-2016-000058

Van Dijk, J. A. G. M. (2020). The digital divide. Polity Press.

Vial, G. (2019). Understanding digital transformation: A review and a research agenda. Journal of Strategic Information Systems, 28(2), 118–144. https://doi.org/10.1016/j.jsis.2019.01.003

Wamala, D., & Augustine, K. (2022). A meta-analysis of telemedicine success in Africa. Journal of Pathology Informatics, 4, 6. https://doi.org/10.4103/2153-3539.91612

Whitelaw, S., Mamas, M. A., Topol, E., & Van Spall, H. G. C. (2020). Applications of digital technology in COVID-19 pandemic planning and response. The Lancet Digital Health, 2(8), e435–e440. https://doi.org/10.1016/S2589-7500(20)30142-4

World Bank. (2022). Digital-in-health: Unlocking the value for everyone. World Bank Group.

World Health Organization. (2007). Everybody's business: Strengthening health systems to improve health outcomes. WHO.

World Health Organization. (2021). Global strategy on digital health 2020–2025. WHO. https://www.who.int/publications/i/item/9789240020924

Yin, R. K. (2017). Case study research and applications: Design and methods (6th ed.). SAGE Publications.

Chapter 2: Africa's Health Sector Landscape

2.1 Overview

This chapter provides a comprehensive analysis of Africa's health sector landscape—the context in which digital health transformation must take place. It traces the historical forces that shaped today's health systems, examines their current state across Africa's five regions using detailed country-level data, and analyzes the key challenges—infrastructure deficits, human resource shortages, financing gaps, the quadruple disease burden, and geographic disparities—that both motivate and constrain digital health transformation. Understanding this landscape is essential for designing digital health interventions that address real needs, operate within real constraints, and avoid repeating past mistakes.

The challenges outlined in this chapter—infrastructure deficits, workforce shortages, financing gaps, disease burden, and geographic disparities—shaped the Digital Health Technology Stack introduced in Chapter 4. The stack organizes digital health architecture into five foundational layers and seven cross-cutting enablers. Each subsequent chapter in this book explores a specific aspect of the transformation agenda prompted by the landscape analysis presented in this chapter.

2.2 Historical Context of Healthcare in Africa

Understanding Africa's current health challenges requires examining the historical forces that have shaped the continent's health systems. The legacy of colonialism, post-independence nation-building struggles, structural adjustment programs, and the recent push toward universal health coverage have all had lasting effects on how health services are organized, financed, and delivered across the continent (Iliffe, 2006). Before colonization, African societies had diverse healing traditions and healthcare systems tailored to local disease patterns and cultural contexts (Feierman & Janzen, 1992).

Colonial health systems, established primarily to serve European settlers and to support a healthy workforce for extractive industries, created dual structures that favored urban areas and European populations while neglecting rural African communities (Turshen, 1984). Mission hospitals provided much of the healthcare available to Africans, shaping patterns of geographic distribution and religious affiliation that persist today (Grundmann, 2005). The colonial focus on vertical disease-control programs —targeting specific diseases such as sleeping sickness, plague, and yellow fever —set a precedent for disease-specific interventions that continued to define African health systems long after independence (Packard, 2016).

The 1960s and 1970s saw most African countries gain independence and launch ambitious efforts to build comprehensive national health systems. The 1978 Alma-Ata Declaration inspired community-based health programs, training for community health workers, and hierarchical referral systems linking village health posts to district hospitals (WHO, 1978; Sanders, 1985). However, the initial hopes following independence were undermined by economic crises, political instability, brain drain, and—most devastatingly—the structural adjustment programs of the 1980s and 1990s, which mandated cuts in public spending and the introduction of user fees for health services (Logie & Woodroffe, 1993; McPake, 1993).

The AIDS epidemic, which peaked in the late 1990s and early 2000s, overwhelmed already fragile health systems. By 2000, HIV/AIDS had become the leading cause of death in sub-Saharan Africa, devastating healthcare workforces and reversing decades of progress (UNAIDS, 2006; Barnett & Whiteside, 2006). The international response—the Global Fund (2002), the US President's Emergency Plan for AIDS and Relief (PEPFAR) (2003), and the Global Alliance for Vaccines and Immunization (GAVI)—mobilized unprecedented resources and achieved significant successes in expanding access to antiretroviral therapy, strengthening disease surveillance, and improving immunization coverage. However, these initiatives also reinforced vertical program structures, creating parallel implementation systems that bypassed national health authorities and distorted workforce allocation (Biesma et al., 2009; Marchal et al., 2009).

From around 2010 to the present, the period has seen greater African control over health plans, increased local health funding, and commitments to universal health coverage. Several countries have made significant progress: Rwanda achieved 91% health insurance coverage through community-based health insurance and performance-based financing (Binagwaho et al., 2014). Ethiopia reduced under-five mortality by 67% through its Health Extension Worker program, which deployed more than 42,000 community health workers (Federal Ministry of Health, Ethiopia, 2020). Ghana pioneered National Health Insurance in sub-Saharan Africa in 2003 (National Health Insurance Authority, Ghana, 2019). Kenya has become a hub for digital health entrepreneurship, with more than 140 digital health startups (Ministry of Health, Kenya, 2021).

Still, major challenges persist—Africa has the lowest per-capita health spending worldwide, critical workforce shortages, infrastructure gaps, and stockouts of essential medicines—creating a complex environment for digital health transformation. Recently, the 2025 restructuring of PEPFAR and the dissolution of US Agency for International Development resulted in an estimated USD 12 billion shortfall in Africa's healthcare financing, exposing the structural vulnerabilities of donor-dependent health systems and accelerating discussions about domestic resource mobilization and health financing sovereignty—dynamics examined in detail in Chapter 17. This funding disruption, along with Africa's rising debt (countries expected to service USD 81 billion in 2025), underscores the urgency of investing in sustainable, domestically driven digital health initiatives.

2.2 Current State of Health Systems Across African Regions

African countries exhibit remarkable diversity in health system performance, reflecting differences in income levels, governance quality, epidemiological profiles, and historical trajectories. Regional patterns highlight both shared challenges and important differences that shape digital health opportunities and challenges. The regional patterns summarized below are directly linked to the foundational layers of the Digital Health Technology Stack: infrastructure readiness, workforce capacity, and the high-value digital priorities for each region, explored in detail across Chapters 7 through 18.

Health expenditure per capita across Africa in 2018 shows dramatic variation, ranging from $18 in Eritrea to $570 in South Africa. The sub-Saharan African average of $129 falls far below high-income country levels of $4,000+. This variation reflects differing income levels and political priorities.

Figure 2.1 Health Expenditure Per Capita Across Africa (2018)

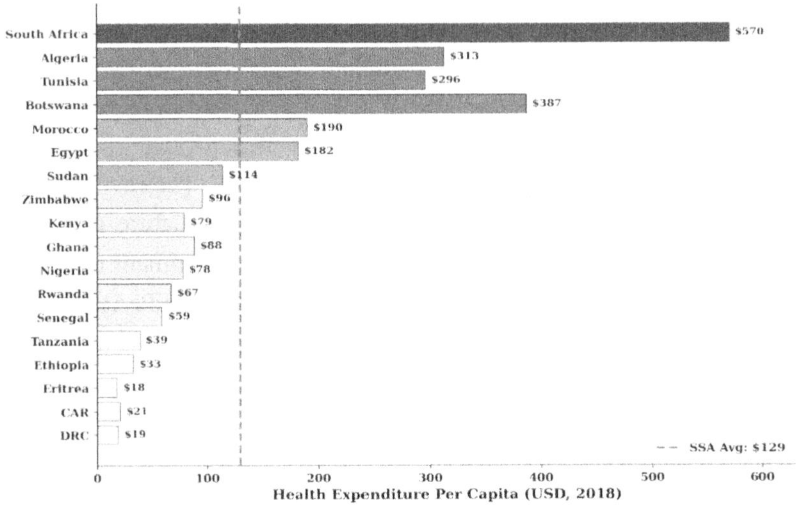

Sources: WHO (2021), Global Health Expenditure Statistics

East Africa

East Africa has a mixed health system landscape, with notable successes alongside ongoing challenges. Rwanda stands out as a regional success story, achieving significant improvements through innovative financing, strong governance, and community-based service delivery. From 2005 to 2020, Rwanda's maternal mortality ratio fell from 750 to 248 per 100,000 live births, while under-five mortality dropped from 152 to 36 per 1,000 live births. The country achieved 91% health insurance coverage through Mutuelle de Santé, supported by performance-based financing, driven by strong political commitment, 45,000 community health workers, and systematic, data-driven decision-making (Binagwaho et al., 2014; Nkurunziza et al., 2021).

Ethiopia made significant progress with its Health Extension Program, deploying over 42,000 Health Extension Workers to deliver community-level primary healthcare. This contributed to a 67% decline in under-five mortality and a rise in contraceptive use from 8% to 41% (2000–2019). However, Ethiopia still faces challenges, including 0.8 physicians per 10,000 people, a per capita health expenditure of $33, and internal disparities influenced by conflict and geographic remoteness. Kenya developed a relatively advanced health system, with rising insurance coverage (28% in 2018) and an innovative digital health ecosystem with more than 140 startups. Nonetheless, it faces significant issues, including high out-of-pocket costs (26%) and stark urban–rural disparities in physician distribution (2.0 versus 0.2 per 10,000).

Table 2.1: Key Health System Indicators for East Africa (2018–2020)

Country	HE/ Cap ($)	Govt HE (% GDP)	OOP (%)	Docs/ 10k	Nurse s/10k	Beds/ 10k	Ins. Cov. (%)
Rwanda	$67	3.1	7	1.3	8.9	16	91
Kenya	$79	2.6	26	2.0	11.6	14	28
Tanzania	$39	3.6	37	0.5	5.3	7	26
Uganda	$41	2.8	39	1.2	13.1	5	4
Ethiopia	$33	3.5	33	0.8	8.7	3	8
Burundi	$21	5.1	32	0.7	5.1	8	6
Djibouti	$117	2.1	22	2.2	15.4	14	25
Somalia	$22	0.5	76	0.3	1.8	--	3
South Sudan	$26	2.2	14	0.8	5.2	9	--

HE = Health Expenditure; OOP = Out-of-Pocket; THE = Total Health Expenditure.

Sources: WHO (2021); World Bank (2021).

East African health systems demonstrate strong innovation ecosystems and rapid adoption of digital service models, especially mobile-enabled interventions and community health worker platforms. However, ongoing primary healthcare challenges—such as facility readiness, medication availability, and referral systems—alongside workforce shortages, particularly in rural areas, limit the impact of digital solutions. Digital tools can enhance coordination and measurement, but they cannot replace missing staff, reliable power, or essential supplies.

West Africa

In West Africa, Nigeria, Africa's most populous country, has a federal health system with significant variation across states and a large private sector that serves an estimated 67% of the population. Despite being Africa's largest economy, Nigeria has struggled to translate economic resources into improvements in its health system. Immunization coverage remains a challenge, and the country has lost 8,500 doctors to the UK alone (General Medical Council UK, 2020). Ghana has been a regional leader since implementing National Health Insurance in 2003, reaching 40% coverage by 2018. Outpatient visits rose from 0.4 to 0.9 per capita, and maternal mortality fell by 57%. Senegal also performed well relative to its income level, with 91% DTP3 immunization coverage and 53% universal health coverage by 2020.

The West African Ebola epidemic of 2014–2016 devastated health systems in Guinea, Liberia, and Sierra Leone, killing 11,310 people and 881 health workers, and significantly set back development progress. However, it also catalyzed investments in health system strengthening and disease surveillance that remain relevant to digital health. The region continues to face security challenges, including Sahel insurgencies and Boko Haram violence, which disrupt health service delivery across multiple countries.

Table 2.2: Key Health System Indicators for Selected Western African Countries (2018–2020)

Country	HE/ Cap ($)	Govt HE (% GDP)	OOP (%)	Docs/ 10k	Nurse s/10k	Beds/ 10k	Ins. Cov. (%)
Nigeria	$78	3.9	77	3.8	15.6	5	5
Ghana	$88	3.4	37	1.7	32.5	9	40
Senegal	$59	4.2	50	0.7	3.1	3	53
Côte d'Ivoire	$70	2.2	44	1.6	8.4	4	10
Mali	$38	3.9	43	1.4	5.8	1	12
Burkina Faso	$44	5.6	30	0.8	6.1	4	8
Niger	$36	5.5	59	0.5	2.9	3	5
Sierra Leone	$78	10.2	68	0.3	2.3	4	11
Liberia	$88	9.5	40	0.4	2.7	8	6

Sources: WHO (2021); World Bank (2021).

Southern Africa

South Africa, the region's economic powerhouse, has a dual health system: a well-resourced private sector serving 16% of the population through medical schemes and an overburdened public sector serving 84%. The country has the world's largest HIV treatment program, with 5.1 million on ART by 2020, and among Africa's highest health expenditures at 8.1% of GDP ($570 per capita). Yet, it faces persistent inequities rooted in apartheid-era spatial segregation and a quadruple disease burden: HIV/TB, maternal/child conditions, non-communicable diseases (51% of deaths), and violence/injuries (homicide rate of 35.9 per 100,000) (Mayosi et al., 2009; UNAIDS, 2020).

The Southern African region has been heavily impacted by HIV/AIDS, with seven of the ten countries worldwide having the highest HIV prevalence rates. However, the widespread ART expansion has transformed AIDS from a fatal disease: across the region, the number of people on ART increased from 2.4 million in 2010 to 9.2 million in 2020, and AIDS-related deaths decreased by 58%, from 350,000 to 148,000 (UNAIDS, 2020). Southern Africa has comparatively higher health spending and more advanced healthcare facilities, but also faces notable inequities and a rising prevalence of NCDs. Digital transformation efforts focus on integrating existing systems, improving interoperability, and shifting toward person-centered, long-term care.

Table 2.3 Key Health System Indicators for Selected Southern African Countries (2018-2020)

Country	Health Expenditure per Capita (USD)	Government Health Expenditure (% GDP)	Out-of-Pocket (% THE)	Physicians per 10,000	Nurses per 10,000	Hospital Beds per 10,000	HIV Prevalence Adults 15-49 (%)
South Africa	$570	8.1	7	9.1	52.7	28	13.5
Botswana	$387	5.9	5	4.6	41.3	18	20.7
Namibia	$456	8.0	6	5.9	40.2	27	8.0
Zimbabwe	$96	6.6	24	1.6	7.2	17	12.1
Zambia	$68	4.9	16	1.9	19.5		

Sources: WHO (2021); World Bank (2021)

Central Africa

Central Africa faces some of the continent's most severe health system challenges. The Democratic Republic of Congo, Africa's second-largest country by land area (2.3 million km^2) and fourth by population (92 million), has a health system ravaged by decades of conflict, mismanagement, and neglect. Despite mineral reserves estimated at $24 trillion, health spending was only $19 per capita in 2018, and only 23% of health facilities have basic electricity and water. The country faces recurrent disease outbreaks, including 14 Ebola epidemics between 1976 and 2022. The Central African Republic has only 37% of its health facilities fully operational, and 63% of the population needs humanitarian health assistance. Chad ranks among Africa's worst for health indicators, with a maternal mortality rate of 1,140 per 100,000, despite its oil wealth (WHO, 2021).

Central Africa faces challenges related to fragility, conflict, and displacement. Digital transformation priorities should therefore emphasize "minimum viable" system functions, including civil registration and vital statistics linkages, immunization registries, resilient surveillance, and offline-capable tools that function despite infrastructure volatility.

Table 2.4 Key Health System Indicators for Selected Countries in Central Africa (2018-2020)

Country	**Health Expenditure per Capita (USD)**	**Government Health Expenditure (% GDP)**	**Out-of-Pocket (% THE)**	**Physicians per 10,000**	**Nurses per 10,000**	**Maternal Mortality Ratio**	**Under-5 Mortality Rate (per 1,000)**
Cameroon	$74	3.2	65	1.3	7.8	529	78
CAR	$21	4.9	42	0.5	2.9	829	110
Chad	$52	4.4	57	0.5	3.4	1,140	117
DRC	$19	1.6	48	0.7	5.9	473	88
Rep. of Congo	$71	2.2	41	1.6	8.5	378	45
Equat. Guinea	$275	2.5	17	4.0	14.7	301	83
Gabon	$293	2.7	22	4.6	44.9	252	47
São Tomé	$134	5.7	31	4.9	40.4	130	16

MMR = Maternal Mortality Ratio per 100,000 live births; U5MR = Under-Five Mortality per 1,000 live births.

Sources: WHO (2021); World Bank (2021).

North Africa

North African health systems differ markedly from those in sub-Saharan Africa in epidemiological profiles, organization, and development trajectories. Tunisia achieved near-universal health coverage (98%) through mandatory social insurance and subsidized care, with 13.0 doctors per 10,000 people and a maternal mortality rate of 43 per 100,000. Morocco expanded health insurance coverage from 33% in 2010 to 90% by 2020 through mandatory insurance and a subsidized Régime d'Assistance Médicale (RAMED) program for people living in poverty, which reduced maternal mortality by 54%. Egypt achieved 78% insurance coverage and reduced maternal mortality to 37 per 100,000, although concerns about quality and equity persist. Algeria has 18.1 doctors per 10,000—one of the highest rates in Africa—but faces inefficiencies and challenges related to non-communicable diseases. Libya's health system deteriorated severely after the 2011 conflict, with 35% of hospitals partially or fully nonfunctional (Rashad & Sharaf, 2015; WHO, 2021).

Table 2.5: Key Health System Indicators for Selected Countries, North Africa (2018–2020)

Country	HE/Cap ($)	Govt HE (% GDP)	OOP (%)	Docs/10k	Nurses/10k	MMR	Ins. Cov.
Egypt	$182	5.3	62	8.1	35.1	37	78
Tunisia	$296	7.3	38	13.0	41.5	43	98
Morocco	$190	5.3	46	7.3	15.1	70	90
Algeria	$313	6.2	27	18.1	20.4	112	85
Libya	$269	4.0	73	20.9	54.3	72	-
Sudan	$114	8.3	73	3.2	8.5	295	16
Mauritania	$55	3.6	37	1.8	6.7	766	13

Sources: WHO (2021); World Bank (2021)

North African systems generally have better infrastructure and a more established public-sector healthcare delivery system. Digital transformation efforts in the region focus on hospital information systems, insurance and payment platforms, e-prescribing, and nationwide health data management. A major challenge is ensuring that digital investments promote equity by narrowing the gap between urban and rural areas.

The regional patterns summarize health system readiness for digital transformation, outlining typical profiles, key constraints, and high-priority digital interventions for each African region.

Table 2.6 presents a comparative snapshot of how African regions differ in health system readiness for digital transformation, showing that readiness is neither uniform nor shaped by distinct institutional, epidemiological, and infrastructural realities.

Table 2.6. Regional Patterns in Health Systems Readiness for Digital Transformation

Region	Typical System Profile	Key Constraints	High-Value Digital Priorities
East Africa	Strong innovation diffusion; PHC expansion efforts	Rural workforce gaps; facility readiness; fragmentation	CHW platforms, interoperable HMIS/HIE, eLMIS, surveillance
West Africa	High emergency exposure; mixed governance	Financing gaps; parallel systems; supply chain fragility	Integrated surveillance, logistics visibility, telehealth
Southern Africa	Higher institutional capacity; high inequality	Referral/quality gaps; system integration complexity	Interoperability, longitudinal care records, lab integration
Central Africa	Fragility and displacement common	Infrastructure volatility; continuity; coordination	Offline-first tools, immunization registries, outbreak analytics
North Africa	More institutionalized; rising NCD burden	Equity across regions; data governance at scale	Hospital digitization, e-prescribing, payment platforms

Source: Author's Analysis

East Africa emerges as a leader in the diffusion of innovation, driven by robust ecosystems for digital health startups and community-based primary healthcare models. Yet it faces persistent rural workforce shortages, uneven facility readiness, and fragmented systems. In contrast, West Africa is marked by frequent exposure to public health emergencies and varying governance capacities across countries, complicating system coherence. Financing gaps and fragmented digital initiatives further weaken resilience.

Southern Africa, with relatively stronger institutional capacity, demonstrates more advanced system structures but still struggles with inequality, referral inefficiencies, and complex integration challenges across legacy systems. Meanwhile, Central Africa has fragile, often crisis-affected health systems, where displacement and instability exacerbate infrastructure weaknesses and coordination challenges. North Africa, by comparison, shows greater institutional maturity and more structured health systems but is increasingly burdened by non-communicable diseases (NCDs) and must address regional disparities and large-scale data governance issues. Digital priorities must be tailored to these regional contexts rather than adopting a one-size-fits-all approach.

- In East Africa, the emphasis needs to be on scaling digital platforms for community health workers (CHWs), interoperable health management information systems (HMIS), health information exchanges (HIE), electronic logistics management systems (eLMIS), and surveillance tools to consolidate fragmented gains.

- West Africa needs to prioritize integrated disease surveillance, end-to-end supply chain visibility, and telehealth solutions to improve access and emergency response.

- Southern Africa needs to focus on deeper system integration, including interoperability frameworks, longitudinal patient records, and laboratory system integration to enhance continuity and quality of care.

- In Central Africa, the most impactful interventions are resilient, offline-first digital tools, immunization registries, and outbreak analytics that function in low-connectivity and crisis settings.

- Finally, North Africa could move toward advanced digitalization by expanding hospital information systems, e-prescribing, and digital payment platforms, reflecting a shift toward efficiency, chronic disease management, and system-wide modernization.

Collectively, digital transformation pathways in Africa should be context-dependent, requiring differentiated strategies aligned with each region's and country's structural realities and health priorities.

2.3 Key Challenges Facing African Health Systems

Despite regional variations and significant progress, African health systems face common challenges that impede performance and constrain progress toward universal health coverage. These challenges are interconnected and mutually reinforcing, requiring comprehensive, systems-level solutions rather than narrow technical fixes.

Infrastructure Deficits

Physical infrastructure deficits are major barriers to healthcare delivery across much of Africa. These deficits define the challenge that Layer 1 of the Digital Health Technology Stack (Chapter 4) addresses. Infrastructure constrains every layer above it: without reliable electricity and connectivity, digital identity systems, interoperability platforms, analytics tools, and clinical applications cannot function. Chapter 7 explores infrastructure solutions in detail, including solar power deployment, satellite connectivity, and cloud computing strategies.

A comprehensive WHO Service Availability and Readiness Assessment across sub-Saharan African countries found that only 28% of health facilities had reliable electricity in 2013–2015, improving modestly to 34% by 2019—meaning two-thirds of facilities still face frequent power outages or lack electricity altogether (Adair-Rohani et al., 2013; WHO, 2020). Rural facilities are significantly worse: in Uganda, only 19% of rural health facilities had reliable electricity, compared to 81% in urban areas; in Tanzania, although 92% of hospitals had electricity, only 39% of rural dispensaries did. These electricity gaps directly affect clinical care—vaccines cannot be properly refrigerated, laboratory tests cannot be processed, and emergency obstetric care is compromised.

Infrastructure availability in African health facilities shows dramatic urban–rural disparities across six critical indicators. Rural facilities lag urban facilities by 33–58 percentage points, with the widest gaps in electricity, Internet connectivity, and availability of essential equipment.

Water access shows similarly concerning patterns: only 55% of sub-Saharan African health facilities have improved water sources, and only 37% have water available within the facility. Only 34% practice functional handwashing with soap and water, contributing to healthcare-associated infections that affect an estimated 15% of hospitalized patients (versus 7% in high-income countries) (WHO & UNICEF, 2020; Allegranzi et al., 2011).

Figure 2.2. Infrastructure Availability in African Health Facilities: Urban vs. Rural Disparities

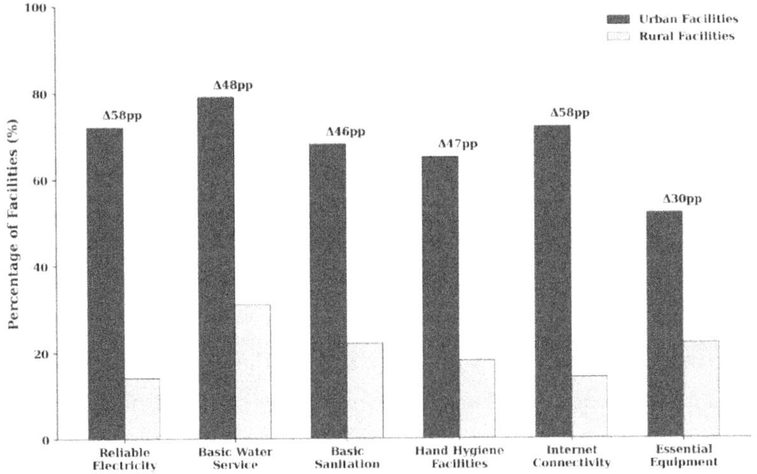

Sources: WHO Service Availability and Readiness Assessment (2020), WHO & UNICEF(2020), Whal et al. (2018)

Telecommunications connectivity remains limited—a 2019 survey found that only 28% of health facilities had functional Internet access, with 72% in urban areas and 14% in rural areas. Geographic access modeling estimates that 420 million people (48% of sub-Saharan Africa's population) live more than one hour's travel time from a hospital, and 210 million (24%) more than two hours away (Ouma et al., 2018; Weiss et al., 2020).

Table 2.7: WASH Services in African Health Facilities in Selected Countries in Africa

Country	Basic Water (%)	Basic Sanitation (%)	Hand Hygiene (%)	Year	Region
Rwanda	71	64	58	2018	East
Ghana	68	61	52	2017	West
Kenya	62	57	46	2018	East
Tanzania	59	50	41	2018	East
Uganda	56	42	35	2018	East
Zambia	53	46	39	2018	Southern
Malawi	47	41	33	2019	Southern
Nigeria	42	38	26	2018	West
Mozambique	41	35	28	2018	Southern
Ethiopia	37	27	22	2016	East
DRC	29	22	17	2017	Central
Chad	21	18	12	2019	Central

Source: WHO & UNICEF (2020)

Human Resource Shortages

Africa faces the world's most severe health workforce crisis. Sub-Saharan Africa accounts for 24% of the global disease burden yet has only 3% of the global health workforce (Anyangwe & Mtonga, 2007). In 2018, the region averaged 13.2 doctors, nurses, and midwives per 10,000 population—far below WHO's minimum benchmark of 23 per 10,000 and the high-income country average of 130 per 10,000 (WHO, 2020). Twenty-four African countries have fewer than one physician per 10,000 population. At current production rates, sub-Saharan Africa will not meet WHO's minimum benchmarks until after 2050. Health worker density (doctors, nurses, and midwives per 10,000 population) shows that Central Africa has the lowest level, while North Africa remains above the global average.

Figure 2.3. Health Worker Density: Africa Regions vs. Global Benchmarks in 2018

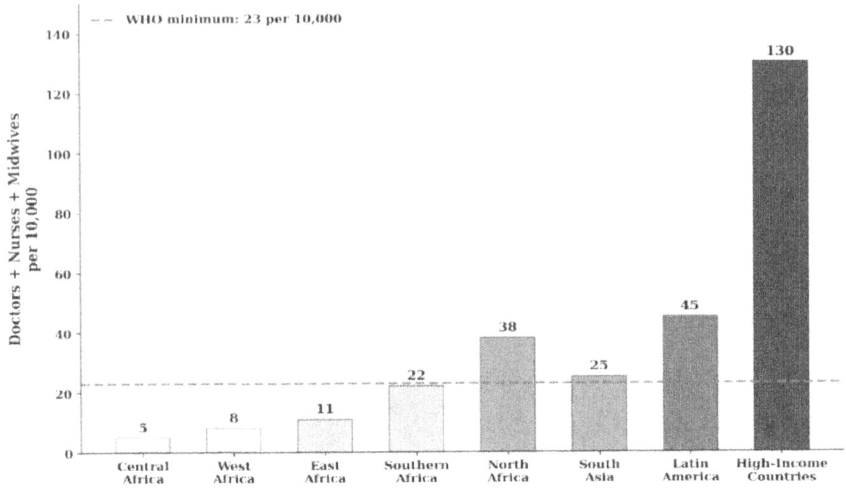

Source: WHO (2020) Global Health Workforce Statistics

Central and West Africa fall well below the WHO minimum threshold of 23 per 10,000, while even Southern Africa's higher density reflects extreme maldistribution between urban and rural areas. Some countries achieved impressive percentage gains from very low baselines; others show stagnation or a decline in the number of physicians per 10,000 people.

Health workers are concentrated in urban areas, with urban–rural physician ratios ranging from 4:1 to 12:1 across African countries. In Kenya, urban areas have 2.0 doctors per 10,000 people compared to 0.2 in rural areas (a 10:1 ratio); in Tanzania, the ratios are 1.2 versus 0.1 (a 12:1 ratio)—even though 60–80% of the population lives in rural regions. International migration further depletes the workforce: an estimated 65,000–70,000 African-trained physicians work in high-income countries (23% of all African-trained physicians), with 23,000 in the US (up 64% since 2010), 17,000 in the UK (up 100%), and 8,500 in Canada. The financial cost is staggering—training these physicians costs roughly $6.5–7 billion, representing a massive subsidy from poor to rich countries (Clemens & Pettersson, 2008; Tankwanchi et al., 2015).

Table 2.8: Physician Density Trends 2010–2018 (per 10,000 population) in Selected Countries

Country	2010	2014	2018	Change	Notes
Ethiopia	0.3	0.5	0.8	167%	Impressive growth but from extremely low base
Tanzania	0.2	0.3	0.5	150%	Doubling still leaves critical shortfall
Malawi	0.2	0.3	0.4	100%	Remains among Africa's lowest physician densities
Rwanda	0.7	1.0	1.3	86%	Strong trajectory with sustained investment
Ghana	1.0	1.4	1.7	70%	Growing but high emigration rate
South Africa	7.7	8.2	9.1	18%	Highest in SSA; urban concentration
Nigeria	3.8	3.8	3.8	0%	Stagnation despite population growth
DRC	0.9	0.8	0.7	-22%	Decline due to conflict and emigration
Tunisia	11.9	12.7	13.0	9%	North Africa's strong training pipeline

Source: WHO (2021).

Urban–rural health disparities across five dimensions in sub-Saharan Africa. Rural areas face substantially worse outcomes and limited service availability, with physician density showing the most extreme ratio (nearly 12:1 urban advantage). These disparities define the equity challenge that digital health must address.

Figure 2.4. Urban-Rural Health Disparities in Sub-Saharan Africa, Multiple Dimensions of Inequality

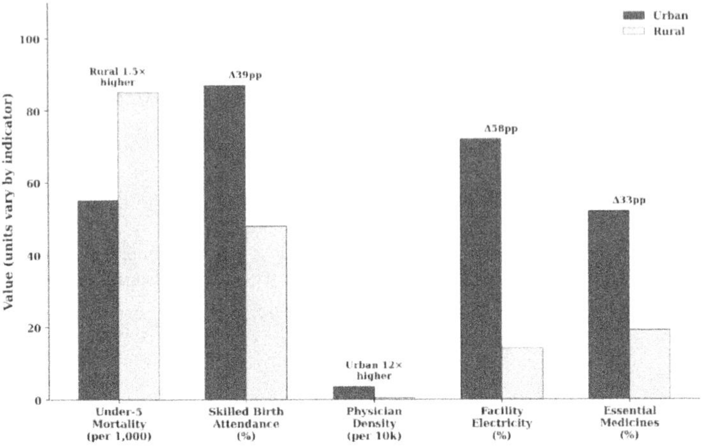

Source: DHS Surveys 2016-2020, WHO SARA (2020), Leslie et al. (2017)

Financing Gaps

Health financing remains grossly inadequate in most African countries—and the landscape has shifted dramatically since 2025. Chapter 17 examines digital health financing in depth, documenting the 2025 disruption that created a USD 12 billion shortfall, analyzing the return on investment for digital health interventions (typically 2–15-fold over five years), and proposing sustainable financing strategies, including domestic resource mobilization, innovative instruments, and lifecycle cost planning. Total health expenditure per capita in sub-Saharan Africa averaged $129 in 2018, up from $74 in 2010 (+74% nominal, +35% real), but remained well below levels in high-income countries ($4,000+) and middle-income countries ($400–800).

As of 2018, only 6 out of 55 AU Member States met the Abuja Declaration target of allocating 15% of national budgets to health. Out-of-pocket payments account for an average of 36% of total health expenditure, with some countries exceeding 70% (Nigeria: 77%; Sudan: 73%), creating financial barriers that push families into poverty—an estimated 15 million Africans are pushed into poverty each year due to catastrophic health expenses (WHO, 2021; Wagstaff et al., 2018). Several low-income countries achieved impressive growth from very low baselines, yet Nigeria's decline is particularly concerning.

Table 2.9: Health Expenditure Trends 2010–2018 in Selected Countries in Africa (current USD per capita).

Country	2010	2014	2018	Change	Key Trend
Ethiopia	$19	$27	$33	74%	Strong growth; remains critically low in absolute terms
Kenya	$53	$68	$79	49%	Steady increase; driven by devolution and insurance expansion
Rwanda	$46	$57	$67	46%	Sustained growth with performance-based financing model
Ghana	$67	$82	$88	31%	NHIS expansion driving some growth; challenges in sustainability
Morocco	$134	$175	$190	42%	Insurance expansion from 33% to 90% driving spending
Egypt	$135	$156	$182	35%	Universal coverage push from 58% to 78% coverage
Nigeria	$80	$85	$78	-2.5%	Stagnation/decline despite Africa's largest economy
South Africa	$566	$607	$570	0.7%	Highest in SSA; NHI reform pending

Source: WHO (2021)

External financing accounts for an average of 24% of total health spending in sub-Saharan Africa, rising to 44% in low-income countries and exceeding 50% in Malawi and Mozambique. Total development assistance for health in Africa peaked at $15.2 billion in 2015 but fell to $14.1 billion in 2019, raising sustainability concerns. Moreover, external funding tends to focus on specific diseases—HIV/AIDS (35%), maternal/child health (22%), malaria (12%)—which leaves other health areas underfunded and creates dependence on vertical programs (Dieleman et al., 2020). Expanding health insurance offers a path forward: Tunisia (98%), Morocco (90%), Rwanda (91%), and Egypt (78%) show that high coverage is achievable, though most sub-Saharan African countries remain below 30%.

Disease Burden: The Quadruple Challenge

Africa faces a unique quadruple burden of disease encompassing communicable diseases, maternal and child health conditions, non-communicable diseases, and injuries. This complex epidemiological landscape places demands on health systems that far exceed available resources and requires diverse clinical skills that most systems lack (Mayosi et al., 2009). In Africa, the quadruple burden of disease is evident when comparing sub-Saharan Africa's cause-of-death distribution with North Africa's. Sub-Saharan Africa retains a high communicable disease burden (38%) while facing a growing NCD challenge (29%). North Africa has undergone a full epidemiological transition, with 78% of deaths from NCDs.

Figure 2.5. The Quadruple Burden of Disease in Africa

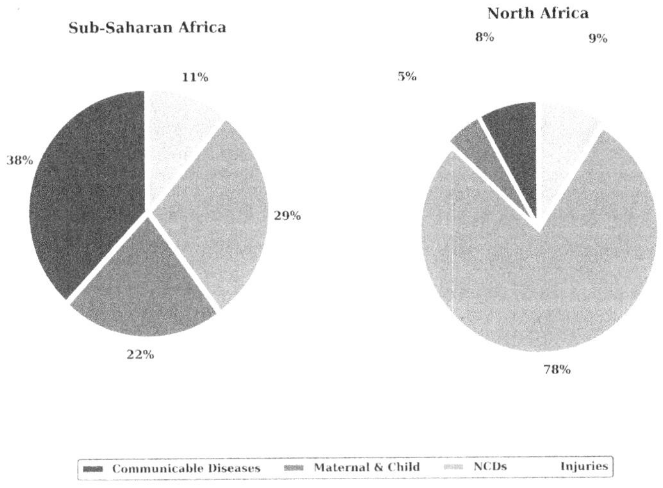

Source: GBD 2019 Disease and Injuries Collaborators (2020)

Communicable diseases still dominate in sub-Saharan Africa. Malaria accounted for 229 million cases and 409,000 deaths in 2019 (94% of global totals), though death rates declined by 30% from 2010 levels. HIV/AIDS has been transformed by the expansion of ART—with 16.9 million people on treatment in 2020 (66% coverage) compared with 6.8 million in 2010 (37%)—resulting in a 51% drop in AIDS deaths, from 950,000 to 470,000. Still, there are 1.5 million new infections each year, and adolescents account for 34% of new cases despite making up only 21% of the population. Tuberculosis caused 565,000 deaths among Africans in 2019, with HIV–TB co-infection (30–60% of TB cases) complicating treatment efforts (WHO, 2020; UNAIDS, 2020).

Figure 2.6. HIV/AIDS in Sub-Saharan Africa: ART Scale-Up and Mortality Rate 2010-2020

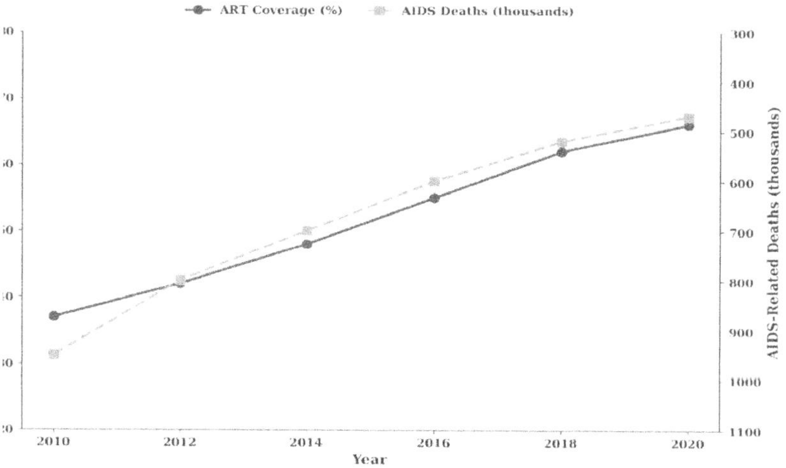

Source: UNAIDS (2020), AIDSinfo

The inverse relationship between ART coverage scale-up and AIDS-related mortality in sub-Saharan Africa (2010–2020) shows that as treatment coverage rose from 37% to 66%, annual deaths fell from 950,000 to 470,000—marking one of Africa's greatest public health achievements, driven by the Global Fund, PEPFAR, and national HIV programs.

Maternal and child health have improved significantly in Africa—under-five mortality dropped by 53%, from 155 to 74 per 1,000 live births (2000–2019), and maternal mortality fell by 38%, from 866 to 534 per 100,000 live births. Top performers include Rwanda (-80% in under-five mortality), Malawi (-76%), and Ethiopia (-67%). However, Africa still accounts for 66% of global maternal deaths, and neonatal mortality (first 28 days) now represents 43% of under-five deaths, underscoring the need for further progress to strengthen newborn care (UNICEF, 2020; WHO, 2019). Under-five mortality trends (2000–2019) for selected African countries, compared with the sub-Saharan African and global averages, show that Rwanda and Malawi achieved remarkable 76–80% reductions, while Nigeria's modest 41% decline demonstrates that conflict, governance challenges, and health system weaknesses constrain progress.

Figure 2.7. Under-Five Mortality Trends in Selected Countries in Africa (2000-2019)

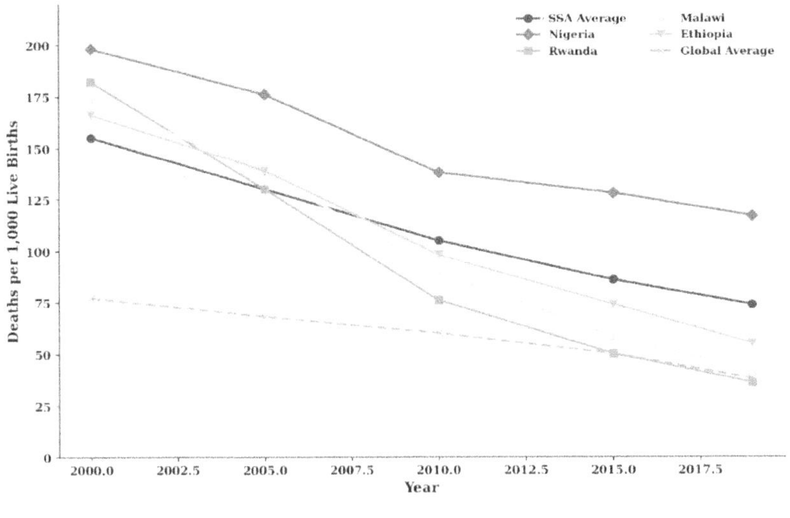

Source: UNICEF (2020)

Non-communicable diseases are rising rapidly, now accounting for 37% of deaths in sub-Saharan Africa and 73–85% in North Africa. Cardiovascular disease mortality rates in sub-Saharan Africa increased by 11% from 2010 to

2019, compared with a 6% decline in high-income countries. Diabetes prevalence rose from 3.1% to 4.7%, and cancer cases are projected to increase by 73% by 2030. Health systems built for acute, episodic care struggle to manage chronic diseases — only 30% of primary care facilities have essential NCD medicines and technologies (WHO, 2018; Kengne et al., 2013).

Injuries from road traffic accidents (313,000 deaths annually, with Africa's rate of 26.6 per 100,000 the highest in the world), interpersonal violence (134,000 deaths), and conflict (22 active armed conflicts in 2020) now account for 11% of deaths.

Geographic and Urban–Rural Disparities

Health outcomes and access to services vary significantly between urban and rural areas and across regions within countries. Rural children face mortality rates 18–40% higher than those of urban children, and rural women are 30–70% less likely to have skilled attendance during childbirth. Urban areas have 4–12 times as many physicians per capita as rural areas, even though 60–80% of the population lives in rural areas. Distance modeling shows that 420 million people live more than 1 hour from a hospital, representing 71% of Chad's population, 64% of the DRC's, and 61% of CAR's (Ouma et al., 2018).

Within-country regional disparities often exceed urban–rural gaps. In Nigeria, under-five mortality rates range from 37 per 1,000 in Lagos to 246 per 1,000 in Jigawa State, a 6.6-fold difference; in Ethiopia, from 39 per 1,000 in Addis Ababa to 133 per 1,000 in Afar, a 3.4-fold difference; and in Kenya, from 22 per 1,000 in Nairobi to 108 per 1,000 in Turkana, a 4.9-fold difference. These disparities reflect historical development patterns, political-economic factors, geographic challenges, marginalized populations, and conflicts.

Meanwhile, rapid urbanization has created urban health challenges: 200 million Africans live in slums, where health outcomes can be worse than in rural areas—in Nairobi, under-five mortality is 18 per 1,000 in affluent neighborhoods versus 151 in slums (Zulu et al., 2011; UN-Habitat, 2020).

Summary and Implications for Digital Health

Africa's health progress (2005–2020) across eight key indicators shows both substantial achievements and areas needing acceleration. Over the past fifteen years, Africa saw a 53% drop in under-five mortality, a 38% decrease in maternal mortality, a 51% decline in AIDS-related deaths, a 30% reduction in malaria deaths, a 74% increase in per capita health spending, and a significant expansion of health insurance, immunization, and facility-based services. However, profound challenges persist: two-thirds of health facilities lack reliable electricity; 420 million people live more than an hour from a hospital; 65,000–70,000 physicians trained in Africa work abroad; health spending averages $129 per capita, compared with $4,000 in high-income countries; and the quadruple disease burden continues to exceed system capacity.

Figure 2.8. Africa's Health Progress (2005-2020)

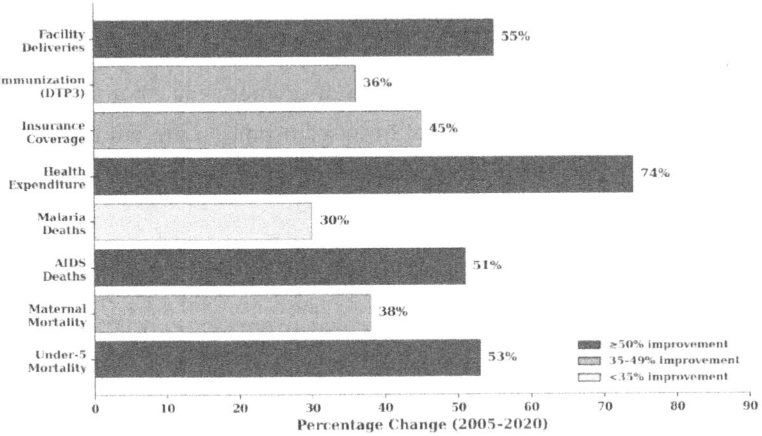

Source: WHO (2021), UNICEF (2020), UNAIDS(2020)

The health challenges outlined in this chapter—infrastructure deficits that leave two-thirds of facilities without reliable electricity, workforce shortages in 24 countries with fewer than 1 physician per 10,000 people, and financing gaps that keep health spending at USD 129 per capita—are compounded by an extraordinary disease burden. This quadruple burden shapes the demand side of the digital health equation: it defines the clinical and public health problems digital tools must address, the range of applications needed, and the potential scale of impact digital health transformation could achieve. The application layer of the Digital Health Technology Stack (Layer 5, Chapter 4) must support interventions across all four disease categories simultaneously—from infectious disease surveillance to chronic disease management platforms, maternal health mHealth tools, and injury registries.

The geographic and urban–rural disparities documented above present perhaps the most compelling case for digital health transformation in Africa. Telemedicine can connect rural patients with specialists hundreds of kilometers away. Mobile health applications can deliver health information and appointment reminders to populations far beyond facility catchment areas. Clinical decision support tools can extend diagnostic capabilities to primary care settings where specialists are scarce. Electronic records can enable care coordination across dispersed facilities. Digital surveillance can detect outbreaks in remote areas before they spread to cities. These are not theoretical possibilities—they are already being demonstrated across the continent.

However, the same disparities that make a case for digital health also constrain its deployment: rural areas with the greatest need for telemedicine often lack the connectivity to support it, and regions with the highest disease burden often have the weakest health informatics workforce. Addressing this paradox—designing digital health solutions that function within the constraints they aim to overcome—is the central design challenge the Digital Health Technology Stack and the implementation roadmap seek to resolve.

2.5 Conclusion

The complex challenges presented in this chapter set the stage for digital health transformation. Digital technologies provide powerful tools: telemedicine to overcome geographic barriers, mobile health to extend reach beyond facility catchment areas, clinical decision support to improve quality in under-resourced settings, electronic records for care coordination, supply chain systems to reduce medicine stockouts, digital surveillance for faster outbreak detection, and online training for workforce development. However, infrastructure deficits (particularly in electricity and connectivity), workforce shortages, and limited funding pose significant obstacles.

Effective digital health transformation requires a realistic assessment of infrastructure limitations, integration with workforce strengthening rather than substitution, sustainable financing models, targeted attention to equity, and prioritizing basic functionality before advancing to more complex systems. These principles are operationalized through the Digital Health Technology Stack introduced in Chapter 4, which provides the architectural framework for the rest of this book. The five foundation layers—infrastructure and connectivity, digital identity and registries, interoperability and data exchange, data management and analytics, and applications and services—define the technical architecture on which digital health systems are built. The seven cross-cutting enablers—digital health strategy, governance and standards, workforce development, research and development, the healthtech ecosystem, regional cooperation and financing and sustainability—define the conditions that determine whether those technical investments succeed or fail. Each challenge documented in this chapter—electricity gaps (Layer 1), the absence of patient identifiers (Layer 2), fragmented health information systems (Layer 3), limited analytical capacity (Layer 4), the workforce crisis (Enabler 3), and financing inadequacy (Enabler 6)—maps directly to a specific element of the technology stack, ensuring that the book's subsequent analysis is grounded in the realities of Africa's health sector landscape.

References

Adair-Rohani, H., Zuber, A., Bonjour, S., Wilburn, S., Kuesel, A. C., Hebert, R., & Fletcher, E. R. (2013). Limited electricity access in health facilities of sub-Saharan Africa. Global Health: Science and Practice, 1(2), 249–261.

Allegranzi, B., Bagheri Nejad, S., Combescure, C., et al. (2011). Burden of endemic health-care-associated infection in developing countries: Systematic review. The Lancet, 377(9761), 228–241.

Anyangwe, S. C., & Mtonga, C. (2007). Inequities in the global health workforce: The greatest impediment to health in sub-Saharan Africa. International Journal of Environmental Research and Public Health, 4(2), 93–100.

Barasa, E. W., Maina, T., & Ravishankar, N. (2017). Assessing the impoverishing effects and factors associated with the incidence of catastrophic health care payments in Kenya. International Journal for Equity in Health, 16(1), 31.

Barnett, T., & Whiteside, A. (2006). AIDS in the twenty-first century: Disease and globalization (2nd ed.). Palgrave Macmillan.

Biesma, R. G., Brugha, R., Harmer, A., Walsh, A., Spicer, N., & Walt, G. (2009). The effects of global health initiatives on country health systems. The Lancet, 373(9681), 2137–2169.

Binagwaho, A., Farmer, P. E., Nsanzimana, S., et al. (2014). Rwanda 20 years on: Investing in life. The Lancet, 384(9940), 371–375.

Clemens, M. A., & Pettersson, G. (2008). New data on African health professionals abroad. Human Resources for Health, 6(1), 1.

Coovadia, H., Jewkes, R., Barron, P., Sanders, D., & McIntyre, D. (2009). The health and health system of South Africa: Historical roots of current public health challenges. The Lancet, 374(9692), 817–834.

Dieleman, J. L., Micah, A. E., Murray, C. J. L., et al. (2020). Global health spending and development assistance for health, 2019. The Lancet, 395(10239), 1811–1829.

Federal Ministry of Health, Ethiopia. (2020). Health Sector Transformation Plan II 2020/21–2024/25. FMOH Ethiopia.

GBD 2019 Diseases and Injuries Collaborators. (2020). Global burden of 369 diseases and injuries in 204 countries. The Lancet, 396(10258), 1204–1222.

General Medical Council UK. (2020). The state of medical education and practice in the UK 2020. GMC.

GSMA. (2021). The mobile economy: Sub-Saharan Africa 2021. GSM Association.

Iliffe, J. (2006). The African AIDS epidemic: A history. Ohio University Press.

Kengne, A. P., June-Rose McHiza, Z., Amoah, A. G. B., & Mbanya, J.-C. (2013). Cardiovascular diseases and diabetes as economic and developmental challenges in Africa. Progress in Cardiovascular Diseases, 56(3), 302–313.

Kruk, M. E., Gage, A. D., Arsenault, C., et al. (2018). High-quality health systems in the SDGs era. The Lancet Global Health, 6(11), e1196–e1252.

Leslie, H. H., Spiegelman, D., Zhou, X., & Kruk, M. E. (2017). Service readiness of health facilities in Bangladesh, Haiti, Kenya, Malawi, and other countries. Bulletin of the WHO, 95(11), 738–748.

Logie, D. E., & Woodroffe, J. (1993). Structural adjustment: The wrong prescription for Africa? BMJ, 307(6895), 41–44.

Mayosi, B. M., Flisher, A. J., Lalloo, U. G., Sitas, F., Tollman, S. M., & Bradshaw, D. (2009). The burden of non-communicable diseases in South Africa. The Lancet, 374(9693), 934–947.

McPake, B. (1993). User charges for health services in developing countries: A review of the economic literature. Social Science & Medicine, 36(11), 1397–1405.

Ministry of Health, Kenya. (2021). Kenya Digital Health Strategic Framework 2021–2025. MOH Kenya.

National Health Insurance Authority, Ghana. (2019). NHIS membership and claims data 2018. NHIA.

Nkurunziza, A., Nshogoza, G., Kateera, F., et al. (2021). Sustaining a national community health worker program: Lessons from Rwanda. Global Health: Science and Practice, 9(Suppl 1), S85–S97.

Ouma, P. O., Maina, J., Thuranira, P. N., et al. (2018). Access to emergency hospital care in sub-Saharan Africa. The Lancet Global Health, 6(3), e342–e350.

Rashad, H., & Sharaf, M. (2015). Catastrophic and impoverishing effects of out-of-pocket health expenditure: New evidence from Egypt. American Journal of Economics, 5(5), 526–533.

Tankwanchi, A. B. S., Vermund, S. H., & Perkins, D. D. (2015). Monitoring sub-Saharan African physician migration. PLOS ONE, 10(4), e0124734.

UNAIDS. (2020). 2020 Global AIDS update: Seizing the moment. Joint United Nations Programme on HIV/AIDS.

UNICEF. (2020). Levels and trends in child mortality: Report 2020. United Nations Children's Fund.

UN-Habitat. (2020). The state of African cities 2018. United Nations Human Settlements Programme.

Wagstaff, A., Flores, G., Hsu, J., et al. (2018). Progress on catastrophic health spending in 133 countries. The Lancet Global Health, 6(2), e169–e179.

Weiss, D. J., Nelson, A., Vargas-Ruiz, C. A., et al. (2020). Global maps of travel time to healthcare facilities. Nature Medicine, 26(12), 1835–1838.

WHO. (2020). World health statistics 2020: Monitoring health for the SDGs. World Health Organization.

WHO. (2021). Global health expenditure database. World Health Organization.

WHO & UNICEF. (2020). WASH in health care facilities: Global baseline report 2019. WHO and UNICEF.

World Bank. (2021). World Development Indicators 2021. World Bank Group.

Zulu, E. M., Beguy, D., Ezeh, A. C., et al. (2011). Overview of migration, poverty and health dynamics in Nairobi City's slum settlements. Journal of Urban Health, 88(Suppl 2), 185–199.

Chapter 3: Digital Technologies for Health Transformation

3.1 Overview of Digital Health Technologies

Digital health encompasses a broad and evolving range of technologies that use digital platforms to deliver, improve, and support health services. The World Health Organization (2019) defines digital health as the field of knowledge and practice focused on developing and using digital technologies to improve health. In Africa, digital health tools have become crucial for overcoming infrastructure challenges, addressing critical human resource shortages, and expanding healthcare access for the underserved population.

The implications of digital health are widely recognized across the continent. Digital health investments in Africa increased by more than 400% in the decade leading up to 2024, reflecting a significant shift in how governments, development partners, and the private sector view technology's role in healthcare delivery (AfDB, 2024). Investment rose from about $92 million in 2015 to about $1.18 billion in 2024, representing more than a tenfold increase. Growth was steady, followed by a sharper acceleration around 2020, indicating rising investor confidence and greater prioritization of digital health.

Figure 3.1. Digital Health Investment Growth (2015-2024)

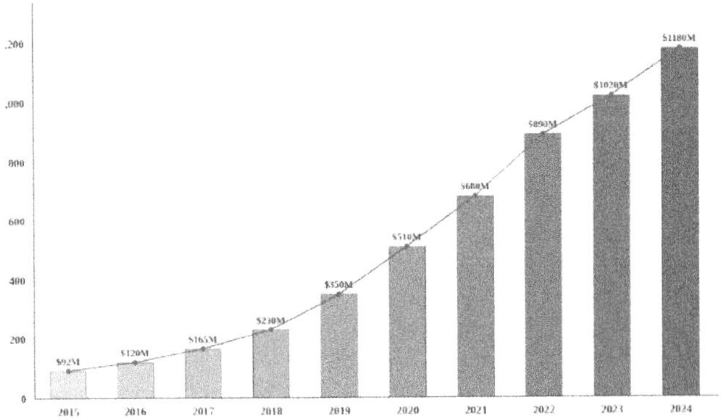

Source: African Development Bank (2020)

There is also an inflection point during the 2020–2022 period, when investments rose sharply from $510 million in 2020 to $890 million in 2022, likely reflecting the COVID-19 pandemic's acceleration of digital health adoption, particularly in telemedicine and health surveillance systems. Growth continued beyond the pandemic, reaching $1.02 billion in 2023 and $1.18 billion in 2024, indicating that digital health is no longer a temporary response but a sustained investment priority. This progress reflects growing recognition of digital health as a critical enabler of health system strengthening, improved service delivery, and resilience, and points to expanding opportunities for innovation and private-sector engagement.

While Africa's digital health ecosystem is rapidly expanding, the continent still lags other regions in overall maturity. North America and Europe lead, with composite digital health scores above 75, fueled by decades of investment in electronic health records, interoperability, regulatory frameworks, and infrastructure. East Asia, led by South Korea, Japan, and Singapore, has leveraged strong government digital strategies to achieve scores near 71.

Figure 3.2. Global Digital Health Maturity Comparison by Region

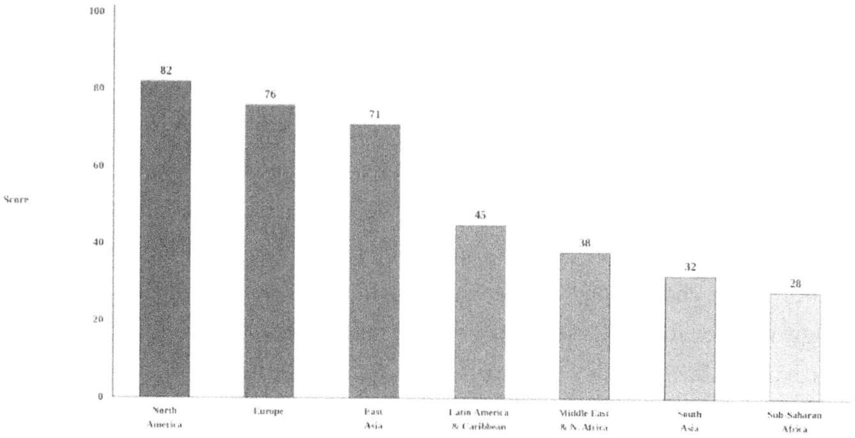

Source: WHO (2023)

Latin America and the Caribbean, with a score of 45, occupy a middle ground, with notable leaders such as Brazil, whose Unified Health System (SUS) digitalization serves as a model for large-scale deployment of public health digital technologies. Africa's composite score of 28 reflects a significant gap but also enormous potential for accelerated growth (WHO, 2023).

The digital health ecosystem is more than just a collection of isolated tools; it's an interconnected network of technologies working together to transform healthcare systems. These technologies range from simple short message service (SMS) interventions accessible on basic feature phones to advanced artificial intelligence (AI) platforms that offer sophisticated computational capabilities. Some of the core technologies that underlie digital health include mobile health solutions, digital payment systems, big data analytics, blockchain for health, Internet of Medical Things, AI and Machine Learning, Telemedicine and telehealth and Electronic Medical Records.

The technologies examined in this chapter operate primarily within Layers 4 and 5 of the digital health technology stack—the Data Management and Analytics Layer and the Applications and Services Layer, as introduced in Chapter 4 (see Figure 4.1). However, their effective deployment depends critically on the foundational layers beneath them: physical infrastructure and connectivity (Layer 1), digital identity and registries (Layer 2), interoperability and data exchange (Layer 3), and the cross-cutting governance, policy, and standards framework that shapes all layers. Readers are encouraged to consult Chapter 4's layer reference model for the architectural context in which these application-layer technologies are situated. While Chapter 4 provides the typological framework for classifying and organizing digital health interventions, this chapter provides the applied detail—examining what each technology is, how it works, where it has been deployed, what global best practices exist, and what policy and regulatory considerations apply.

3.2 Mobile Health (mHealth) Solutions

Mobile health applications operate within the Applications and Services Layer (Layer 5) of the digital health technology stack, serving as the primary interface through which patients and community health workers interact with the broader digital health ecosystem. As discussed in Chapter 4 (Section 4.6, Patient Engagement and Empowerment Tools), mHealth applications depend on the connectivity infrastructure of Layer 1 and, when integrated with clinical systems, draw upon the interoperability standards of Layer 3.

Mobile health, commonly referred to as mHealth, is one of the most transformative digital health innovations in Africa. With mobile phone penetration reaching about 85% in sub-Saharan Africa by 2024 (GSMA, 2024), the continent has a unique asset for health service delivery that bypasses the need for extensive fixed-line or broadband infrastructure. mHealth leverages mobile devices—from basic feature phones capable of SMS to advanced smartphones—to deliver health information, facilitate remote monitoring, support frontline health workers, and enable access to care for populations previously out of reach of formal health systems.

3.2.1 Categories of mHealth Applications

SMS-Based Health Information Systems

Short message service applications remain the most widely used mHealth interventions in Africa, primarily because they work on any mobile phone and incur minimal data costs. These systems serve multiple functions: delivering health education messages, sending appointment reminders, issuing medication adherence prompts, and transmitting disease surveillance data from community health workers to district health offices. Research by Aranda Jan et al. (2014) found that SMS reminder systems improved antiretroviral therapy adherence by 12–18% among HIV patients in Kenya and South Africa, making SMS a cost-effective intervention with significant clinical outcomes.

South Africa's MomConnect program demonstrates the potential of SMS-based systems on a national scale. Launched in 2014, MomConnect has enrolled over 2.5 million pregnant women who receive timely health messages throughout pregnancy and the postnatal period (South African National Department of Health, 2023). In West Africa, Ghana's Mobile Technology for Community Health (MOTECH) initiative deployed SMS and interactive voice response (IVR) to reach populations with low literacy, delivering health information in local languages (Grameen Foundation, 2019).

Mobile Applications for Health Service Delivery

Smartphone applications have expanded mHealth capabilities far beyond simple text messaging. Mobile apps now support clinical decision-making at the point of care, enable patients to self-manage chronic conditions, facilitate maternal and child health tracking during pregnancy and early childhood, and strengthen disease surveillance through real-time reporting. In Rwanda, the Babyl platform (formerly Babylon Health Rwanda) provides virtual consultations to more than 2 million registered users, delivering scalable digital primary care in a country where the physician-to-population ratio remains among the lowest globally (Babyl Rwanda, 2023).

The reach of mobile health applications extends far beyond Africa. In India, the Aarogya Setu app, developed during the COVID-19 pandemic, became one of the most downloaded health apps worldwide, combining contact tracing with telemedicine referrals and reaching over 200 million users within months (Government of India, 2021). India has built a Digital Public Infrastructure (DPI)—identity, registries, consented data exchange, and interoperability—on top of which many mobile services can operate. DPI creates a much more scalable model than launching isolated apps. In Latin America, Brazil's e-SUS platform has digitized primary care records for its public health system, supporting over 150 million citizen records and demonstrating how mobile-first strategies can be integrated into universal health coverage plans (Brazilian Ministry of Health, 2022).

In Singapore, mHealth use is widespread, and the national platform HealthHub integrates records, appointments, prescriptions, and trusted public information into a single citizen-facing interface. Singapore shows that the public uses mHealth more consistently when the service is unified, government-supported, and transaction-focused rather than merely informational. Users turn to mHealth when it helps them accomplish specific tasks: book, refill, view, pay, or share.

Community Health Worker Digital Platforms

Digital platforms on tablets and smartphones have fundamentally changed how community health workers (CHWs) operate across Africa. These platforms enable CHWs to register patients digitally, collect structured health data during household visits, access clinical decision-support algorithms, coordinate referrals to higher levels of care, and report data to district health management teams in near real time. The CommCare platform, developed by Dimagi, has been deployed in more than 50 countries, including extensive implementations in Ethiopia, Mozambique, and India, and has supported over 500,000 frontline health workers (Dimagi, 2024).

In the East African Community, the use of CHW digital tools has been supported by regional policy frameworks that recognize community health workers as integral members of the health workforce. Kenya's community health strategy explicitly incorporates digital tools for CHWs. At the same time, Ethiopia's Health Extension Program—one of the largest CHW programs globally—has progressively integrated digital reporting using the District Health Information Software (DHIS2) platform (Ethiopian Federal Ministry of Health, 2021).

3.2.2 mHealth Impact and Scale

The scale and impact of mHealth interventions in Africa have been substantial, though unevenly distributed. North Africa (91%) and Southern Africa (88%) have the highest mobile penetration rates, followed by East Africa (82%) and West Africa (78%), while Central Africa (55%) remains significantly behind (GSMA, 2024). A similar pattern is evident in mHealth service reach, with Southern Africa (42 per 1,000) leading, followed by East Africa (38) and North Africa (35), while West Africa (29) and Central Africa (15) trail (WHO, 2023). Overall, regions with stronger digital infrastructure tend to have higher levels of mHealth service availability and use.

However, the relationship is not perfectly proportional, indicating that connectivity alone is insufficient to drive mHealth scale. For instance, despite having the highest mobile penetration, North Africa does not lead in mHealth reach, suggesting that other factors—such as policy environments, health system integration, digital literacy, and innovation ecosystems—play a crucial role. While mobile connectivity is a necessary foundation for digital health, meaningful impact requires complementary investments in governance, service design, and user adoption.

Figure 3.3. Mobile Phone Penetration and MHealth Reach (2024)

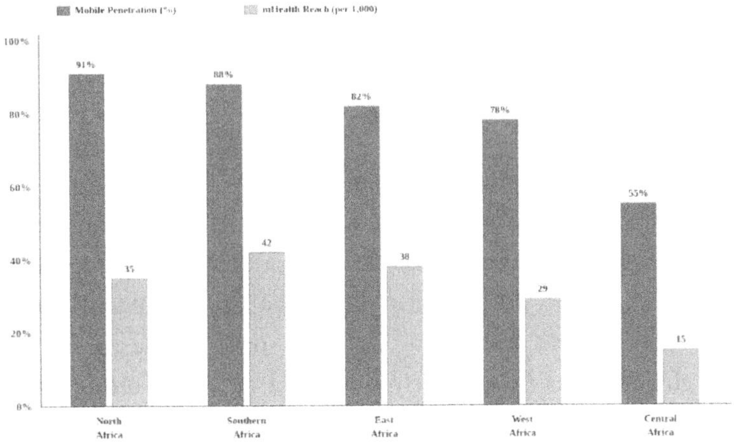

Sources: GSMA (2024), WHO (2023)

Leading mHealth Programs in Africa

Initiatives such as MomConnect in South Africa and Text4Baby Nigeria focus on maternal and child health, reaching millions of women and improving antenatal attendance and health literacy. Babyl in Rwanda has expanded access to virtual consultations for more than 2 million users, easing pressure on health facilities. Platforms like CommCare, operating in more than 50 countries with more than 500,000 community health workers, highlight the role of digital tools in strengthening frontline service delivery and improving data quality.

Other targeted interventions include mPedigree in Ghana and Nigeria, which has enabled over 10 million drug verifications to combat counterfeit medicines, WelTel in Kenya, which has improved HIV treatment adherence by 12–18%, and mTrac in Uganda, which supports nationwide real-time disease surveillance. Collectively, the table illustrates the breadth of mHealth applications—from service delivery and behavior change to supply chain integrity and public health monitoring—and underscores their growing impact on health outcomes and system efficiency across the continent.

Table 3.1. Leading mHealth Platforms in Africa

Program	**Country**	**Focus Area**	**Users/Reach**	**Key Outcome**
MomConnect	South Africa	Maternal & child health	2.5M+ pregnant women	Improved antenatal
Babyl	Rwanda	Virtual consultations	2M+ registered users	Reduced facility congestion
CommCare	50+ countries	CHW digital	500,000+ CHWs	Enhanced data
mPedigree	Ghana,	Drug	10M+ verifications	Reduced
WelTel	Kenya	HIV adherence	10,000+ patients	12–18% adherence
Text4Baby	Nigeria	Prenatal/postnatal	500,000+ women	Improved health
mTrac	Uganda	Disease surveillance	All districts nationally	Real-time outbreak

Source: Data compiled from program reports, peer-reviewed literature, and organizational impact assessments (2023–2024).

Countries should prioritize mHealth systems for primary health care settings where transactions are simple, frequent, and high-value—such as appointment reminders, antenatal care and immunization follow-ups, medication adherence, remote triage, chronic disease monitoring, community health worker support, and referrals—while also developing the underlying health data and interoperability infrastructure. Emphasis should be placed on a PHC-centered mHealth architecture built around a secure digital health identity, or, when appropriate, a Unified Patient Identifier linked to national ID systems; provider and facility registries; interoperable patient summaries; e-prescribing; referral and follow-up tools; teleconsultation services for remote and underserved areas; and reimbursement or public financing rules for approved digital services.

3.3 Electronic Health Records and Health Information Systems

Electronic health records (EHR) and health information systems (HIS) span multiple layers of the digital health technology stack. EMR/EHR systems operate within the Applications and Services Layer (Layer 5), while the aggregate reporting and analytical functions of HMIS platforms extend into the Data Management and Analytics Layer (Layer 4). Both depend on the Digital Identity and Registries Layer (Layer 2) for patient identification and the Interoperability and Data Exchange Layer (Layer 3) for cross-system communication. Chapter 4 (Section 4.3.1) examines the architectural dimensions of EMR systems and their role within the technology stack; this section provides detailed examples of specific platforms, deployment experiences, and implementation lessons.

Figure 3.4. Electronic Health Record Adoption Rates in Selected African Countries (2024)

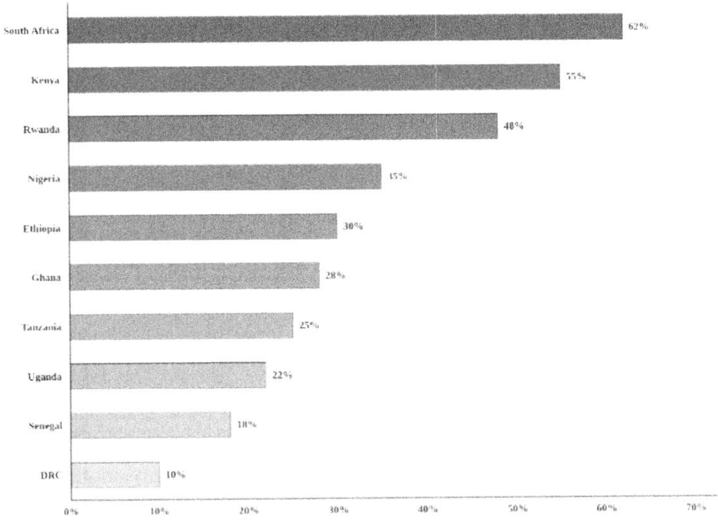

Source: WHO (2024)

Electronic Health Records and Health Management Information Systems constitute the backbone of digital health infrastructure. EMRs manage individual patient records and clinical workflows, while HMIS platforms manage aggregate reporting, planning, surveillance, financing, and performance management. HMIS answers questions like how many, where, trends, stock-outs, performance, and let EMRs answer who, what care, what medication, what diagnosis, and what follow-up.

These systems digitize patient records, clinical workflows, and health data management, enabling improved care coordination, more informed clinical decision-making, and robust monitoring of health system performance (Katurura & Cilliers, 2018). However, EHR adoption in Africa remains uneven, shaped by disparities in infrastructure, human resources, political will, and funding.

3.3.1 Open-Source EHR Platforms

Open-source platforms have been pivotal to EHR expansion across Africa, lowering cost barriers and enabling local customization. OpenMRS, developed at the Regenstrief Institute and Partners in Health, has become one of the most widely deployed open-source medical record systems on the continent, with active implementations in Kenya, Rwanda, Uganda, Mozambique, and other countries. The platform's modular architecture allows implementers to adapt it to local clinical workflows, language requirements, and reporting needs (Mamlin et al., 2006).

In Southern Africa, South Africa's National Health Insurance (NHI) reforms have identified EHR integration as a foundational requirement, and the government is investing in systems to link patient records across the public health network. The country's Health Patient Registration System (HPRS) is one of the continent's largest patient identification projects, aiming to create a master patient index for the public sector (South African National Department of Health, 2023).

3.3.2 District Health Information Software 2

The District Health Information Software 2 (DHIS2) is one of Africa's most consequential digital health achievements. Developed at the University of Oslo with significant contributions from African institutions, DHIS2 is now the world's largest health management information system platform, deployed in more than 80 countries and used by more than 47 African countries as their primary national health information system (HISP, 2024). The platform captures routine health facility data, supports disease surveillance, tracks supply chain logistics, and generates analytical reports.

DHIS2's success offers important lessons for deploying digital health solutions in resource-limited settings. Its open-source model reduced licensing costs. Its web-based architecture minimized hardware requirements. Its configurable design allowed each country to adapt the system to local reporting structures without custom software development. During the COVID-19 pandemic, multiple African countries adopted DHIS2 to track cases, manage contact tracing data and monitor vaccine distribution, demonstrating the platform's adaptability to emergent needs (DHIS2, 2021).

International Insight: EHR Systems Across Global Regions

The European Union's eHealth Digital Service Infrastructure (eHDSI) project enables cross-border sharing of patient summaries and electronic prescriptions among EU member states. The European Health Data Space Regulation entered into force on 26 March 2025 and will be implemented in phases. EU countries are expected to exchange core priority data, such as patient summaries and ePrescriptions, and, by March 2031, broader categories of data, such as lab results, images, and discharge reports, should be operational (European Commission, 2022).

In Southeast Asia, Thailand's universal coverage scheme features a national EHR backbone that connects more than 10,000 public health facilities. In the Caribbean, the Pan American Health Organization (PAHO) has supported EHR deployments aligned with the HL7 FHIR standard across several small island developing states, demonstrating that even resource-limited health systems can achieve digital interoperability through coordinated adoption of standards (PAHO, 2023).

The global practice shows that OpenMRS is the world's leading open-source medical records system, with no license fees or vendor lock-in. Bahmni is a common hospital-focused stack built around OpenMRS, including labs, billing, and other modules, and is specifically designed for low-resource environments. The advantages of open-source practices are clear: lower licensing costs, less vendor lock-in, greater local customization, multilingual support, and a better fit for low-resource settings. However, open source is not inherently sustainable, which is an equally important consideration. Beyond infrastructure, open-source adaptation requires skilled software engineers to maintain and customize the tool for local settings.

Table 3.2. Major Open-Source EHR Platforms Deployed in Africa

Platform	Country examples	Primary Features	Distinguishing Characteristics
OpenMRS	Kenya, Rwanda, Uganda, Mozambique	Patient records, clinical workflows, reporting	Modular, large global community, HIV/TB focus
DHIS2	40+ African countries	Aggregate data, surveillance, analytics	National-scale HMIS, WHO-endorsed
OpenELIS	Côte d'Ivoire, Haiti, Vietnam	Lab information management	Laboratory workflow specialization
GNU Health	Cameroon, Argentina, Jamaica	EHR, hospital management, public health	Integrated socioeconomic determinants
Bahmni	Sierra Leone, Bangladesh, India	Integrated hospital system	Built on OpenMRS with enhanced user

Source: Information drawn from platform documentation, implementation studies, and organizational reports.

The experience indicates that building a layered digital health ecosystem with: a unique patient identity approach; registries for facilities, providers, terminology, and medicines; interoperable EMRs at the point of care; a national HMIS for aggregate reporting; and a health information exchange or interoperability layer that connects them is critical to a national digital health ecosystem.

3.4 Telemedicine and Telehealth Platforms

Telemedicine—the delivery of healthcare services via communications technology—addresses one of Africa's most pressing challenges: the critical shortage of healthcare professionals, particularly specialists, and the difficulty of delivering care across vast distances and in remote communities. The COVID-19 pandemic was a watershed moment for telemedicine adoption on the continent, demonstrating both its feasibility and its value in maintaining continuity of health services during crises (Nachega et al., 2021).

3.4.1 Models of Telemedicine in Africa

Telemedicine in Africa uses several models, each tailored to the continent's specific challenges and opportunities. Synchronous telemedicine, which involves real-time video or audio consultations between patients and providers, has expanded significantly with improved mobile broadband coverage, especially in urban and peri-urban areas. Asynchronous or store-and-forward models, in which clinical data such as medical images, lab results, or patient histories are sent for later review by a specialist, are particularly useful in areas with limited bandwidth or where time zone differences make live consultations difficult.

Nigeria's mDoc and Kenya's Daktari Africa are innovative telemedicine startups that have adapted international telemedicine models to local contexts. In Southern Africa, the Vula Mobile app connects primary care providers in rural areas with specialists across more than 30 medical disciplines and has facilitated over 200,000 clinical consultations since its launch (Vula Mobile, 2023). In Central Africa, where the availability of specialist physicians is among the lowest globally, teleconsultation networks supported by organizations such as the African Center for Global Health and Social Transformation (ACHEST) have linked rural clinics to specialists at regional hospitals.

Figure 3.5. Telemedicine Adoption Growth: Africa vs. Global Average

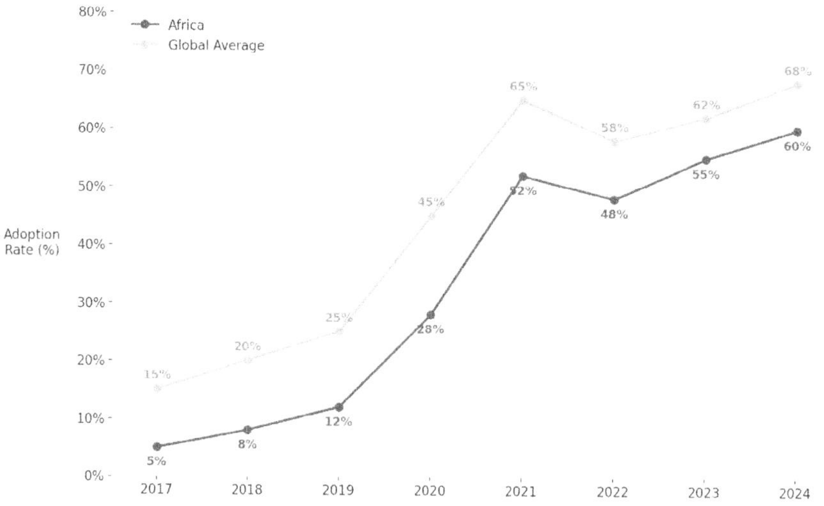

Source: Nachega et 1l. (2021)

3.4.2 Regulatory and Policy Frameworks

The rapid expansion of telemedicine has outpaced regulatory development in most African countries. As of 2024, fewer than 15 African nations had enacted comprehensive telemedicine-specific legislation or regulatory frameworks, creating legal uncertainty regarding clinical liability, cross-border practice, data protection, and reimbursement (WHO AFRO, 2023). South Africa, Kenya, and Nigeria have made progress in developing telemedicine guidelines, yet harmonized regional frameworks remain elusive.

Across the globe, telemedicine is used as a routine channel of care for low-risk, high-volume, and follow-up services, while reserving in-person care for patients who need physical examinations, procedures, or higher-acuity assessments. The most mature systems pair telemedicine with e-prescribing, shared records, triage, referral pathways, reimbursement rules, and clear safety protocols, rather than running it as a standalone video app. WHO's implementation guidance and the OECD's 2025 review point in the same direction (WHO, 2019; OECD, 2025): telemedicine works best when it is integrated into routine care pathways, financed predictably, and governed by clear rules on privacy, quality, continuity, and equity.

Four models of telemedicine are available globally.

- First, provider-embedded telemedicine, in which the patient's usual clinic or hospital offers phone or video visits within its standard EHR and scheduling workflow.
- Second, national or publicly backed telehealth platforms are often used for triage, primary care access, rural outreach, and urgent, low-acuity care.
- Third, specialty telemedicine networks for stroke, mental health, dermatology, ICU support, and remote monitoring.
- Fourth, hybrid marketplace models in which private telemedicine vendors operate under public reimbursement or licensing frameworks.

Countries typically combine these models and regulate them so that telemedicine complements the broader health system rather than fragmenting it. Consistent best practices in regulation include requiring clinician licensure and accountability; defining which cases are appropriate for telemedicine; setting minimum standards for identity, privacy, documentation, and consent; integrating telemedicine with prescribing and referral rules; establishing reimbursement parity or at least predictable reimbursement for appropriate use; requiring escalation to in-person care when clinically necessary; and avoiding "text-only diagnosis" or one-click prescribing for first-time or complex cases. In terms of implementation, countries start with high-value use cases, embed telemedicine in routine clinical workflows, train staff, support digital inclusion, monitor quality and safety, and connect telemedicine to interoperable records and patient-access tools.

In Latin America, the most significant development is the shift toward telehealth as a digital public good, not merely a commercial platform. Brazil is a clear example: telehealth received a permanent national legal basis under Law No. 14,510/2022, which covers both public and private systems

(Government of Brazil, 2022) and multiple regulated health professions. Brazil's Resolution 2.314/2022 from the Federal Council of Medicine significantly expanded the legal basis for telemedicine practice, while Colombia's Law 2015 of 2020 established a comprehensive telehealth regulatory framework (MinSalud Colombia, 2020). The most useful lesson from Latin America is that telemedicine scales more effectively when governments provide common building blocks, open standards, and public implementation support, especially in rural and underserved areas.

Singapore has one of the more tightly regulated models in Asia. Under the Healthcare Services Act framework and the 2024 joint circular (Ministry of Health Singapore, 2024), telemedicine providers must meet licensing requirements, governance obligations, clinical suitability guidelines, and advertising restrictions. The circular also requires real-time video for first-time patients to establish the doctor-patient relationship, prohibits the delivery of teleconsultations solely via self-service text questionnaires, and outlines protocols specifying which patients, conditions, and medications are appropriate for telemedicine. This stands as one of the clearest examples worldwide of a safety-first telemedicine rule set.

These global experiences show that African countries should incorporate telemedicine into an integrated health system. The ideal setup should include provider-embedded video and phone tools, interoperable records, e-prescribing, secure messaging, triage, remote monitoring for selected conditions, clear licensure and clinical-suitability rules, predictable reimbursement, accessibility requirements, and strong privacy protections. Countries should adopt a hybrid model that uses standard clinic and hospital systems for routine telehealth visits, alongside publicly supported national or regional telehealth access points for underserved populations and after-hours care.

Africa should also move toward risk-based regulations that allow simple cases to be managed remotely, while requiring video, identity verification, documentation, and swift escalation for initial visits, controlled medicines, vulnerable patients, or higher-risk conditions. The most effective implementation strategy is to begin with primary care follow-up, mental health services, specialist outreach, hospital-at-home programs, and remote monitoring, then expand telemedicine based on evidence on safety, equity, patient experience, and cost.

3.5 Artificial Intelligence and Machine Learning in Healthcare

Artificial intelligence and machine learning operate across the Data Management and Analytics Layer (Layer 4) and the Applications and Services Layer (Layer 5) of the technology stack. AI-powered analytics depend on data flowing through the Interoperability Layer (Layer 3), and their governance falls under the cross-cutting Governance, Policy, and Standards framework. Chapter 4 briefly introduces clinical decision support systems (Section 4.3.3); this section provides a comprehensive treatment of AI/ML applications, governance frameworks, and global regulatory developments.

Artificial intelligence and machine learning technologies are increasingly applied to healthcare challenges across Africa, offering potential solutions for disease diagnosis, treatment optimization, drug discovery, and improved health system efficiency. While adoption remains in relatively early stages compared to high-income settings, AI and ML applications have demonstrated promising results across multiple domains, and a growing ecosystem of African AI researchers and startups is driving context-appropriate innovation (Wahl et al., 2018).

3.5.1 Disease Diagnosis and Medical Imaging

AI-powered diagnostic tools are among the most advanced and promising applications in African digital health. Computer vision algorithms trained to analyze medical images have shown particular promise in settings where specialist physicians are scarce. In East Africa, AI has been validated in multiple studies for automating chest X-ray reading for tuberculosis screening, with some algorithms achieving sensitivity and specificity comparable to those of expert radiologists (Qin et al., 2019). The CAD4TB algorithm, developed with contributions from African research institutions, has been deployed in screening programs across South Africa, Kenya, Tanzania, and other African countries.

In ophthalmology, AI-based retinal imaging analysis for diabetic retinopathy screening has been piloted in Kenya and South Africa, where the technology enables non-specialist health workers to capture fundus images that are then analyzed by machine-learning algorithms to identify patients who require referral to ophthalmologists. These applications are particularly valuable on a continent where the ophthalmologist-to-population ratio may exceed 1:500,000 in some countries (International Agency for the Prevention of Blindness, 2022).

3.5.2 Predictive Analytics and Public Health Surveillance

Machine learning models are used to predict disease outbreaks, optimize resource allocation, and inform public health interventions across Africa. During the COVID-19 pandemic, predictive models helped several African countries anticipate case surges and plan the deployment of healthcare resources. The Africa Center for Disease Control and Prevention (Africa CDC) integrated AI-driven analytics into its continental surveillance platforms, improving the speed and granularity of epidemiological intelligence (Africa CDC, 2022).

In Nigeria, the eHealth Africa platform uses machine learning algorithms to analyze routine immunization data, identify communities at risk of vaccine-preventable disease outbreaks, and optimize microplanning for vaccination campaigns. Similar predictive analytics tools have been deployed in malaria control programs across East and West Africa, where machine learning models integrate climate data, population movement patterns, and historical case data to forecast transmission intensity and guide intervention targeting (Zinszer et al., 2020).

Across the globe, the use of AI and machine learning is expanding for specific, high-value problems—clinical decision support, imaging, triage, workflow automation, surveillance, and population-risk analytics—while keeping safety, ethics, governance, and human oversight at the center. WHO's guidance stresses that AI in health should be people-centered, equitable, and embedded in health systems, not treated as a stand-alone technology project. WHO also warns that generative and multimodal models require robust governance of validation, transparency, privacy, and accountability before they are used in care. The Organization for Economic Co-operation and Development makes a similar point: the opportunity is large, but so are the risks; countries need coordinated policy, evidence, and incident learning rather than ad hoc deployment.

Across countries, AI-in-health programs typically begin with risk-based regulation, high-quality, representative data, local clinical validation, procurement rules, post-market monitoring, interoperability, and workforce training. The best-performing systems do not start by asking "Where can we use AI?" but rather "Which health-system bottleneck are we solving, with what evidence, under what safeguards?"

The EU AI Act (Regulation 2024/1689) entered into force in August 2024, with AI literacy obligations taking effect in February 2025 and high-risk rules for AI embedded in regulated products taking effect later. It is the most comprehensive regulation addressing AI-related health risks. Many clinical AI tools are classified as high risk and must meet requirements for risk management, data quality, transparency, and human oversight.

In Latin America, PAHO frames AI as a tool for modernizing health systems and services but insists it must be guided by both technical and ethical standards (PAHO, 2024). It has published eight guiding principles for AI in public health, launched an AI in Public Health Readiness Assessment Toolkit with the Inter-American Development Bank in 2024, and in 2025 added workforce-oriented AI training through its Virtual Campus. The regional pattern is less about isolated hospital pilots and more about readiness assessment, ethical guidance, and workforce capability-building at scale. That is a strong model for the Global South because it begins with system readiness before large-scale deployment.

India offers another important model from the Global South: the use of AI in health as part of a broader public digital health and service-delivery ecosystem. Official statements from the Ministry of Health report AI solutions linked to public platforms such as e-Sanjeevani, including clinical decision support and tools for diabetic retinopathy and chest X-ray classification. India has also issued ethical guidance for AI in biomedical research and healthcare through the Indian Council of Medical Research. The lesson from India is that AI works best when it is connected to national digital health infrastructure, telehealth platforms, and public health priorities, rather than sitting in isolated innovation labs.

African countries need not develop AI governance frameworks in isolation; instead, adapt global best practices while ensuring alignment with national and continental values, data sovereignty principles, and the African Union's data policy framework (European Commission, 2024; OECD, 2023).

- First, countries must avoid copying the most expensive or most hyped models. The AU's Continental AI Strategy, endorsed in 2024 (African Union, 2024), provides a high-level commitment to an Africa-centric, development-focused, ethical, and equitable approach.

- Second, countries should prioritize high-impact, low-regret use cases. These include AI for disease surveillance and outbreak intelligence, radiology and pathology decision support in settings where specialists are scarce, maternal and child health risk stratification, supply chain forecasting, claims and fraud analytics, and workflow support in overstretched facilities. These applications better align with Africa's current health-system pressures than a rush into frontier consumer AI. WHO AFRO has emphasized the importance of using AI for risk prediction ahead of public health events, suggesting that health security is one of the most practical entry points.

- Third countries should establish the prerequisites before scaling: interoperable data systems, data governance, digital IDs where appropriate, cloud and connectivity strategy, procurement standards, and workforce capability in health informatics, epidemiology, and AI oversight. Without these foundations, countries risk buying opaque tools trained on non-representative data that perform poorly, thereby widening inequality and locking them into external vendors.

- Fourth, countries need to establish national AI-for-health frameworks within ministries of health. These frameworks will be essential for classifying use cases by risk, requiring human oversight for clinical applications, validating models locally, linking AI procurement to interoperability and data standards, prioritizing public health and workforce-saving use cases, and investing in local research, regulatory capacity, and national datasets.

3.6 Internet of Medical Things (IoMT)

The Internet of Medical Things spans the Physical Infrastructure and Connectivity Layer (Layer 1)—where devices and sensors reside—and the Applications and Services Layer (Layer 5), where the data they generate is processed and acted upon. IoMT devices also rely on the Interoperability Layer (Layer 3) for data transmission standards and on the Governance Layer for device regulation and cybersecurity. This technology domain is not addressed separately in Chapter 4's typology but intersects multiple categories, including digitalization of clinical care (Section 4.3) and public health surveillance (Section 4.4).

The Internet of Medical Things (IoMT) is the interconnected ecosystem of medical devices, software applications, and health systems that collect, transmit, and analyze health data via networked technologies. IoMT devices include wearable health sensors, remote patient monitoring equipment, smart diagnostic instruments, and connected hospital infrastructure. In Africa, IoMT adoption is accelerating, driven by falling device costs, expanding mobile network coverage, and growing recognition of the value of remote monitoring in bridging geographic barriers to care (Gatouillat et al., 2018).

3.6.1 Wearable and Remote Monitoring Technologies

Wearable devices and remote monitoring technologies are increasingly used in African healthcare, particularly for chronic disease management and maternal health. Low-cost pulse oximeters, blood pressure monitors, and glucometers that transmit data via Bluetooth to mobile phones allow patients in rural areas to share vital signs with clinicians without traveling to distant health facilities.

In South Africa, remote monitoring programs for hypertension management have significantly improved blood pressure control among enrolled patients (Bobrow et al., 2016).

Maternal health is a particularly impactful domain for IoMT in Africa. Portable fetal heart rate monitors, such as the Moyo device developed in collaboration with Laerdal Global Health and deployed across multiple East African countries, provide continuous fetal monitoring during labor, enabling earlier detection of fetal distress and reducing stillbirth rates. In West Africa, solar-powered diagnostic devices for off-grid health facilities address the dual challenges of unreliable electricity and limited access to equipment (Laerdal Global Health, 2023).

3.6.2 Smart Diagnostics and Point-of-Care Devices

Point-of-care diagnostic devices linked to digital platforms are a rapidly growing segment of IoMT in Africa. These devices enable laboratory-quality testing at the community level, reducing turnaround times and improving clinical decision-making. The GeneXpert platform, primarily known for tuberculosis diagnosis, exemplifies how connected diagnostic devices can transmit results in real time to national surveillance systems, improving both individual patient management and public health monitoring (Cepheid, 2023).

Global practices indicate that IoMTs are treated as part of a connected care model built on interoperability, reimbursement or procurement pathways, device regulation, clinical governance, cybersecurity, and data-sharing infrastructure. The lesson is that successful deployment of IoMTs depends less on the devices themselves and more on the surrounding system. OECD notes that Remote Patient Monitoring can reduce hospital use and costs in some pilots (OECD, 2025), but adoption remains limited where reimbursement, digital skills, and health-sector digitalization are weak. WHO's digital health strategy similarly frames IoT, virtual care, remote monitoring, and assistive technologies as useful only when embedded in broader health-system transformation (WHO, 2020).

The focus should therefore be on building the foundations that make IoMT useful: patient identity, facility connectivity, interoperable records, device regulation, cybersecurity, clinical workflows, and maintenance capacity. Medical devices can be integrated into digital health systems to improve monitoring and diagnostics, but this integration depends on ICT infrastructure and broader digital health capacity.

- First, use Remote Patient Monitoring and connected devices in high-value, lower-complexity settings: maternal care follow-up, hypertension and diabetes management, oxygen saturation and cardiac monitoring for referral patients, and selected hospital-at-home models in urban areas.

- Second, prioritize smart diagnostics where specialist shortages are acute, such as connected ultrasound, digital radiology, and lab-linked diagnostic instruments.

- Third, build a connected hospital infrastructure focused on interoperability and asset management before attempting to build fully automated smart hospitals.

This should be accompanied by clear reimbursement or public procurement pathways; interoperability standards; regulations for connected and software-enabled medical devices; clinicians' and biomedical engineers' capacity; and resources for maintenance, power, connectivity, and replacement cycles. Without these, wearables and RPM programs remain pilots.

3.7 Blockchain for Health Data Management

Blockchain technology—a distributed, immutable ledger system—offers potential solutions to persistent challenges in African health systems, including health data security, system interoperability, pharmaceutical supply chain integrity, and patient control over personal health information. Although blockchain applications in healthcare remain largely in pilot or early deployment stages across Africa, the technology's core attributes of decentralization, transparency, and tamper resistance make it well suited to environments where institutional trust may be limited and infrastructure fragmented (Kuo et al., 2017). Potential applications range from patient identity management and health data security to drug supply chain verification and clinical trial data integrity.

Drug Supply Chain Verification

Counterfeit and substandard medicines pose one of the most compelling use cases for blockchain in African healthcare. The WHO estimates that 1 in 10 medical products in low- and middle-income countries is substandard or falsified, with sub-Saharan Africa disproportionately affected (WHO, 2017). Blockchain-based track-and-trace systems can create tamper-proof records of a drug's journey from manufacturer to patient, enabling verification at every point in the supply chain.

Ghana's mPedigree, now operating across multiple African and Asian countries, pioneered mobile-based drug authentication, enabling consumers to verify medication authenticity via SMS. The platform has been enhanced with blockchain capabilities to enable end-to-end supply chain transparency.

Health Data Security

In countries with fragmented national health information systems, where data breaches pose growing risks, blockchain offers a framework for securing health data while enabling controlled sharing across institutions. Blockchain-based patient identity systems can create portable, verifiable health credentials that work across providers and even across borders, addressing the challenge of patient identification in health systems where unique national identifiers may not yet be universally deployed.

Insurance Claim Processing

Blockchain has been explored as a means to improve transparency, efficiency, and trust in health insurance claims processing, particularly in contexts where fraud, delays, and fragmented verification systems are prevalent. Using distributed ledgers and smart contracts, claims can be automatically validated against eligibility rules and service records, enabling faster adjudication and reducing administrative overhead.

In Africa, however, most applications remain small and at the pilot or proof-of-concept stage, with limited integration into national insurance systems. Blockchain adds value primarily in multi-actor, low-trust environments, but only when foundational systems—such as digitized claims data, interoperable health information systems, and clear regulatory frameworks—are in place. Without them, blockchain risks increasing complexity rather than solving inefficiencies, suggesting that countries should prioritize system readiness before scaling such solutions.

Clinical Trials and Data Integrity

Blockchain is increasingly seen as a powerful tool for maintaining data integrity, transparency, and auditability in clinical trials, especially in multi-site and cross-border studies. Immutable, timestamped records enable secure tracking of data changes, build trust among stakeholders, and support regulatory compliance. It also facilitates innovations such as dynamic consent, which allows participants to control how their data is used while ensuring traceability for researchers and regulators.

In Africa, where clinical trials are expanding, blockchain offers a promising way to strengthen credibility and trust in global research collaborations, yet implementation remains limited. Most efforts remain conceptual or pilot-based, constrained by gaps in digital infrastructure, regulatory systems, and integration with existing trial management platforms.

Patient Identity Management and Health Records

Blockchain has proven most relevant in Africa for managing patient identities and securely sharing health records, addressing persistent issues such as fragmented records, lack of unique identifiers, and limited interoperability. By enabling decentralized, secure, and patient-controlled identities, blockchain allows individuals to control access to their data while ensuring consistency and traceability across providers. This is especially valuable in areas with mobile populations and weak civil registration systems. Although several pilots and research efforts show promise, large-scale adoption remains limited due to challenges such as integration with national ID systems, data protection frameworks, scalability, and user acceptance.

Blockchain in health has spurred numerous pilots, prototypes, and policy discussions at the international level, with a few mature, routine implementations. Systematic reviews consistently show that the most common applications include health records and personal health records, consent and identity management, pharmaceutical and device supply-chain traceability, clinical trial and research data integrity, insurance and claims automation, and vaccine or health certificates. At the same time, the literature indicates that many implementations remain proof-of-concept rather than scaled national infrastructure, mainly due to governance, interoperability, privacy, cost, and performance issues.

Estonia is the best-known example: its digital health ecosystem uses the KSI blockchain (e-Estonia, 2025) primarily as an integrity and audit layer to protect e-health records and detect tampering, rather than storing full clinical records directly on-chain. In Latin America, a notable regional example is LACPASS, supported by PAHO, HL7, and LACChain (PAHO, 2023), which focuses on interoperable digital health certificates and trusted cross-border exchange. Singapore's HealthCerts, developed by GovTech and the Ministry of Health (GovTech Singapore, 2022), is one of the clearest real-world cases of blockchain adding value in health: it uses blockchain-enabled verifiable documents for tamper-proof vaccination certificates, especially for cross-border verification. South Korea has also piloted blockchain-enabled personal health data platforms, such as MyHealthData (Ministry of Health and Welfare, Republic of Korea, 2023), in which blockchain is used to verify data integrity and support user control over data exchange among institutions.

Global experience shows that blockchain can address trust problems by providing capabilities conventional databases do not readily offer: tamper-evident audit trails, multi-party verification without requiring full trust in a single operator, portable verifiable credentials, and provenance tracking across fragmented supply chains. This suggests that African countries should treat blockchain as a complementary trust layer rather than the foundation of the entire digital health system. The priority should be digital public infrastructure for health: reliable identifiers, standards-based EMRs and HMIS, interoperable health information exchange, consent frameworks, cybersecurity, and governance. Once those foundations exist, blockchain can be useful in a few high-value areas: medicine and vaccine supply-chain traceability, verifiable credentials for cross-border health services or public health certificates, consent and audit logging for health data sharing, and clinical research integrity in multicountry studies.

3.8 Big Data Analytics in Public Health

Big data analytics sits squarely within the Data Management and Analytics Layer (Layer 4) of the technology stack, transforming raw data flowing through the Interoperability Layer (Layer 3) into actionable insights for decision-makers. Chapter 4 (Section 4.9) introduces the research and data analytics platform category within the typology; this section provides a detailed treatment of analytical methods, data sources, and global frameworks for the secondary use of health data.

Big data analytics involves processing and analyzing large, complex, and often heterogeneous datasets to derive actionable insights for health system decision-making. In public health, big data sources include electronic health records, disease surveillance systems, mobile health data, social media content, environmental and climate sensor data, satellite imagery, and, increasingly, genomic data. Advanced analytical methods, including machine learning, natural language processing, and spatial analytics, enable population health monitoring, disease outbreak prediction, health system performance assessment, and evidence-based policymaking (Mooney & Pejaver, 2018).

3.8.1 Disease Surveillance and Outbreak Prediction

Big data analytics have strengthened disease surveillance across Africa, enabling faster detection and more targeted responses to outbreaks. The Integrated Disease Surveillance and Response (IDSR) framework, implemented with WHO support in most African countries, has increasingly integrated digital data sources and analytical tools. During the Ebola outbreaks in West Africa (2014–2016) and the Democratic Republic of Congo (2018–2020), data analytics platforms helped track transmission chains, model outbreak trajectories, and allocate response resources (WHO AFRO, 2020).

The use of anonymized mobile phone data for analyzing population mobility during disease outbreaks has been pioneered in several African settings. In collaboration with mobile network operators, researchers in Senegal, Kenya, and South Africa have used aggregated call detail records to track population movements and predict the geographic spread of infectious diseases, including cholera, malaria, and COVID-19 (Wesolowski et al., 2015). These approaches raise important questions about data privacy and the ethical use of telecommunications data for public health—questions that African data governance frameworks are beginning to address.

3.8.2 Climate-Health Linkages and Environmental Analytics

Africa's disproportionate vulnerability to climate change makes a compelling case for integrating environmental big data into health analytics. Machine learning models that combine satellite-derived environmental data (rainfall patterns, vegetation indices, temperature anomalies) with epidemiological data have improved the precision of malaria early warning systems in the Sahel and East Africa.

Across these regions, experience with big data analytics in health is far more advanced and practical than with blockchain. The dominant pattern is not a single "big data platform," but a gradual build-out of linked health datasets, interoperable digital health systems, public-health surveillance dashboards, and secondary use frameworks that enable the analysis of data from clinical care, insurance claims, registries, laboratories, and population systems for policy, planning, research, and service improvement. Europe is advancing this most explicitly through the European Health Data Space (EHDS) (European Commission, 2022), which is designed to enable both primary use of electronic health data and secondary use for research, innovation, public health, and policymaking.

The EU's approach is evolving from isolated hospital analytics to a governed ecosystem in which health data can be reused across borders for public-interest purposes, science, innovation, and regulatory work. This shift underscores Europe's focus on rules, access bodies, interoperability, and the secure reuse of electronic health data at scale, rather than on AI pilots alone.

In practice, the European lesson is that analytics becomes powerful only when legal frameworks, data stewardship, and shared infrastructure are built together.

In Latin America and the Caribbean, PAHO's work on health information systems emphasizes integrating data from multiple sources (PAHO, 2023) and using digital tools to apply them ethically and generate strategic information for public health. PAHO also maintains regional health data platforms with long-running indicator series and disaggregation tools. Its digital transformation agenda explicitly highlights real-time dashboards, outbreak detection, and analytics to support evidence-based health policy.

The main application areas are quite similar across different regions.

- The first is public health surveillance and outbreak detection, including dashboards, syndromic surveillance, epidemic intelligence, and emergency response.

- The second is health system planning and performance management, where analytics are used for budgeting, capacity planning, target tracking, utilization analysis, and service quality monitoring.

- The third is clinical and population health management, especially in risk stratification, chronic disease management, and care gap identification.

- The fourth encompasses research and the secondary use of health data, with linked datasets supporting innovation, policy analysis, regulatory science, and health technology assessment.

- The fifth involves claims, financing, and efficiency analytics, particularly in insurance-based systems such as those in South Korea and other countries with comprehensive administrative data.

The best path is to build on reliable routine data, including civil registration and vital statistics, interoperable EMRs and HMIS, and laboratory and supply-chain data, and to support health information exchange and clear governance for privacy and data use. Once these are in place, analytics can deliver high value in disease surveillance, maternal and child health tracking, workforce deployment, essential medicine management, insurance analytics, and district-level planning.

3.9 Digital Payment Systems for Healthcare

Digital payment systems for healthcare operate within the Applications and Services Layer (Layer 5) of the technology stack, but their effectiveness depends on the Digital Identity Layer (Layer 2) for beneficiary verification and the Interoperability Layer (Layer 3) to connect payment flows with clinical and insurance systems. Chapter 4 (Section 4.10) introduces digital health financing as one of the eight intervention categories; this section provides applied detail on mobile money platforms, health wallets, and global payment integration models.

Mobile money and digital payment platforms have fundamentally transformed financial transactions across Africa, and healthcare increasingly uses them for health financing, insurance premium collection, and service fee payments. M-Pesa, launched in 2007 in Kenya by Safaricom and Vodafone, demonstrated the viability of mobile-based financial services and subsequently expanded across the region, inspiring other payment platforms across the continent (Jack & Suri, 2014). By 2024, Africa hosted more than 200 active mobile money platforms and over 800 million registered accounts, making it the world's most dynamic mobile money ecosystem (GSMA, 2024).

3.9.1 Mobile Money for Health Financing

Healthcare increasingly uses mobile money for various financing functions. National health insurance schemes in Kenya, Ghana, and Tanzania accept premium payments via mobile money, significantly reducing transaction costs and improving collection rates among informal-sector workers and rural populations who lack access to traditional banking services. In Ghana, the National Health Insurance Authority integrated mobile money payments into its premium collection system, resulting in a 15% increase in enrollment among previously hard-to-reach populations (Ghana NHIA, 2023).

Community-based health financing mechanisms have also adopted digital payments. Village savings and loan associations (VSLAs) in Uganda, Malawi, and several other countries use mobile money to pool health savings and pay for health services, creating digitized community health financing models that improve transparency, reduce cash-handling risks, and generate data for financial planning (UNCDF, 2022).

3.9.2 Digital Health Wallets and Microinsurance

Innovative digital health wallet products are emerging across Africa, combining elements of health savings accounts, microinsurance, and mobile money. Products such as M-TIBA in Kenya create digital health wallets that allow individuals to save specifically for healthcare, receive employer or donor contributions, and pay participating health providers directly. These platforms generate valuable data on healthcare spending patterns and enable mechanisms to extend financial protection to populations outside formal insurance schemes (PharmAccess Foundation, 2023).

Table 3.3. Digital Payment Platforms for Healthcare in Africa

Platform	Country	Health Application	Scale	Impact
M-Pesa	Kenya, Tanzania	Insurance premiums, provider payments	50M+ users (Kenya)	Reduced transaction costs
M-TIBA	Kenya	Health savings wallet	5M+ users	Dedicated health savings
MTN MoMo	Ghana, Uganda	NHIS premium collection	Regional coverage	Improved enrollment rates
Airtel Money	Malawi, Uganda	Health facility fee payment	Multi-country	Reduced cash handling

Source: Data drawn from operator reports, published case studies, and organizational documentation (2023–2024).

Across Asia, Latin America, the Caribbean, and Europe, digital payment systems in healthcare have evolved from simple cashless transactions into integrated components of broader digital health and financial ecosystems. In Asia, countries such as India, China, Thailand, and Indonesia demonstrate how real-time payment systems, digital identity, and health platforms can be tightly integrated. Systems such as the Unified Payments Interface and PromptPay enable instant, low-cost payments at the point of care, often linked to national health insurance and digital health records. Similarly, platforms such as Alipay and WeChat Pay integrate healthcare payments with broader digital services, creating seamless user experiences.

Latin America's Pix instant payment system in Brazil has been integrated into the public health system for fee collection and provider reimbursement, reaching more than 150 million users (Central Bank of Brazil, 2023). In South and Southeast Asia, India's Unified Payments Interface (UPI) has been linked to the Ayushman Bharat health insurance scheme, enabling cashless hospital transactions for more than 500 million beneficiaries (Reserve Bank of India, 2023; National Health Authority India, 2024). In the Caribbean, Jamaica's JAM-DEX central bank digital currency pilot includes a health payment use case (Bank of Jamaica, 2023). Africa's mobile money ecosystem is arguably more advanced than many of these systems in terms of population coverage and grassroots adoption, suggesting that integrating mobile money with health financing is a strategic opportunity for the continent (World Bank, 2023; Reserve Bank of India, 2023).

3.10 Conclusion

The digital technologies examined in this chapter—from mobile health applications reaching millions of users to emerging AI diagnostic systems—collectively represent a transformative force for African healthcare systems. Each technology addresses specific health system challenges while contributing to a broader digital health ecosystem that, when functioning cohesively, can fundamentally reshape how healthcare is delivered, financed, and experienced across the continent.

However, the transformative potential of these technologies can be realized only when implementation is grounded in several cross-cutting themes. Infrastructure development, including reliable electricity and Internet connectivity, remains a prerequisite for most digital health interventions. Interoperability standards ensure that disparate systems can exchange data and work together rather than creating new information silos. Data governance frameworks, including privacy protections and ethical data-use policies, are essential to maintaining public trust. Digital literacy among health workers and communities determines whether technologies are adopted, used effectively, and sustained over time. Sustainable financing models ensure that digital health investments are not dependent solely on external donor funding but are integrated into national health budgets. Finally, enabling policy environments provide the regulatory clarity and institutional support needed for digital health innovations to scale responsibly.

More importantly, Africa does not need to develop these technologies and frameworks in isolation. Global experience offers valuable models for adaptation. The continent's unique strengths—including its mobile money ecosystem, its young and digitally engaged population, and the flexibility afforded by the relative absence of legacy systems—position it to innovate in ways other regions cannot. The challenge is to translate these advantages into sustained, equitable progress in digital health transformation.

References

Africa CDC. (2022). Digital transformation strategy for Africa's public health: Annual progress report. Africa Centers for Disease Control and Prevention.

African Development Bank. (2020). Digitalization of healthcare in Africa: A decade of growth. African Development Bank Group.

Aranda-Jan, C. B., Mohutsiwa-Dibe, N., & Loukanova, S. (2014). Systematic review on what works, what does not work and why of the implementation of mobile health (mHealth) projects in Africa. BMC Public Health, 14, 188. https://doi.org/10.1186/1471-2458-14-188

Babyl Rwanda. (2023). Annual impact report 2023. https://www.babyl.rw

Bobrow, K., Farmer, A. J., Springer, D., Shany, T., Myers, B., Powell, J., ... & Levitt, N. (2016). Mobile phone text messages to support treatment adherence in adults with high blood pressure. Circulation, 133(6), 592–600. https://doi.org/10.1161/CIRCULATIONAHA.115.017530

Brazilian Ministry of Health. (2022). e-SUS: National primary care information system annual report. Ministério da Saúde.

Cepheid. (2023). GeneXpert connectivity and data management solutions. Cepheid/Danaher Corporation.

DHIS2. (2021). COVID-19 response: How countries used DHIS2 for pandemic surveillance and vaccine management. University of Oslo.

Dimagi. (2024). CommCare: Global impact report. https://www.dimagi.com

Ethiopian Federal Ministry of Health. (2021). Health sector digital transformation plan (2021–2025). Federal Democratic Republic of Ethiopia.

European Commission. (2022). eHealth Digital Service Infrastructure: Progress Report on Cross-Border Health Data Exchange. European Commission.

European Commission. (2024). Regulation (EU) 2024/1689 laying down harmonized rules on artificial intelligence (AI Act). Official Journal of the European Union.

Gatouillat, A., Badr, Y., Massot, B., & Sejdic, E. (2018). Internet of medical things: A review of recent contributions dealing with cyber-physical systems in medicine. IEEE Internet of Things Journal, 5(5), 3810–3822. https://doi.org/10.1109/JIOT.2018.2849014

Ghana NHIA. (2023). National Health Insurance Authority annual report 2022/2023. Republic of Ghana.

Government of India. (2021). Aarogya Setu: Digital health technology for COVID-19 response. Ministry of Electronics and Information Technology.

Grameen Foundation. (2019). Mobile Technology for Community Health (MOTECH): Ghana implementation final report. Grameen Foundation.

GSMA. (2023). The mobile economy: Sub-Saharan Africa 2023. GSM Association.

GSMA. (2024). The state of mobile Internet connectivity 2024. GSM Association.

HISP. (2024). DHIS2 global implementation map and statistics. Health Information Systems Programme, University of Oslo.

International Agency for the Prevention of Blindness. (2022). Africa WOphthalmology Workforce Report. IAPB.

Jack, W., & Suri, T. (2014). Risk sharing and transaction costs: Evidence from Kenya's mobile money revolution. American Economic Review, 104(1), 183–223. https://doi.org/10.1257/aer.104.1.183

Katurura, M. C., & Cilliers, L. (2018). Electronic health record system in the public health care sector of South Africa: A systematic literature review. African Journal of Primary Health Care & Family Medicine, 10(1), e1–e8. https://doi.org/10.4102/phcfm.v10i1.1746

Kuo, T. T., Kim, H. E., & Ohno-Machado, L. (2017). Blockchain distributed ledger technologies for biomedical and health care applications. Journal of the American Medical Informatics Association, 24(6), 1211–1220. https://doi.org/10.1093/jamia/ocx068

Laerdal Global Health. (2023). Moyo fetal heart rate monitor: Impact assessment 2018–2023. Laerdal Global Health.

Mamlin, B. W., Biondich, P. G., Wolfe, B. A., Fraser, H., Jazayeri, D., Allen, C., ... & Tierney, W. M. (2006). Cooking up an open source EMR for developing countries: OpenMRS—A recipe for successful collaboration. AMIA Annual Symposium Proceedings, 529–533.

Medical Council of India. (2020). Telemedicine practice guidelines: Enabling registered medical practitioners to provide healthcare using telemedicine —Board of Governors, Medical Council of India.

Mooney, S. J., & Pejaver, V. (2018). Big data in public health: Terminology, machine learning, and privacy. Annual Review of Public Health, 39, 95–112. https://doi.org/10.1146/annurev-publhealth-040617-014208

Nachega, J. B., Atteh, R., Ihekweazu, C., Sam-Agudu, N. A., Adejumo, P., Nsanzimana, S., ... & Zumla, A. (2021). Contact tracing and the COVID-19 response in Africa. American Journal of Tropical Medicine and Hygiene, 104(4), 1179–1187. https://doi.org/10.4269/ajtmh.21-0073

OECD. (2023). Artificial intelligence in health: State of the art and future directions. Organisation for Economic Co-operation and Development.

Pan American Health Organization. (2022). Digital health in the Americas: Telemedicine regulatory landscape. PAHO/WHO.

Pan American Health Organization. (2023). EHR implementation in the Caribbean: Lessons from FHIR-based deployments. PAHO/WHO.

PharmAccess Foundation. (2023). M-TIBA digital health wallet: Impact and lessons learned. PharmAccess Foundation.

Qin, Z. Z., Sander, M. S., Rai, B., Titber, C. N., Suber, S., Pervaiz, A., ... & Creswell, J. (2019). Using artificial intelligence to read chest radiographs for tuberculosis detection: A multi-site evaluation. Scientific Reports, 9, 15434. https://doi.org/10.1038/s41598-019-51503-3

Reserve Bank of India. (2023). UPI ecosystem: Annual report on digital payments infrastructure—Reserve Bank of India.

Sondaal, S. F., Browne, J. L., Amoakoh-Coleman, M., Borgstein, A., Miltenburg, A. S., Verwijs, M., & Klipstein-Grobusch, K. (2016). Assessing the effect of mHealth interventions in improving maternal and neonatal care in low- and middle-income countries: A systematic review. PLoS ONE, 11(5), e0154664. https://doi.org/10.1371/journal.pone.0154664

South African National Department of Health. (2023). National digital health strategy 2023–2028. Republic of South Africa.

UNCDF. (2022). Village savings and loan associations in the digital era: Mobile money integration for health financing. United Nations Capital Development Fund.

UNECA. (2022). Blockchain for health supply chain management in Africa: A technical assessment. United Nations Economic Commission for Africa.

USAID. (2023). Famine Early Warning Systems Network (FEWS NET): Health-climate integration framework. United States Agency for International Development.

Vula Mobile. (2023). Impact report: Telemedicine consultations in Southern Africa 2016–2023. Vula Mobile.

Wahl, B., Cossy-Gantner, A., Germann, S., & Schwalbe, N. R. (2018). Artificial intelligence (AI) and global health: How can AI contribute to health in resource-poor settings? BMJ Global Health, 3(4), e000798. https://doi.org/10.1136/bmjgh-2018-000798

Wesolowski, A., Buckee, C. O., Engel, L., Metcalf, C. J. E., Schoning, S., Zuber, M., ... & Tatem, A. J. (2015). Connecting mobility to infectious diseases: The promise and limits of cell phone data. Journal of Infectious Diseases, 214(suppl_4), S414–S420. https://doi.org/10.1093/infdis/jiw273

WHO. (2017). WHO global surveillance and monitoring system for substandard and falsified medical products. World Health Organization.

WHO. (2022). Global strategy on human resources for health: Workforce 2030 progress report. World Health Organization.

WHO. (2023). Global digital health monitor: Regional assessment 2023. World Health Organization.

WHO AFRO. (2020). Integrated disease surveillance and response in the African Region: Community-based surveillance progress report. WHO Regional Office for Africa.

WHO AFRO. (2023). Telemedicine in the WHO African Region: Policy and regulatory landscape assessment. WHO Regional Office for Africa.

World Bank. (2023). Global Findex Database 2022: Financial inclusion, digital payments, and resilience in the age of COVID-19. World Bank Group.

World Health Organization. (2019). WHO guideline: Recommendations on digital interventions for health system strengthening. WHO Press.

World Health Organization. (2020). Global strategy on digital health 2020–2025. WHO Press.

Zinszer, K., Verma, A. D., Charland, K., Brewer, T. F., Brownstein, J. S., Sun, Z., & Buckeridge, D. L. (2020). A scoping review of malaria forecasting: Past work and future directions. BMJ Open, 10(7), e029736. https://doi.org/10.1136/bmjopen-2019-029736

Chapter 4: Typologies of Digital Health Applications

4.1 Introduction

The digital health landscape encompasses a wide array of technologies, applications, and interventions that span the entire health system—from individual patient care to population health management, from clinical diagnostics to supply chain logistics, and from health worker education to health research. This diversity, while representing enormous potential, also creates challenges in understanding, comparing, and coordinating digital health efforts across countries and organizations. A clear typology—a systematic framework for categorizing digital health interventions—provides essential structure for analyzing the current landscape, identifying gaps, and planning strategic investments.

This chapter presents a comprehensive typology of digital health, building on frameworks developed by the World Health Organization (WHO, 2018; WHO, 2023), the International Telecommunication Union (ITU, 2021), and the African Union, while also considering the realities of health systems across Africa and the broader Global South. The typology organizes digital health interventions into eight major categories based on their primary purpose and target users, recognizing that many interventions span multiple categories. Before exploring these categories, the chapter introduces the digital health technology stack—a fundamental conceptual model that describes the layered structure underpinning all digital health systems. This technology stack model will serve as a recurring reference throughout the rest of this book, providing readers with a consistent lens for understanding how different applications connect to shared infrastructure, data standards, and governance frameworks.

4.2 The Digital Health Technology Stack

Understanding how digital health applications are built, deployed, and interconnected requires a conceptual model that transcends individual products and vendors. The digital health technology stack provides this model. Analogous to the technology stacks used in software engineering—where layers of hardware, middleware, and applications work together to deliver services—the digital health technology stack describes the hierarchical architecture on which all digital health efforts rest. Each layer depends on the layers beneath it; weaknesses at any level can cascade upward, affecting the applications end users interact with and rely on.

The concept of a technology stack has become increasingly common among global health architects and policymakers. The WHO's revised Classification of Digital Interventions, Services and Applications in Health (CDISAH) emphasizes that digital health interventions do not exist in isolation but are embedded within digital services and applications, which, in turn, depend on enabling infrastructure (WHO, 2023). Similarly, the concept of Digital Public Infrastructure (DPI)—comprising digital identity, data exchange layers, and payment systems—has emerged as a foundational paradigm for national digital health strategies, particularly in low- and middle-income countries (Sharma et al., 2023).

This section presents a digital health technology stack that will serve as a reference framework throughout this book. The model comprises five foundation layers and seven cross-cutting enablers. From bottom to top, the five foundation layers are: (1) the Physical Infrastructure and Connectivity Layer; (2) the Digital Identity and Registries Layer; (3) the Interoperability and Data Exchange Layer; (4) the Data Management and Analytics Layer; and (5) the Application and Services Layer. Seven cross-cutting enablers operate vertically across all five foundation layers: Digital Health Skills and Workforce; Research and Development; the HealthTech Ecosystem; Digital Health Strategy; Governance, Policy, and Standards; Regional Cooperation; and Financing and Sustainability. Figure 4.1 illustrates this layered model, with the foundation layers on the left and the enablers on the right.

4.2.1 Layer 1: Physical Infrastructure and Connectivity

The foundational layer of the digital health technology stack comprises the physical hardware, network connectivity, power supply, and cloud or on-premise computing infrastructure on which all digital health systems depend.

This layer includes telecommunications networks (broadband, mobile, and satellite), data centers and cloud computing platforms, end-user devices (smartphones, tablets, workstations, point-of-care devices), and the electrical power that powers them.

Infrastructure availability varies widely across and within countries. In Sub-Saharan Africa, mobile network coverage has expanded rapidly, reaching about 84% of the population by 2023, yet meaningful broadband connectivity remains limited in rural areas (GSMA, 2024). The rise of cloud computing has reduced the need for on-premises server infrastructure, enabling countries to deploy scalable health information systems without heavy capital investment. Amazon Web Services, Microsoft Azure, and Google Cloud each offer healthcare-specific solutions with regional data residency options, though data sovereignty concerns remain paramount in many jurisdictions (Aalpha, 2026).

Figure 4.1. The Digital Health Technology Stack: Five Foundation Layers and Seven Cross-Cutting Enablers

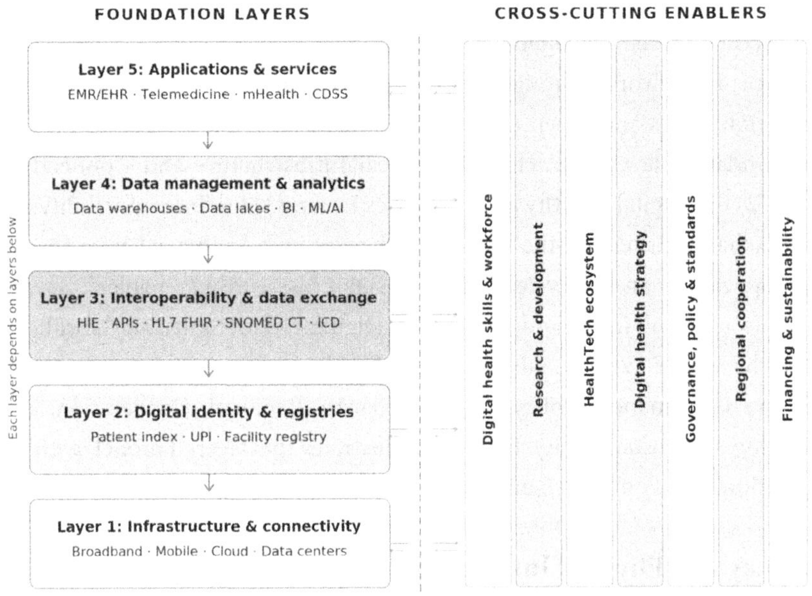

Source: Adapted from WHO (2023), Aalpha (2026), and the author's elaboration.

Singapore's Synapxe (formerly IHiS) provides an instructive example of how a national health technology agency manages the infrastructure layer. Synapxe operates a unified healthcare technology stack that integrates cloud platforms such as Azure with established solutions like HealthHub, the country's patient-facing digital health portal (Synapxe, 2023). Australia's approach to infrastructure illustrates a federated model: the Australian Digital Health Agency manages the national My Health Record system, which connects a diverse ecosystem of state-based hospital systems, private general practitioners, and pathology laboratories through a shared national infrastructure (Australian Digital Health Agency, 2024).

4.2.2 Layer 2: Digital Identity and Registries

Effective digital health systems require the ability to uniquely identify patients, health workers, and health facilities. This layer includes master patient indices, health worker and facility registries, and digital identity systems that authenticate users across platforms. Without a reliable identity infrastructure, data cannot be reliably linked across encounters and institutions, undermining the value of digitalization.

India's Ayushman Bharat Digital Mission (ABDM) is one of the most ambitious implementations of health identity infrastructure. Built on the Aadhaar biometric identification system, ABDM assigns every citizen a 14-digit Ayushman Bharat Health Account (ABHA) number, enabling interoperable health records across public and private providers. As of March 2024, more than 568 million ABHA accounts had been created, and over 350 million health records were linked to the digital ecosystem (Balsari et al., 2024). Estonia takes a different approach, using its national e-ID system—held by virtually all residents—as the authentication backbone for its Estonian Health Information System (EHIS). Nearly 100% of residents have a digital health record, and approximately 99% of prescriptions are issued electronically (Groenewegen et al., 2018; e-Estonia, 2025).

In Africa, countries have pursued varied approaches to health identity. Rwanda's Community-Based Health Insurance (CBHI) scheme includes a unique beneficiary identification system integrated with the national EMR platform. Nigeria's National Health Insurance Authority has begun issuing digital health insurance identification cards linked to a biometric database. These identity layers are essential prerequisites for the interoperability functions described in the next section.

4.2.3 Layer 3: Interoperability and Data Exchange

The interoperability layer enables different health information systems to communicate, exchange, and meaningfully use shared data. This layer comprises health information exchange (HIE) platforms, application programming interfaces (APIs), messaging standards (such as HL7 and Fast Healthcare Interoperability Resources (FHIR)), and terminology services (such as Systematized Nomenclature of Medicine -- Clinical Terms (SNOMED CT), International Classification of Diseases (ICD), and Logical Observation Identifiers, Names and Codes (LOINC)). Without robust interoperability, digital health systems become silos—generating data that cannot be shared across facilities, programs, or jurisdictions.

Estonia's X-Road exemplifies the highest standard for national interoperability infrastructure. Originally developed in the early 2000s as a secure data exchange platform for all government services, X-Road enables Estonia's health information systems to exchange data securely while preserving a decentralized structure: data remains with the original custodian and is shared on demand through encrypted, digitally signed transactions (e-Estonia, 2025). X-Road now connects over 929 institutions, supports more than 3,000 digital services, and has been adopted or adapted by over 20 countries, including Finland and Iceland, and, more recently, through pilot implementations in Chile, Australia, and South Africa (Nortal, 2024; NIIS, 2023).

In Africa, DHIS2 has become the de facto platform for routine health data exchange, deployed in 47 countries. However, DHIS2 primarily supports aggregate-level data reporting. Individual-level data exchange—critical for care coordination—requires additional interoperability infrastructure.

Rwanda's national Health Information Exchange, which connects the national EMR system to laboratory, pharmacy, and insurance systems, demonstrates how African countries can build interoperability infrastructure on existing platforms (Rwanda Biomedical Center, 2022). The Open Health Information Exchange (OpenHIE) framework provides an architectural blueprint that several African countries have adopted to guide their interoperability strategies.

Figure 4.2. Interoperability Architecture: How Health Information Systems Connect Through a Health Information Exchange

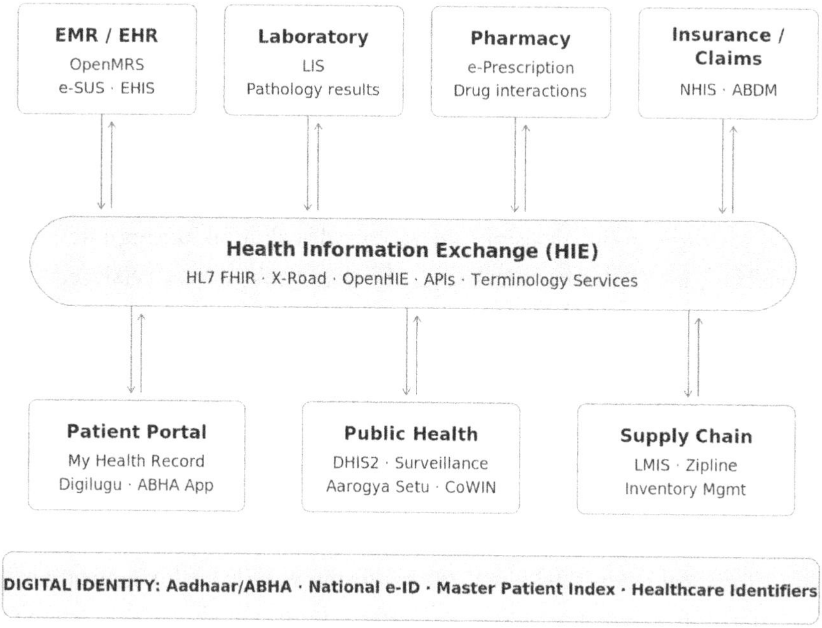

Source: Adapted from OpenHIE Architecture and the author's elaboration.

4.2.4 Layer 4: Data Management and Analytics

The data management and analytics layer encompasses data warehouses, data lakes, business intelligence tools, machine learning platforms, and analytical pipelines that transform raw health data into actionable insights. It converts data flowing through the interoperability layer into dashboards, reports, predictive models, and decision-support outputs.

Advanced analytics capabilities are increasingly central to health system performance. South Africa's Health Data Research Network connects researchers with de-identified health data while safeguarding privacy, enabling local researchers to generate evidence rather than relying exclusively on international collaborators (South African Medical Research Council, 2022). Brazil's Unified Health System (SUS) aggregates data from more than 5,400 municipalities via the e-SUS platform, feeding national dashboards that monitor primary care coverage and disease burden across the country's vast and diverse territory (Ministério da Saúde do Brasil, 2022).

The COVID-19 pandemic highlighted both the power and the limitations of health data analytics in low- and middle-income settings. India's CoWIN platform, originally developed to manage COVID-19 vaccination registration and scheduling for more than a billion citizens, generated vast datasets that informed real-time policy decisions on vaccine distribution, dosing intervals, and coverage gaps (Balsari et al., 2024). The platform's success catalyzed the expansion of India's digital health data infrastructure under ABDM.

4.2.5 Layer 5: Applications and Services

The application layer is the most visible component of the digital health technology stack—it is where clinicians, patients, administrators, and public health officials directly interact with digital health tools. This layer includes electronic medical records, telemedicine platforms, mobile health applications, clinical decision support systems, laboratory information systems, supply chain management software, e-learning platforms, and many other applications described in the typology presented later in this chapter.

Applications at this layer draw on all the lower layers for connectivity, identity, interoperability, and analytics. The eight categories of digital health interventions presented in Section 4.2 operate entirely within this application layer, though their effectiveness depends critically on the maturity of the layers beneath them. A telemedicine application, for example, requires reliable connectivity (Layer 1), authenticated user identities (Layer 2), access to patient records from other systems (Layer 3), and analytical capabilities for clinical decision support (Layer 4).

Latin America provides compelling examples of application-layer innovation. Colombia's 1DOC3 telemedicine platform has reached millions of users by delivering doctor consultations via WhatsApp and other common messaging platforms, effectively leveraging existing consumer infrastructure to bridge the digital divide (1DOC3, 2025). Chile's TRAINFES platform enables remote electrostimulation therapy for patients with neurological disorders and has served more than 10,000 patients who would otherwise lack access to rehabilitation centers (TRAINFES, 2024). Brazil's Mevo, a digital prescription platform, secured nearly USD 20 million in venture funding in late 2024 to scale mobile prescription access nationwide (GHI, 2025).

4.2.6 Cross-Cutting Enablers: From Governance to Ecosystem

The revised technology stack model distinguishes between five foundation layers—the technical architecture on which digital health systems are built—and seven cross-cutting enablers that shape the conditions for success across all layers. The seven cross-cutting enablers are digital health skills and workforce development, research and development priorities, the healthtech ecosystem, regional cooperation, and financing and sustainability. Each enabler operates vertically across all five foundation layers, and weaknesses in any one can undermine investments across the entire stack.

Enabler 1: Digital Health Skills and Workforce. Digital health systems are only as effective as the people who design, implement, manage, and use them. This enabler encompasses the health informatics workforce (system architects, data engineers, interoperability specialists), the clinical workforce's digital literacy (the ability to use EMRs, telemedicine platforms, and Clinical Decision Support Systems effectively), and the managerial workforce's capacity to use data for decision-making. Africa faces an acute shortage of health informatics professionals. HELINA's Digital Health Applied Leadership Program, operating in Burkina Faso, Rwanda, and Zambia, is one of the few dedicated continental capacity-building initiatives (HELINA, 2025). Without sustained investment in digital health skills, countries risk deploying systems that cannot be maintained locally, creating dependence on external technical assistance. This enabler will be examined in greater depth in Chapter 11.

Enabler 2: Research and Development Priorities. Digital health innovation requires a research ecosystem that generates evidence on what works, adapts global technologies to local contexts, and develops Africa-specific solutions to Africa-specific challenges. This enabler, among others, encompasses health informatics research, clinical validation of AI tools in African populations, implementation science for digital health interventions, and issues concerning the development of African datasets to train machine learning models. The Africa CDC's Digital Strategy (2024) and WHO AFRO's research agenda for digital health provide continental frameworks, while institutions such as the African Institute for Mathematical Sciences (AIMS) and university-based health informatics programs in Ethiopia, Kenya, Nigeria, and South Africa are building research capacity. This enabler will be examined in Chapter 12.

Enabler 3: HealthTech Ecosystem. The healthTech ecosystem comprises private-sector companies, startups, social enterprises, and innovation hubs that develop, deploy, and maintain digital health products and services. Africa's healthTech ecosystem has expanded rapidly: digital health investment on the continent grew from about $92 million in 2015 to about $1.18 billion in 2024 (African Development Bank, 2020). A strong ecosystem requires supportive regulatory frameworks, access to risk capital, procurement pathways that enable innovative products to reach the public health sector, and mechanisms for public-private partnerships. Countries such as Kenya, Nigeria, Rwanda, and South Africa have developed particularly vibrant healthTech ecosystems that are developing locally relevant innovations. This enabler will be examined in Chapter 13.

Enabler 4: Digital Health Strategy. A national digital health strategy provides the vision, roadmap, and coordination mechanism that aligns digital health investments with health system priorities. The WHO/ITU National eHealth Strategy Toolkit (2012) identifies strategy as foundational. By 2024, over 80% of African countries had developed or were developing national digital health strategies (WHO, 2023). However, the existence of a strategy document does not guarantee implementation. The most effective strategies—such as those of Rwanda, Estonia, and Australia—are living documents linked to investment plans, implementation timelines, accountability mechanisms, and regular reviews. In this model, digital health strategy is distinct from governance because strategy sets direction and priorities, while governance provides the rules and institutional arrangements for execution. A country may have excellent governance frameworks but lack strategic coherence, or vice versa. Both are necessary. This enabler will be examined in Chapter 14.

Enabler 5: Governance, Policy, and Standards. This enabler encompasses data protection legislation, health data standards and policies, cybersecurity frameworks, ethical guidelines for artificial intelligence, institutional oversight arrangements, and the regulatory environment for digital health products and services. Australia's governance of its My Health Record system illustrates the complexity involved: the My Health Records Act 2012 established privacy provisions, and the 2025 Health Legislation Amendment transitioned the system to a "share by default" framework (Australian Government, 2025). The EU's GDPR has profoundly shaped digital health governance globally, and the EHDS regulation creates a unified framework for the primary and secondary use of health data (European Commission, 2022). In Africa, over 40 countries have enacted data protection legislation, but health-sector-specific frameworks and enforcement capacity remain underdeveloped. This enabler will be examined in Chapter 15.

Enabler 6: Regional Cooperation. Digital health transformation in Africa and the broader Global South cannot be achieved by individual countries acting in isolation. Regional cooperation—encompassing cross-border data exchange agreements, harmonized regulatory frameworks, shared digital public goods, joint capacity-building initiatives, and coordinated responses to transnational health threats—is a critical enabler that spans all five foundation layers of the technology stack. At the infrastructure layer, regional cooperation enables shared connectivity investments, such as the African Union's Program for Infrastructure Development in Africa (PIDA), which includes transnational broadband backbone networks that reduce costs for individual countries. At the identity and registries layer, cross-border patient identification and health worker credentialing facilitate labor mobility and continuity of care for migrant and refugee populations.

At the interoperability layer, harmonizing regional standards—such as adopting common health data exchange protocols across economic communities like the East African Community (EAC) and the Economic Community of West African States (ECOWAS)—enables surveillance data sharing and coordinated epidemic response, as demonstrated during the COVID-19 pandemic and subsequent Ebola outbreaks. The Africa Center for Disease Control and Prevention (Africa CDC) has catalyzed regional digital health cooperation through initiatives including the Continental Health Information Exchange framework, the Partnership for African Vaccine Manufacturing (PAVM) digital tracking systems, and the Saving Lives and Livelihoods program, which leveraged digital tools to coordinate vaccine deployment across 55 African Union Member States.

Similarly, the African Union's Digital Transformation Strategy for Africa (2020–2030) and the Smart Africa Alliance provide continental frameworks that promote harmonized approaches to digital health governance, data protection, and innovation ecosystems. Beyond Africa, regional cooperation models such as the European Health Data Space, the Nordic eHealth collaboration, and ASEAN's Digital Health Development Framework offer instructive parallels. Without deliberate regional cooperation, countries risk building incompatible systems that cannot support the cross-border disease surveillance, health workforce mobility, and shared learning that effective health systems increasingly require. This enabler will be examined in Chapter 16.

Enabler 7: Financing and Sustainability. Sustainable digital health transformation requires predictable, long-term financing that covers not only initial capital investments but also the recurrent operational costs of maintaining systems, connectivity, workforce, and governance over time. As documented in Chapter 7 (Section 7.6), Africa's digital health infrastructure investment gap is estimated at $6.3 billion over five years. Fewer than 20% of African countries include dedicated budget lines for health information system maintenance in their national health budgets (WHO, 2022). The transition from donor-funded pilot projects to domestically financed national systems remains one of the most persistent challenges in African digital health. This enabler will be examined in Chapter 17.

4.2.7 Interconnections across the Stack

The five foundation layers of the technology stack are deeply interdependent. A failure at the infrastructure layer—such as unreliable electricity or connectivity—undermines every layer above it, regardless of how sophisticated the applications may be. Similarly, weaknesses in any of the seven cross-cutting enablers cascade across the entire stack: poor governance can make technically sound systems legally unsustainable; insufficient financing can leave partially built infrastructure unused; skills shortages can prevent sophisticated systems from being fully utilized. In the remaining chapters of this book, the technology stack model will be used to situate specific digital health interventions within their broader architectural context. Chapters 7 through 10 examine each foundation layer in depth, while subsequent chapters (11 through 17) focus on the enablers that determine whether investments in the foundation layers succeed.

4.3 Framework for Categorizing Digital Health Interventions

Effective typologies balance comprehensiveness and simplicity, capturing the diversity of interventions while remaining practical for planning and communication. The framework presented here builds on WHO's Classification of Digital Health Interventions (WHO, 2018), which was updated in 2023 as the Classification of Digital Interventions, Services and Applications in Health (CDISAH). It is adapted to the contexts addressed in this book and strengthened through consultation with regional experts and analysis of existing implementations.

4.3.1 Principles for Classification

Several principles guide this classification framework.

- First, categories are defined by primary purpose and target users rather than by specific technologies. A single technology platform—such as a smartphone application—might serve multiple purposes across categories.

- Second, the framework recognizes that most sophisticated digital health systems integrate multiple types of interventions. A comprehensive electronic health record system, for instance, includes digitalization of clinical care, administrative functions, and research capabilities.
- Third, the typology accommodates innovations emerging across income contexts alongside established intervention types from high-income settings.

The WHO's CDISAH organizes digital health interventions along three axes: the health system challenges addressed, the digital health interventions deployed, and the digital applications and services through which they are delivered (WHO, 2023). This three-axis model helpfully distinguishes between what a technology does (its intervention function) and the platform through which it operates (its application type). Building on this conceptual foundation, the typology presented in this chapter organizes interventions into eight functional categories that closely map to health system building blocks.

The framework also recognizes varying levels of maturity. Countries at early stages of digitalization may prioritize foundational interventions, such as health information systems, while more advanced countries deploy sophisticated applications, such as AI-powered diagnostics. Neither approach is inherently superior; appropriateness depends on the health system context, infrastructure availability, and strategic priorities (Labrique et al., 2018).

4.3.2 The Eight Categories of Digital Health Interventions

This typology classifies digital health interventions into eight major categories, each primarily operating within the Application and Services Layer (Layer 5) of the technology stack while drawing on the foundational layers described above. Figure 4.3 illustrates these eight categories and their relationships.

1. Clinical Care Digitalization: Technologies supporting direct patient care, including electronic medical records, clinical decision support, digital diagnostics, and telemedicine.

2. Public Health and Surveillance Systems: Digital tools for disease surveillance, outbreak detection, immunization tracking, and population health monitoring.

3. Health Administration and Management Systems: Digital solutions for health facility management, human resources, financial management, and strategic planning.

4. Patient Engagement and Empowerment Tools: Technologies that enable patients to access health information, manage conditions, communicate with providers, and participate in care decisions.

5. Medical Education and Training Platforms: Digital tools for health worker education, continuing professional development, and clinical skill development.

6. Supply Chain and Logistics Management: Systems for managing pharmaceutical supplies, medical equipment, vaccines, and other health commodities.

7. Research and Data Analytics Platforms: Infrastructure and tools for health research, data science, and evidence generation.

8. Digital Health Financing and Payment Systems: Technologies enabling health insurance, payment processing, and financial transactions related to health services.

Each category includes multiple specific interventions that vary in technological sophistication and implementation complexity. The following sections examine each category in detail and provide examples from implementations across Africa, Europe, Latin America, Asia, Canada, and Australia.

Figure 4.3 The Eight Categories of Digital Health Interventions.

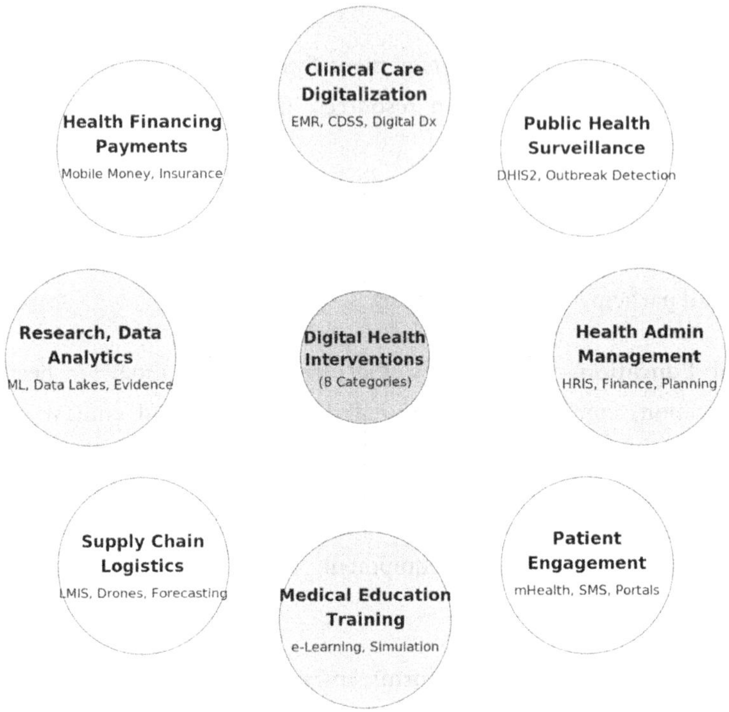

Source: Adapted from WHO Classification of Digital Health Interventions (WHO, 2018; WHO, 2023) and Author's Elaboration.

4.4 Clinical Care Digitalization

Clinical care digitalization uses technologies that directly support healthcare delivery at the point of care. These interventions aim to improve clinical decision-making, care quality, efficiency, and patient safety. In terms of technology infrastructure, clinical care applications (Layer 5) are among the most complex, requiring strong connectivity (Layer 1), reliable patient identification (Layer 2), seamless interoperability with laboratory and pharmacy systems (Layer 3), and increasingly, analytical capabilities for clinical decision support (Layer 4). Clinical digitalization typically begins with basic electronic health records and progressively incorporates more advanced features, such as clinical decision support, digital diagnostics, and integrated care coordination (Fritz et al., 2015).

4.4.1 Electronic Medical Records

Electronic medical records or electronic health records form the foundation of digitalization in clinical care, replacing paper-based documentation with systems that capture, store, and retrieve patient health information. Implementations vary widely in scope and sophistication—from basic patient registration and visit documentation systems to comprehensive platforms that integrate laboratory results, medication orders, imaging reports, and clinical notes.

OpenMRS is the most widely used EMR platform in Sub-Saharan Africa, implemented in over 6,000 healthcare facilities across 25 countries (OpenMRS, 2023). Originally developed for HIV care in Kenya, OpenMRS has evolved into a flexible platform that supports diverse clinical workflows. Its open-source architecture enables customization to meet local needs while adhering to core interoperability standards. Rwanda's nationwide EMR rollout, covering all 502 public health facilities, demonstrates successful large-scale implementation with OpenMRS as the foundation (Rwanda Biomedical Center, 2022).

Comparative experiences across diverse health systems reveal similar patterns. Brazil's e-SUS system, part of the Unified Health System (SUS), provides free EMR software to municipal health systems nationwide, mirroring open-source initiatives in Africa. The system supports more than 5,400 municipalities, demonstrating that open-source EMRs can achieve national scale in a large and diverse country (Ministério da Saúde do Brasil, 2022). Australia's My Health Record system takes a different approach: rather than replacing local clinical systems, it provides a national shared health summary that aggregates key information—such as medications, allergies, immunizations, pathology results, and hospital discharge summaries—from various provider systems into a single, consumer-controlled record accessible to patients and authorized providers (Australian Digital Health Agency, 2024). The 2025 legislative reform mandating that pathology and diagnostic imaging services upload results by default marks a significant shift from voluntary to mandatory data sharing (Australian Government Department of Health, 2025).

Estonia's approach demonstrates what is possible when EMR systems are integrated into a mature national digital infrastructure. Almost every Estonian resident has a digital health record accessible through the national patient portal, Digilugu. Healthcare providers nationwide access a unified health history via the X-Road data exchange layer, and about 99% of prescriptions are processed electronically (e-Estonia, 2025; Groenewegen et al., 2018). Achieving this level of integration took nearly two decades, reflecting sustained political commitment, consistent investment, and an enabling legal framework.

4.4.2 Telemedicine and Virtual Care

Telemedicine has become one of the fastest-growing areas of digital healthcare worldwide, largely driven by the COVID-19 pandemic. This technology enables both real-time (synchronous) and store-and-forward (asynchronous) consultations among patients and providers, as well as among generalists and specialists, helping remove geographic barriers to care.

In Latin America, telemedicine adoption patterns vary significantly across countries. Chile, Ecuador, and Uruguay have been regional leaders, with Chile reporting telemedicine use in about 65% of hospitals and a 900% increase in telehealth consultations during the pandemic (Nieblas et al., 2022; Saigí-Rubió, 2023). The Colombian platform 1DOC3 demonstrates how telemedicine can be delivered through user-friendly channels: it provides doctor consultations via WhatsApp and other messaging apps, using AI-powered triage to reduce wait times and costs, and reaches millions of users, even in remote areas (1DOC3, 2025).

Australia's experience with telehealth during the pandemic was transformative. Between March 2020 and July 2022, 118.2 million Medicare-subsidized telehealth services were delivered to 18 million patients by more than 95,000 practitioners (Australian Digital Health Agency, 2022). The permanent integration of telehealth items into the Medicare Benefits Schedule represents a policy shift from emergency response to structural reform. India's eSanjeevani telemedicine platform, developed under the ABDM umbrella, has facilitated tens of millions of teleconsultations nationwide, providing free access to specialists for patients in rural areas who would otherwise travel long distances for care (National Health Authority, 2024).

4.4.3 Clinical Decision Support Systems

Clinical decision support systems (CDSS) augment healthcare providers' decision-making by delivering alerts, reminders, diagnostic suggestions, treatment guidelines, and drug interaction checks. In resource-constrained settings, where healthcare workers often manage high patient volumes with limited specialist support, CDSS can significantly improve care quality and safety. Mobile-based CDSS tools have spread across Africa and South Asia, enabling community health workers and primary care providers to follow evidence-based protocols even in remote areas (Watkins et al., 2018). As artificial intelligence and machine learning capabilities mature, CDSS are shifting from rule-based systems to probabilistic and predictive models that can suggest diagnoses from symptom clusters, identify high-risk patients, and optimize treatment pathways.

4.5 Public Health and Surveillance Systems

Public health and surveillance systems enable population-level health monitoring, outbreak detection, immunization tracking, and program evaluation. These systems aggregate data from multiple sources—health facilities, laboratories, and community health workers—to provide situational awareness for public health decision-makers. Experience with epidemics, including Ebola, cholera, and COVID-19, has driven substantial investment in digital surveillance infrastructure worldwide (Africa CDC, 2022).

DHIS2 (District Health Information Software 2) is the leading health surveillance tool across Africa and much of the Global South, with 47 African countries and more than 100 countries worldwide using it for routine health data reporting. Originating in post-apartheid South Africa through collaboration with the University of Oslo, DHIS2 was designed as an open-source, flexible platform for managing health data. Its development was heavily influenced by a participatory, user-centered approach led by the Health Information Systems Programme (HISP), which fostered local ownership and customization. Over time, DHIS2 evolved into a global public good recognized by the World Health Organization, with Africa remaining central to its development and to leadership in open-source health systems.

DHIS2 has transformed health information management by significantly improving data availability, timeliness, and quality. Reporting rates have risen substantially, and real-time dashboards now support decision-making across all levels of the health system. Built-in validation tools have improved data accuracy, while user-friendly analytics have made data accessible to frontline health workers, managers, and policymakers. These capabilities proved especially vital during health emergencies such as COVID-19, enabling rapid tracking and response.

Despite these successes, challenges persist. Infrastructure limitations, especially in rural areas, constrain real-time data use, and gaps in human capacity hinder system utilization and data analysis. Fragmentation across health programs also requires ongoing integration efforts. However, continuous adaptations—such as offline functionality, expanded training programs, and system integration—have bolstered DHIS2's resilience. The platform is evolving to incorporate advanced features, including interoperability with electronic health records, machine learning, and geospatial analytics, positioning it as a key part of Africa's future digital health ecosystems.

India's experience during the COVID-19 pandemic demonstrates how surveillance systems can be rapidly deployed at the population level. The Aarogya Setu mobile application, developed for COVID-19 contact tracing, achieved 240 million downloads and later evolved into a national health and wellness application integrated with the ABDM ecosystem (Sharma et al., 2023). The CoWIN platform managed vaccine registration and administration for more than 1.78 billion doses, generating real-time dashboards that informed distribution decisions across the country's vast geography (Balsari et al., 2024). Both platforms are now being repurposed: Aarogya Setu as a comprehensive health services application and CoWIN as an immunization management system supporting India's universal immunization program.

4.6 Health Administration and Management Systems

Digital health administration and management systems support core operational functions essential to health system performance, including human resource management, financial management, facility operations, and strategic planning. Although less visible than clinical systems, effective administration directly affects the quality and efficiency of service delivery.

Human resource information systems (HRIS) track the deployment, qualifications, training, and performance of health workers. In countries facing severe health worker shortages, HRIS enables evidence-based workforce planning and equitable distribution. Ghana's HRIS, integrated with payroll systems, has improved workforce data quality and reduced ghost workers on government payrolls (Ghana Health Service, 2021). India's e-Hospital application, developed by the National Informatics Center, provides a Hospital Management Information System (HMIS) for government hospitals on a Software-as-a-Service (SaaS) model, covering functions from patient registration to laboratory management to bed occupancy tracking across more than 268 hospitals nationwide (National Health Authority, 2024).

4.7 Patient Engagement and Empowerment Tools

Patient engagement tools empower individuals to actively participate in their healthcare by providing access to health information, self-management support, communication with providers, and shared decision-making. Mobile health (mHealth) apps dominate this category, leveraging high smartphone penetration to reach patients outside healthcare facilities.

SMS-based systems are the most widely deployed patient engagement approach in low-resource settings, delivering appointment reminders, medication adherence prompts, health education messages, and test result notifications via basic mobile phones. Kenya's M-TIBA platform integrates patient engagement with health financing, enabling individuals to save for healthcare, access health information, and schedule clinic appointments via mobile phones (Safaricom Health, 2022).

In higher-income settings, patient portals connected to national health record systems offer more comprehensive engagement. Estonia's Digilugu patient portal enables citizens to view their full medical history, see who has accessed their records, and manage their health data—a transparency feature central to building and maintaining public trust in digital health systems (e-Estonia, 2025). Australia's My Health Record system offers similar patient-facing access through the My Health mobile app, enabling consumers to view medications, pathology results, vaccination history, and electronic prescriptions (Australian Digital Health Agency, 2024).

India's ABHA mobile app, developed under ABDM, serves as a personal health record system that allows individuals to securely store, view, and manage health records from multiple providers on a single platform, including records from ABDM-linked hospitals, labs, and pharmacies (Balsari et al., 2024). The Latin American mental health landscape has also seen notable innovation in patient engagement, with platforms such as Brazil's Zenklub launching AI-powered therapy-matching tools and Colombia's 1DOC3 expanding into behavioral health services across the region (GHI, 2025).

4.8 Medical Education and Training Platforms

Digital platforms for medical education and training address critical capacity constraints by providing scalable, accessible learning opportunities for healthcare providers at all levels. E-learning, simulation, telemedicine-enabled supervision, and virtual reality training complement traditional education and are especially valuable given health workforce shortages and the uneven geographic distribution of training institutions across the Global South.

The African Field Epidemiology Network (AFENET) delivers digital training programs that reach thousands of public health professionals each year. Medical schools are increasingly integrating online components, enabling students in resource-constrained settings to access high-quality educational content (AFENET, 2023).

4.9 Supply Chain and Logistics Management

Supply chain and logistics management systems track pharmaceutical stocks, medical supplies, vaccines, and equipment from central warehouses to service delivery points. Stock-outs of essential medicines remain a critical challenge across Africa and in many parts of Asia and Latin America; digital systems enable improved forecasting, inventory management, and more efficient distribution (Barrington et al., 2010).

Rwanda's early adoption of comprehensive supply chain management systems demonstrates impact at the national level. By integrating logistics management information systems across pharmaceuticals, medical supplies, and vaccines, Rwanda achieved remarkable improvements in stock availability and reduced waste. The system generates automated orders based on consumption patterns and stock levels, enabling just-in-time delivery to health facilities (Rwanda Ministry of Health, 2021). Zipline's drone delivery network, initially deployed in Rwanda and later expanded to Ghana, Nigeria, and other countries, is an innovation in last-mile delivery of health commodities. Using autonomous drones to deliver blood products, vaccines, and essential medications to remote health facilities, Zipline demonstrates that technological solutions can bypass infrastructure gaps in the physical connectivity layer of the technology stack.

4.10 Research and Data Analytics Platforms

Research and data analytics platforms provide infrastructure and tools for health research, data science, and evidence generation. As health systems generate increasing amounts of digital data, analytics capabilities become crucial for turning data into actionable insights. Advanced analytics, including machine learning, provide opportunities for predictive modeling, pattern recognition, and optimization (Beam & Kohane, 2018).

National health research platforms aggregate data from multiple sources—health facilities, surveys, vital registration, and disease surveillance—enabling analyses that are impossible with any single data source. South Africa's Health Data Research Network connects researchers with de-identified health data while maintaining privacy protections (South African Medical Research Council, 2022). Brazil's growing AI ecosystem is noteworthy: the country leads Latin America in developing an AI strategy focused on health research, and AI initiatives are improving diagnostics in oncology and pathology (IMARC, 2024). Throughout the region, integrating AI into health research marks a frontier with great potential but also raises important equity implications, as access to the necessary computational infrastructure and expertise for AI development remains highly concentrated in a few institutions and countries.

4.11 Digital Health Financing and Payment Systems

Digital health financing and payment systems are increasingly important, especially in areas where individuals pay out of pocket for healthcare and where traditional insurance infrastructure is underdeveloped. These technologies enable mobile health insurance enrollment and claims processing, digital payments for health services, health savings wallets, and electronic voucher systems.

Kenya's M-TIBA platform, built on the M-Pesa mobile money infrastructure, enables users to save money earmarked for healthcare and pay providers directly through their mobile phones. This combination of financial technology and health technology—often called "fintech for health"—demonstrates how existing digital payment infrastructure can be repurposed to address health financing challenges. India's Ayushman Bharat scheme, the world's largest publicly funded health insurance program, relies on digital infrastructure for beneficiary identification, hospital enrollment, claims processing, and fraud detection. Digitalization of claims processing has accelerated reimbursements and improved transparency, although challenges related to digital literacy and connectivity in rural areas remains.

4.12 Conclusion

This chapter presents two complementary frameworks for understanding digital health: the five-layer, seven cross-cutting enablers digital health technology stack and the eight-category typology of digital health interventions. The technology stack provides a structural model for understanding how individual digital health applications depend on and connect to the broader system architecture. The typology—covering clinical care, public health surveillance, health administration, patient engagement, medical education, supply chain, research analytics, and health financing—organizes the diverse landscape of digital health interventions into functional categories that support planning, benchmarking, and communication.

The international examples presented throughout this chapter reveal several cross-cutting insights.

- First, the most successful digital health ecosystems—Estonia, India, Rwanda, Australia, and Brazil—have deliberately invested in the foundational layers of the technology stack, particularly digital identity and interoperability, rather than focusing exclusively on end-user applications.

- Second, governance and legislative frameworks increasingly distinguish countries that achieve sustainable, scaled digital health systems from those that remain in pilot mode.

- Third, open-source platforms and open standards have proven essential for achieving scale and avoiding vendor lock-in, as demonstrated by the global adoption of OpenMRS, DHIS2, FHIR, and X-Road.

Most critically, this chapter establishes that digital health interventions cannot be understood in isolation from their technological, institutional, and political contexts. The chapters that follow will examine specific intervention categories in greater depth, consistently situate them within the technology stack framework introduced here, and draw on the growing body of evidence from implementations worldwide.

References

1DOC3. (2025). Telemedicine platform: Connecting patients with doctors across Latin America. 1DOC3.

Aalpha. (2026). Healthcare technology stack – 2026: All you need to know. Aalpha Information Systems.

AFENET. (2023). Digital training platforms for public health workforce development. African Field Epidemiology Network.

Africa CDC. (2022). Africa CDC surveillance strategy 2022–2027. Africa Centres for Disease Control and Prevention.

Australian Digital Health Agency. (2022). Telehealth. Australian Digital Health Agency.

Australian Digital Health Agency. (2024). My Health Record: Statistics and implementation report. Australian Digital Health Agency.

Australian Government Department of Health. (2025). Health Legislation Amendment (Modernizing My Health Record—Sharing by Default) Act 2025. Commonwealth of Australia.

Balsari, S., Sesia, P., & Patnaik, S. (2024). India's evolving digital health strategy. npj Digital Medicine, 7, Article 285. https://doi.org/10.1038/s41746-024-01279-2

Barrington, J., Wereko-Brobby, O., Ward, P., Mwafongo, W., & Kungulwe, S. (2010). SMS for Life: A pilot project to improve anti-malarial drug supply management in rural Tanzania using standard technology. Malaria Journal, 9(1), 298. https://doi.org/10.1186/1475-2875-9-298

Beam, A. L., & Kohane, I. S. (2018). Big data and machine learning in health care. JAMA, 319(13), 1317–1318. https://doi.org/10.1001/jama.2017.18391

Bhatia, R. S., Desveaux, L., & Bhyat, R. (2024). The Connected Care for Canadians Act: An important step toward interoperability of health data. Canadian Medical Association Journal, 196(48), E1383–E1388. https://doi.org/10.1503/cmaj.241161

Canada Health Infoway. (2024). Infoway Centre for Clinical Innovation in Digital Health: Launch announcement. Canada Health Infoway.

CMA & Canada Health Infoway. (2024). 2024 National Survey of Canadian Physicians: Digital health perspectives. Canadian Medical Association.

e-Estonia. (2025). X-Road: Secure data exchange layer. e-Estonia.

European Commission. (2022). Proposal for a regulation on the European Health Data Space. COM(2022) 197 final.

Fritz, F., Tilahun, B., & Dugas, M. (2015). Success criteria for electronic medical record implementations in low-resource settings: A systematic review. Journal of the American Medical Informatics Association, 22(2), 479–488. https://doi.org/10.1093/jamia/ocu038

Ghana Health Service. (2021). Human Resource Information System Implementation Report: Ghana Health Service

GHI. (2025). Latin America's healthtech revolution is underway. Global Health Intelligence.

Groenewegen, A., Tsereteli, N., & Tuvike, P. (2018). Ten years of the e-health system in Estonia. In CEUR Workshop Proceedings (Vol. 2336). MMHS.

GSMA. (2024). The mobile economy: Sub-Saharan Africa 2024. GSMA.

IMARC. (2024). Latin America telehealth market: Size and forecast to 2033. IMARC Group.

International Telecommunication Union. (2021). Digital health technology assessment framework. ITU.

Labrique, A. B., Wadhwani, C., Williams, K. A., Lamptey, P., Hesp, C., Luk, R., & Aerts, A. (2018). Best practices in scaling digital health in low and middle-income countries. Globalization and Health, 14(1), 103. https://doi.org/10.1186/s12992-018-0424-z

Manya, A., Braa, J., Øverland, L. H., Titlestad, O. H., Mumo, J., & Nzioka, C. (2020). National rollout of District Health Information Software (DHIS 2) in Kenya, 2011–2018. BMC Health Services Research, 20(1), 1–9. https://doi.org/10.1186/s12913-020-05402-z

Ministério da Saúde do Brasil. (2022). e-SUS Atenção Básica: Relatório de implementação nacional. Ministry of Health, Brazil.

National Health Authority. (2024). Ayushman Bharat Digital Mission: Implementation update. Government of India.

Nieblas, B., Okoye, K., Carrión, B., Mehta, N., & Mehta, S. (2022). A narrative review of telemedicine in Latin America during the COVID-19 pandemic. Healthcare, 10(7), 1361. https://doi.org/10.3390/healthcare10071361

NIIS. (2023). X-Road community report. Nordic Institute for Interoperability Solutions.

Nortal. (2024). X-Road: Estonia's digital backbone. Nortal Group.

OpenMRS. (2023). Global implementations and impact report. OpenMRS Inc.

Rwanda Biomedical Center. (2022). National Health Information Exchange: Implementation and impact report. RBC.

Rwanda Ministry of Health. (2021). Integrated pharmaceutical and medical supplies management system evaluation. Republic of Rwanda.

Safaricom Health. (2022). M-TIBA: Expanding access to quality healthcare. Safaricom PLC.

Saigí-Rubió, F. (2023). Promoting telemedicine in Latin America in light of COVID-19. Revista Panamericana de Salud Pública, 47, e17. https://doi.org/10.26633/RPSP.2023.17

Sharma, R. S., Rohatgi, A., Jain, S., & Singh, D. (2023). The Ayushman Bharat Digital Mission (ABDM): Making of India's digital health story. CSI Transactions on ICT, 11, 3–9. https://doi.org/10.1007/s40012-023-00375-0

South African Medical Research Council. (2022). Health Data Research Network strategic plan. SAMRC.

Synapxe. (2023). Healthcare tech stack and solutions stack: Faster and safer deployment of new healthtech. Synapxe.

TRAINFES. (2024). Remote rehabilitation platform: Impact report. TRAINFES Chile.

Watkins, J. O., Goudge, J., Gómez-Olivé, F. X., & Griffiths, F. (2018). Mobile phone use among patients and health workers to enhance primary healthcare. BMC Medical Informatics and Decision Making, 18(1), 67. https://doi.org/10.1186/s12911-018-0672-8

WHO. (2018). Classification of digital health interventions v1.0: A shared language to describe the uses of digital technology for health (WHO/RHR/18.06). World Health Organization.

WHO. (2023). Classification of digital interventions, services and applications in health (2nd ed.). World Health Organization.

WHO/ITU. (2012). National eHealth strategy toolkit. World Health Organization and International Telecommunication Union.

Chapter 5: Emerging Technologies and Future Implications

5.1. Introduction

The trajectory of digital health in Africa extends far beyond the technologies currently shaping healthcare delivery. A new generation of frontier innovations, such as edge computing, robotic surgery, and quantum computing platforms, presents both extraordinary opportunities and formidable challenges for African health systems. These technologies are not merely incremental improvements on existing tools; they represent qualitative shifts in what is technically possible, economically viable, and clinically transformative in healthcare.

Understanding these emerging technologies, their potential applications, implementation requirements, and implications for health equity is essential groundwork for strategic planning and investment decisions that will shape Africa's health future over the next two decades. This chapter examines six interconnected technology domains: genomics and precision medicine; robotics in surgery and care delivery; virtual and augmented reality for medical training; quantum computing for drug discovery; nanotechnology in diagnostics and treatment; and edge computing for real-time health monitoring. For each domain, the analysis situates African developments within the global technology landscape and draws on comparative experiences from Europe, Asia, and Latin America to highlight pathways, pitfalls, and adaptable models.

As discussed in Chapter 4, the digital health technology stack—comprising five foundational layers and seven cross-cutting enablers—provides the architectural framework for understanding these emerging technologies. Genomics, robotics, and quantum computing primarily operate within the Applications and Services Layer (Layer 5), but their successful deployment depends heavily on the foundational layers beneath them—especially physical infrastructure and connectivity (Layer 1) and interoperability and data exchange (Layer 3)—as well as on cross-cutting enablers, including governance, policy, standards, digital health skills and workforce, and financing and sustainability. Connectivity infrastructure, such as broadband and mobile networks, is covered separately in the infrastructure chapters of this book; therefore, this chapter focuses on the six application-layer technology domains rather than on innovations in telecommunications infrastructure.

Critically, the chapter argues that Africa's engagement with emerging health technologies must be guided not by technological determinism—the belief that adopting the newest technologies automatically leads to progress—but by strategic intentionality focused on health equity, sustainability, and system strengthening. Technologies must be evaluated for their ability to address the continent's priority health needs outlined in Chapter 2, their feasibility within existing infrastructure and resource constraints, and their potential to reduce, rather than exacerbate, health disparities.

Figure 5.1. Projected Adoption Timelines for Emerging Health Technologies in Africa

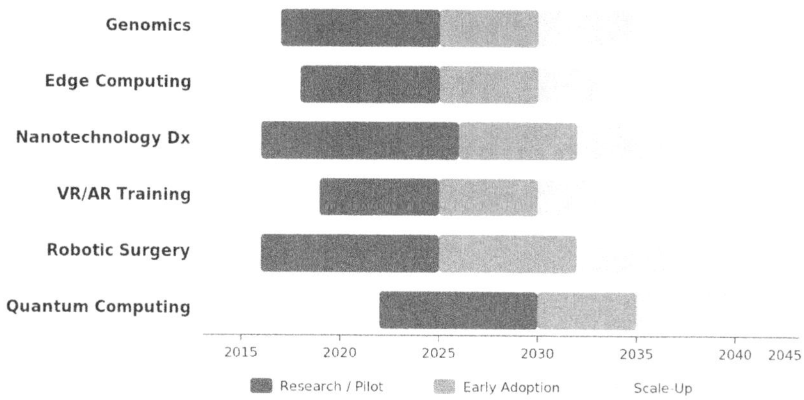

Source: Author's Analysis Based on Literature Review and Industry Reports (2024).

5.2 Genomics and Precision Medicine

Genomics and precision medicine mark a paradigm shift from standardized, one-size-fits-all healthcare to personalized approaches grounded in each patient's unique genetic profile, environmental exposures, and lifestyle factors. In Africa, genomic medicine is especially important—and urgent—because it is both a major scientific strength and a key source of biomedical inequality: African populations harbor more genetic diversity than all other continental populations combined, yet they remain drastically underrepresented in the global genomic databases that inform drug development, diagnostic test design, and clinical guidelines (Sirugo et al., 2019).

Figure 5.2. Comparative Genomic Research Infrastructure: Africa versus the Global South Average Across Key Capacity Indicators (2024).

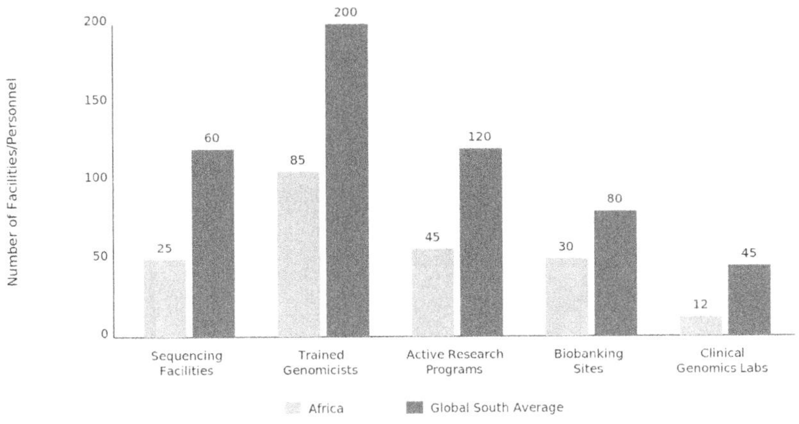

Source: Data Compiled from Initiative Reports, Published Literature, and Organizational Assessments (2022–2024)

This underrepresentation has tangible clinical consequences. Medications developed and dosed using pharmacogenomic data, primarily from European populations, may be ineffective or even dangerous for African patients whose drug-metabolizing enzyme variants differ significantly. Genetic diagnostic tests calibrated to non-African reference genomes yield higher rates of false positives and variants of uncertain significance when applied to African patients. Precision oncology protocols developed without African tumor genomic data may overlook actionable mutations that are more common in African cancer subtypes. Bridging this genomic equity gap is not only a scientific imperative but also a matter of health justice.

5.2.1 Continental Genomic Research Initiatives

The Human Heredity and Health in Africa (H3Africa) initiative, launched in 2010 with funding from the National Institutes of Health and the Wellcome Trust, is the continent's most comprehensive genomic research program. H3Africa has established genomic research capacity in 32 African countries, generated genomic data from more than 100,000 African participants, trained hundreds of African genomics scientists, and built critical bioinformatics infrastructure, including the H3ABioNet computational biology network. The initiative has yielded discoveries with immediate clinical relevance, including the identification of novel genetic variants associated with HIV disease progression, tuberculosis susceptibility, sickle cell disease severity, and cardiovascular disease risk in African populations (Mulder et al., 2018).

The Africa Pathogen Genomics Initiative (Africa PGI), launched in 2020 by the Africa Centre for Disease Control and Prevention, is a complementary investment in pathogen genomics rather than human genomics. Initially established to build SARS-CoV-2 sequencing capacity across the continent, Africa PGI has created sustainable infrastructure for genomic surveillance of tuberculosis, HIV drug resistance, antimalarial resistance, and other priority pathogens. South African genomic surveillance laboratories identified the Beta and Omicron SARS-CoV-2 variants, demonstrating world-class African genomic capacity and underscoring the continent's potential to contribute to, rather than merely consume, global genomic knowledge (Nkengasong et al., 2022).

5.2.2 Pharmacogenomics and Clinical Applications

Pharmacogenomics—the study of how genetic variation influences drug response—offers the most immediately actionable clinical applications in African healthcare. African populations show substantial diversity in drug-metabolizing enzymes, with direct implications for medication safety and efficacy. For example, the CYP2B6 genetic variant, significantly more prevalent in African than in European populations, profoundly affects efavirenz metabolism. Efavirenz is the most widely prescribed non-nucleoside reverse transcriptase inhibitor for HIV treatment across Africa. Depending on their CYP2B6 genotype, some patients reach toxic drug concentrations on standard dosing, while others achieve subtherapeutic levels, contributing to adverse effects and treatment failure. Implementing pharmacogenomic-guided antiretroviral selection could improve outcomes for millions of patients across the continent (Drögemöller et al., 2021).

Cancer genomics applications address Africa's growing burden of malignancies while recognizing that cancer genomic profiles vary significantly between African and non-African populations. In African women, for example, breast cancer more often presents as aggressive triple-negative subtypes with distinct genomic characteristics compared with European populations. The African Cancer Genomics Initiative is systematically sequencing tumor genomes from African cancer patients to build the evidence base for precision oncology approaches tailored to African populations. South Africa has begun implementing clinical tumor sequencing for selected cancer patients, enabling targeted therapy selection based on individual tumor genetics—though access remains concentrated in major academic centers (Sengayi-Muchengeti et al., 2020).

Global Genomics Landscape: Comparative Developments

India's IndiGen program has sequenced more than 10,000 Indian genomes to build population-specific pharmacogenomic reference data, directly informing drug-dosing guidelines for the Indian population—a model Africa could follow. Brazil's involvement in the Human Variome Project has produced clinically actionable genomic data for its highly admixed population, with relevance for African-descent populations in the Americas. The European Union's 1+ Million Genomes Initiative aims to connect genomic data across member states for research and clinical use, demonstrating the value of cross-border genomic data sharing. In the Caribbean, Jamaica's sickle cell genomics program, supported by the National Health Fund, has generated pharmacogenomic data directly relevant to African populations because of shared genetic ancestry (Government of India, 2021; European Commission, 2022; PAHO, 2023).

5.2.3 Implementation Challenges

Implementing genomics medicine in Africa faces significant challenges. The continent has fewer than 100 medical geneticists and even fewer certified genetic counselors, creating severe human capacity constraints for clinical genomic services. Although genome sequencing costs are falling quickly, they still range from $500 to $1,000 per sample, making routine clinical use unaffordable for most African health systems. The bioinformatics infrastructure needed to process and interpret genomic data requires ongoing investment in computing resources and trained analysts. Ethical issues related to genetic data governance, including consent, data sovereignty, benefit-sharing, and the risk of genetic discrimination, require strong regulatory frameworks that most African countries have yet to establish (Wonkam et al., 2021).

Table 5.1. Key African Genomics Initiatives and Their Impact

Initiative	Scope	Focus	Key	Countries
H3Africa	32 countries	Human genomics, disease susceptibility	100,000+ genomes sequenced	Pan-African
Africa PGI	Continental	Pathogen genomic surveillance	Identified Omicron variant	All AU members
African Cancer Genomics	Regional	Tumor sequencing, precision oncology	Population-specific cancer profiles	South Africa, Nigeria, Ghana
MalariaGEN	Global/ African	Malaria parasite and host genomics	Drug resistance mapping	20+ African countries
H3ABioNet	Pan-African	Bioinformatics infrastructure	Trained 500+ bioinformaticians	32 countries

Source: Data Compiled from Initiative Reports, Published Literature, and Organizational Assessments (2022–2024).

5.3 Robotics in Surgery and Care Delivery

Robotic systems in healthcare fall into three broad categories: surgical robots that enable minimally invasive procedures with enhanced precision, service robots that assist with patient care logistics and infection control, and rehabilitation robots that support physical therapy and recovery. Although robotic healthcare applications remain far more limited in Africa than in high-income regions, a growing number of implementations demonstrate that robotic technologies can address critical African healthcare challenges, including specialist shortages, surgical capacity constraints, and care delivery efficiency in under-resourced settings (Agholor et al., 2021).

Figure 5.3. Distribution of Robotic Surgical Systems Across the Africa (2024)

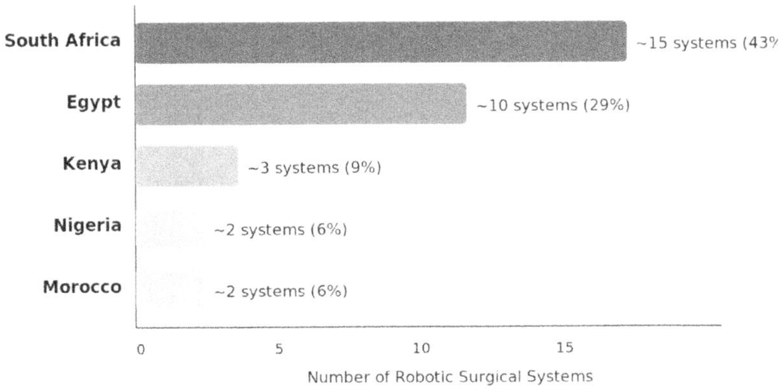

Source: Data Compiled from Institutional Reports and Published Literature (2022–2024)

5.3.1 Robotic Surgery in African Hospitals

Robotic surgical systems, such as Intuitive Surgical's da Vinci platform, enable surgeons to perform complex procedures through small incisions using articulated robotic arms controlled from a console. They provide magnified three-dimensional visualization, tremor reduction, and enhanced dexterity in confined anatomical spaces. Evidence from high-income countries consistently shows that robotic surgery leads to less blood loss, shorter hospital stays, fewer wound complications, and faster patient recovery compared with traditional open surgery. However, the high initial costs of \$1–2.5 million, plus annual maintenance contracts of \$100,000–\$200,000, create financial barriers that profoundly shape the equity of access in African health systems (Intuitive Surgical, 2023).

Africa's robotic surgery landscape remains concentrated in three countries. South Africa has about 15 robotic surgical systems, distributed across major private and academic hospitals in Johannesburg, Cape Town, Pretoria, and Durban, performing over 3,000 robotic procedures annually—primarily in urology, gynecology, and general surgery. Egypt operates about 10 systems, concentrated in Cairo's leading hospitals. Kenya acquired its first da Vinci system in 2021 at the Aga Khan University Hospital in Nairobi. Nigeria and Morocco each have a small number of installations. These systems primarily serve affluent patient populations who can afford the high costs of robotic surgery, raising important questions about whether investing in robotic surgery is appropriate for health systems struggling to provide basic surgical access (Kimani et al., 2022).

5.3.2 Telesurgery and Remote Robotic Procedures

Telesurgery—where a surgeon operates a robotic system from a distant location—arguably represents the most transformative robotic application in the African context, as it could enable specialist surgeons in major urban centers to perform complex procedures on patients in remote regions without transferring patients. However, telesurgery demands robust, ultra-low-latency connectivity (ideally below 10 milliseconds), which remains a current technical limitation in most African settings. South African researchers have conducted experimental remote robotic procedures over dedicated fiber connections. As advanced connectivity infrastructure expands, telesurgery pilots are expected to increase. The convergence of robotics and advanced telecommunications could fundamentally alter the geography of surgical access on the continent (Sterbenz et al., 2021).

5.3.3 Service and Rehabilitation Robotics

Beyond the operating room, service robots for hospital logistics and rehabilitation robots for patient recovery are finding nascent applications in African healthcare. During the COVID-19 pandemic, some African hospitals deployed service robots for contactless medication delivery, supply transport, and patient screening, reducing staff exposure to infectious patients. Kenyatta National Hospital in Nairobi implemented service robots for supply logistics, demonstrating efficiency gains and reduced infection risk. In rehabilitation, specialized centers in South Africa have implemented robotic therapy systems that show promising outcomes for stroke and spinal cord injury recovery, though the costs of $30,000–$200,000 per system limit adoption to a handful of facilities (Tavakoli et al., 2020; Díaz et al., 2020).

Global Perspective: Robotics in Healthcare Across Regions

Japan leads global healthcare robotics deployment, with over 5,000 robotic surgical systems in use and widespread use of care robots in elderly care facilities—driven by the country's aging population and government-subsidized adoption programs. India has adopted a tiered approach: major private hospital chains operate robotic surgery programs, while public hospitals increasingly access shared robotic facilities through hub-and-spoke models. In Latin America, Brazil's Hospital das Clínicas in São Paulo operates the largest robotic surgery program in the Southern Hemisphere, with training programs extending to other Latin American countries. Trinidad and Tobago has deployed robotic surgery through public-private partnerships, demonstrating that even smaller health systems can access advanced surgical technology through innovative financing arrangements. These models suggest pathways to expand access to robotic surgery in Africa beyond the current concentration in private urban facilities (Ministry of Health, Labour and Welfare of Japan, 2023; Brazilian Society of Robotic Surgery, 2023).

Canada's experience in surgical simulation offers valuable insight. Montreal-based OSSimTech has developed the Sim-Ortho platform, which simulates open orthopedic surgery with lifelike haptic force feedback and auditory cues for bone drilling, cutting, and implant placement (DelveInsight, 2025). This focus on realistic tactile training for procedures that remain primarily open is particularly relevant to the African surgical context, where most surgical training occurs in open procedures. VirtaMed, a Swiss-based company with partnerships across European academic centers, has developed the RoboS platform for robotic surgery simulation training, enabling surgeons to develop console skills in risk-free virtual environments before operating on patients (VirtaMed, 2024). The global surgical simulation market, valued at USD 373 million in 2024, is projected to reach USD 666 million by 2032, reflecting growing recognition that simulation-based training can help address surgical capacity challenges worldwide (DelveInsight, 2025).

Australia's Royal Australasian College of Surgeons has integrated simulation-based assessments into its training pathways, providing a regulatory model for how surgical training bodies can officially recognize Virtual Reality and simulation skills. In Africa, where the Colleges of Surgeons of East, Central, and Southern Africa (COSECSA) and the West African College of Surgeons (WACS) serve as the main surgical training institutions, formal recognition of simulation-based competencies could accelerate access to high-quality surgical training beyond the traditional operating theater. The hub-and-spoke model used in India—where several public hospitals share a robotic surgical facility—is especially applicable to Africa, with costly robotic systems located in regional referral centers and expanded access through rotations and telesurgery, potentially maximizing the benefits of limited investments.

5.4 Virtual and Augmented Reality for Medical Training

Virtual reality (VR) and augmented reality (AR) technologies offer transformative approaches to medical education and clinical training, addressing critical challenges that have long constrained the quality and reach of health professional education in Africa. These challenges include limited opportunities for clinical exposure during training, severe shortages of cadavers for anatomy instruction, inadequate access to simulation facilities, and the geographic concentration of advanced training centers in a small number of urban institutions. VR creates fully immersive, computer-generated environments where learners practice clinical skills in realistic scenarios without requiring physical simulation equipment or exposure to actual patients. AR overlays digital information—such as anatomical structures, clinical data, and procedural guidance—onto real-world views, enhancing educational experiences and potentially supporting clinical practice through real-time information display (Pottle, 2019).

Figure 5.4. Current and Projected Adoption Rates of VR/AR Across African Medical Education Domains (2024 vs. 2028)

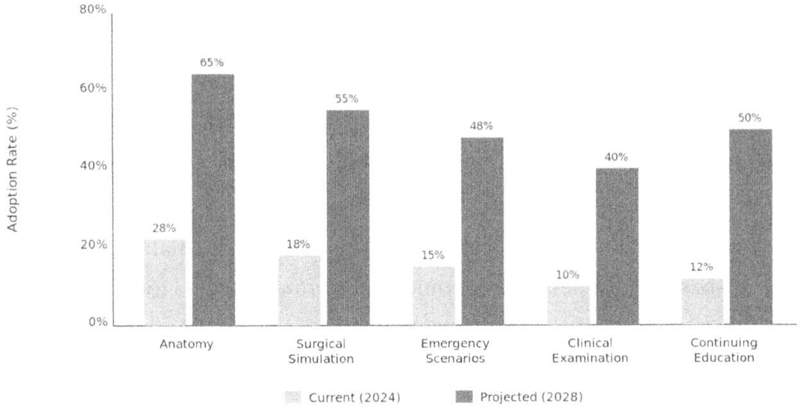

Source: Author's Analysis Based on Institutional Surveys and Published Literature (2024)

5.4.1 Anatomy and Surgical Simulation

The most immediate applications of VR in African medical education address two of the continent's most persistent training constraints: cadaver scarcity and limited access to surgical simulation. Many African medical schools face severe cadaver shortages—the University of Lagos, for example, has approximately one cadaver for every 70 medical students, compared with international recommendations of one per 10–20 students. High-fidelity anatomical VR platforms enable students to explore three-dimensional human anatomy from any angle, perform virtual dissections, and interact with labeled anatomical structures across all body systems, providing unlimited, repeatable access to detailed anatomical learning without the need for preserved specimens (Moro et al., 2021).

Surgical skills training through VR extends this principle to procedural education, enabling trainees to repeatedly practice operations in risk-free simulated environments before operating on patients. VR surgical simulators recreate operating room settings with haptic feedback that provides realistic tactile sensations of tissue handling, instrument manipulation, and procedural steps. Published evidence shows that VR-trained surgeons perform procedures faster and with fewer errors than their traditionally trained counterparts—findings with significant implications for Africa, where surgical training bottlenecks stem from limited capacity for specialist mentorship and high clinical service demands that constrain dedicated teaching time. Several African medical schools have implemented VR surgical training programs, including the University of Cape Town, Makerere University in Uganda, and the University of Nairobi (Pulijala et al., 2020).

5.4.2 Clinical Scenario Training and Continuing Education

Beyond anatomy and surgery, VR-based clinical scenario training places learners in psychologically realistic patient-care situations that demand diagnostic reasoning, treatment decision-making, and interprofessional communication under time pressure. Emergency medicine scenarios enable practice of resuscitation protocols, trauma management algorithms, and critical triage decisions in high-stress virtual environments—addressing the limited emergency medicine training opportunities at many African hospitals, where emergency departments lack dedicated teaching programs. Rwanda's national medical simulation strategy incorporates VR emergency scenarios that can be deployed at district hospitals without physical simulation centers, demonstrating how VR can democratize access to training previously available only at referral institutions (Gordon et al., 2020).

Continuing medical education (CME) through VR and AR is a particularly high-value application for Africa, where practicing clinicians in rural and remote areas face substantial barriers to accessing the periodic training updates essential for maintaining clinical competence. Kenya's Virtual Medical Education platform delivers VR-based CME modules covering topics ranging from updated surgical techniques to rare disease diagnosis, accessible via standalone VR headsets at county hospitals. This model addresses the practical reality that rural healthcare providers often cannot leave their posts for multi-day training courses at distant urban centers, and that the clinical knowledge most needed in rural practice—emergency obstetrics, trauma management, pediatric emergencies—is precisely the knowledge most challenging to maintain without regular refresher training (Kyaw et al., 2019).

Regional Innovations: VR/AR in Medical Education Beyond Africa

The European Union's Erasmus+ program has funded multi-institutional VR medical education networks across member states, enabling the development of shared content and cross-border virtual clinical placements. In India, the National Medical Commission has recognized VR simulation as an acceptable component of surgical training assessments, thereby providing regulatory legitimacy and encouraging institutional investment. Brazil's Hospital Israelita Albert Einstein operates one of Latin America's largest VR medical simulation centers, producing Portuguese-language content that is shared across Lusophone countries, including Mozambique and Angola. In the Caribbean, the University of the West Indies has developed VR clinical training modules that specifically address tropical medicine scenarios—a content-development approach directly relevant to African institutions facing similar disease burdens (European Commission, 2023; National Medical Commission of India, 2022; UWI, 2023).

5.5 Quantum Computing and Its Potential in Drug Discovery

Quantum computing harnesses the principles of quantum mechanics—superposition, entanglement, and quantum interference—to perform calculations that are fundamentally intractable for even the most powerful classical computers. Unlike classical computers, which process information as binary bits in states of 0 or 1, quantum computers use quantum bits (qubits) that can exist in superposition, representing both 0 and 1 simultaneously and enabling parallel exploration of vast solution spaces. For pharmaceutical research and healthcare, quantum computing promises to simulate molecular interactions with unprecedented accuracy, potentially compressing drug development timelines from the current average of 10–15 years to as few as 2–3 years, while identifying treatments for diseases that have resisted conventional drug discovery approaches (Bova et al., 2021).

5.5.1 Applications in Drug Discovery

The primary healthcare application of quantum computing is molecular simulation and optimization for drug discovery. Classical computers struggle to accurately model molecules beyond simple compounds because computational complexity increases exponentially with molecular size—a phenomenon known as the exponential wall. A modest protein with 100 amino acids would require more classical computing operations to simulate accurately than there are atoms in the observable universe. By contrast, quantum computers naturally model quantum-mechanical systems, potentially enabling accurate simulations of complex biomolecular interactions, including protein folding, drug-receptor binding dynamics, and pharmacokinetic pathways (Cao et al., 2018).

In Africa, quantum computing holds particular promise for neglected tropical diseases (NTDs) and other conditions that disproportionately affect African populations yet receive insufficient investment from the pharmaceutical industry because of limited commercial returns. Diseases such as schistosomiasis, African trypanosomiasis (sleeping sickness), leishmaniasis, and drug-resistant malaria collectively affect hundreds of millions of people across the continent, yet attract only a fraction of the research funding directed toward diseases prevalent in high-income markets. Quantum computing could enable academic institutions, public-sector research organizations, and initiatives such as the Drugs for Neglected Diseases initiative (DNDi) to computationally identify promising drug candidates without the massive laboratory infrastructure and funding that characterize traditional pharmaceutical research (Ranasinghe & Kruger, 2020).

5.5.2 Healthcare Optimization Applications

Beyond drug discovery, quantum optimization algorithms have potential applications in healthcare logistics and resource allocation—areas where African health systems face acute challenges. Quantum optimization could dramatically improve vaccine distribution routing across complex logistics networks spanning thousands of delivery points, healthcare facility placement modeling to maximize population coverage under budget constraints, treatment protocol optimization that incorporates patient-specific factors, and supply chain management for essential medicines. While these applications require quantum computers substantially more powerful than currently available systems, optimization is expected to be among the earliest commercially viable domains for quantum computing (Ajagekar et al., 2022).

5.5.3 Africa's Quantum Readiness

Africa's direct quantum computing hardware capacity remains negligible, with no quantum computers currently operational on the continent. However, cloud-based quantum computing platforms—including IBM Quantum, Google Quantum AI, Amazon Braket, and Microsoft Azure Quantum—provide remote access to quantum processors, enabling African researchers to experiment with quantum algorithms and develop quantum applications without local hardware. Some African universities, including the University of KwaZulu-Natal, the University of the Witwatersrand, and Stellenbosch University, have established quantum computing research programs focused on algorithm development, quantum machine learning, and potential healthcare applications (Ekert et al., 2020).

Industry experts predict that quantum computers capable of transformative drug discovery applications may emerge in the early to mid-2030s, though some optimization applications could arrive sooner. For healthcare in Africa, the most practical way to benefit from quantum computing is through cloud-based access to quantum processing for specific, well-defined problems, rather than deploying local quantum computers. Preparing for this future requires building quantum literacy among African computational scientists, identifying priority healthcare problems suitable for quantum solutions, and ensuring African researchers are ready to apply quantum computing to the continent's health challenges from the earliest stages of the technology's development.

5.6 Nanotechnology in Diagnostics and Treatment

Nanotechnology—the engineering of materials and devices at the nanometer scale (1–100 nanometers, where one nanometer equals one billionth of a meter)—enables fundamentally new approaches to disease diagnosis, drug delivery, and therapeutic intervention. At the nanoscale, materials exhibit properties radically different from those of their bulk counterparts: they can cross biological barriers that conventional drugs cannot penetrate, target specific cell types or tissues with high precision, respond to environmental stimuli such as pH or temperature changes, and interact with biological molecules at the molecular level. These capabilities create opportunities for more effective, less toxic therapies and for ultra-sensitive diagnostic tests deployable in resource-limited settings characteristic of much of African healthcare (Patra et al., 2018).

5.6.1 Diagnostic Nanotechnology

Diagnostic nanotechnology applications show particular promise for point-of-care testing in African settings where centralized laboratory infrastructure is limited and sample transport is unreliable. Lateral flow assays using gold nanoparticles—similar in design to rapid pregnancy tests—enable rapid disease detection from fingerstick blood samples without electricity, refrigeration, trained lab technicians, or expensive analytical equipment. The visual color change caused by nanoparticle aggregation in the presence of target biomarkers produces results that are readable by community health workers or even patients themselves (Jahanban-Esfahlan et al., 2020).

Quantum dots—semiconductor nanocrystals with tunable fluorescence—represent an advanced diagnostic nanotechnology with transformative potential for healthcare in Africa. Because quantum dots of different sizes emit light at distinct wavelengths (colors), they enable multiplexed diagnostics that can detect multiple diseases simultaneously from a single patient sample. In African clinical settings, where patients often present with overlapping symptoms from multiple infections—such as HIV, tuberculosis, and malaria—multiplexed quantum dot diagnostics could identify all conditions from a single blood draw. This approach improves diagnostic accuracy while reducing the number of tests required, the volume of blood collected, and the overall cost per diagnostic episode (Petryayeva et al., 2019).

5.6.2 Therapeutic Nanotechnology and Drug Delivery

Therapeutic nanotechnology focuses primarily on targeted drug delivery systems that concentrate medications at disease sites while minimizing systemic exposure, thereby reducing side effects and potentially enhancing therapeutic efficacy. Liposomal formulations—drugs encapsulated in nanoscale lipid vesicles—protect drugs from enzymatic degradation, prolong their circulation time in the bloodstream, and preferentially accumulate in tumors or sites of infection through the enhanced permeability and retention effect. Several liposomal drugs have received regulatory approval and are in clinical use globally, including liposomal amphotericin B for invasive fungal infections and liposomal doxorubicin for cancer treatment (Mitchell et al., 2021).

In Africa, liposomal formulations of antifungal, antiparasitic, and antimicrobial drugs could transform treatment of high-burden conditions across the continent. Liposomal amphotericin B, for instance, has dramatically improved survival rates for cryptococcal meningitis—a leading cause of death among HIV-positive individuals in Africa—while reducing the severe kidney toxicity associated with conventional amphotericin B. Antimicrobial nanotechnology, including silver nanoparticle wound dressings developed by South African researchers and effective against drug-resistant bacteria, addresses the growing threat of antimicrobial resistance across the continent (Franci et al., 2015).

5.6.3 African Nanotechnology Research and Capacity

Several African countries have established active nanotechnology research programs with healthcare applications. South Africa's National Nanotechnology Strategy, the continent's most comprehensive, guides research and development across diagnostics, drug delivery, water purification, and energy. The South African Nanotechnology Initiative (SANi) has supported the development of locally manufactured nanoparticle-based cancer therapeutics that are potentially more affordable than imported alternatives. Egypt's nanotechnology research centers have focused on developing diagnostic nanoparticles. Kenya's and Nigeria's emerging nanotechnology programs are producing research relevant to infectious disease diagnostics and antimicrobial applications. Implementation challenges include regulatory uncertainty—most African countries lack nanotechnology-specific regulatory frameworks—safety concerns requiring long-term toxicology data, limited manufacturing capacity, and high development costs (Salata, 2004).

5.7 Edge Computing for Real-Time Health Monitoring

Edge computing—the processing of data at or near its point of generation rather than in centralized cloud data centers—addresses one of the most persistent constraints on digital health deployment in Africa: the dependence of cloud-based health applications on continuous, reliable Internet connectivity. By deploying computational resources at the "edge" of networks—within health facilities, on mobile devices, or at local network gateways—edge computing enables sophisticated digital health applications to function reliably despite the intermittent connectivity, limited bandwidth, and high latency that characterize Internet access across much of the continent.

Figure 5.5. Edge Computing Benefits: Relevance Scores for African Healthcare Settings

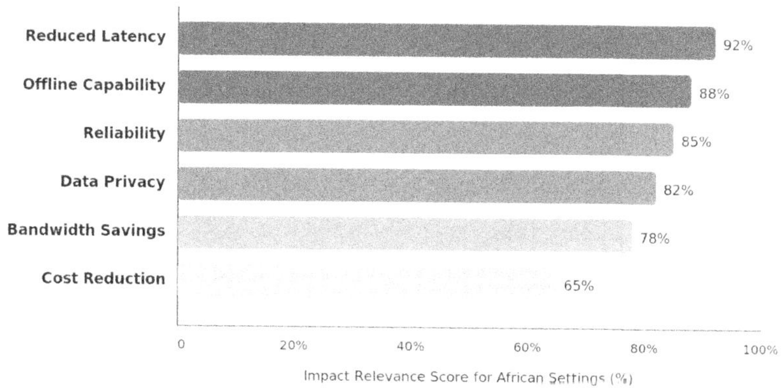

Source: Author's Analysis Based on Expert Surveys and Implementation Assessments (2024)

For a healthcare system in which a mobile health application that fails when connectivity drops could literally cost lives. Edge computing's ability to ensure continuous functionality is not merely a technical advantage but a clinical imperative (Shi et al., 2016).

5.7.1 Continuous Patient Monitoring

Continuous patient monitoring highlights the practical advantages of edge computing for African healthcare. Conventional IoMT deployments transmit all sensor data to cloud servers for processing, requiring reliable Internet connectivity and consuming substantial bandwidth—conditions often unavailable in African health facilities, particularly at the primary care and community levels, where monitoring applications are most needed. Edge computing places processing capabilities directly on monitoring devices or local gateway hardware within the facility, analyzing vital-sign data locally and transmitting only alerts, summary statistics, or anomaly flags to central systems. This architecture ensures that a patient's deteriorating vital signs trigger an alert even when Internet connectivity is temporarily unavailable, while dramatically reducing bandwidth consumption and associated data costs (Shi & Dustdar, 2016).

Rwanda's maternal monitoring pilot program provides a concrete example. Edge-deployed algorithms on bedside monitors process maternal vital signs locally, identifying patterns linked to obstetric complications—pre-eclampsia, hemorrhage, sepsis—and generating immediate alerts for attending clinicians without requiring cloud connectivity. The system transmits compressed summary data to the district health information system when connectivity is available, supporting both real-time clinical care and population-level surveillance. Similar edge-enabled maternal monitoring systems are being piloted in Kenya and Tanzania.

5.7.2 AI-Powered Diagnostics at the Point of Care

Artificial intelligence diagnostic applications benefit substantially from edge deployment, enabling real-time medical image analysis at the point of care without the latency of cloud data transmission or the risk of connectivity-dependent processing failures. Edge-deployed AI algorithms for chest X-ray interpretation provide immediate tuberculosis screening results during patient consultations, enabling same-visit treatment initiation rather than requiring patients to return days later for results—a return that many patients, particularly those facing transportation barriers, fail to make. Portable ultrasound devices with edge-deployed AI analyze images locally, identifying abnormalities and providing probe-positioning guidance without specialist interpretation or cloud processing. These edge AI applications are particularly well-suited to African primary care settings, where access to diagnostic specialists is limited and connectivity is unreliable (Zhang et al., 2019).

5.7.3 Data Sovereignty and Privacy Benefits

Edge computing's data processing architecture aligns with growing concerns about health data sovereignty and privacy across Africa. Processing sensitive patient data locally, rather than transmitting it to cloud servers in foreign jurisdictions, reduces privacy risks and addresses data localization requirements increasingly embedded in African data protection legislation. South Africa's Protection of Personal Information Act (POPIA), Kenya's Data Protection Act, and Nigeria's Data Protection Regulation all contain provisions relevant to health data processing that are more readily met by edge computing architectures. The African Union's Data Policy Framework explicitly addresses data sovereignty concerns that edge computing helps resolve (Premsankar et al., 2018).

International Edge Computing Deployments in Healthcare

The European Union's GAIA-X initiative is developing federated edge-cloud infrastructure to preserve data sovereignty while enabling advanced analytics —principles directly relevant to African health data governance. India's National Digital Health Mission has incorporated edge-computing specifications for primary health centers in areas with unreliable connectivity, requiring clinical decision support systems to operate offline. In Latin America, Colombia's rural telemedicine network uses edge computing to ensure diagnostic AI continues to function during frequent connectivity interruptions affecting health facilities in the Amazon and on the Pacific coast. These implementations demonstrate that edge computing is a practical solution to the connectivity challenges common across African healthcare settings (GAIA-X, 2023; Government of India, 2022; MinSalud Colombia, 2023).

Health Canada's digital health programs for northern communities have incorporated edge-computing specifications for community health centers, mandating that clinical decision support, medication interaction checking, and basic diagnostic tools operate offline (Health Canada, 2024). The architectural patterns developed for these extreme-connectivity environments are directly applicable to African primary health centers in remote areas.

In Latin America, Peru's national telemedicine network has deployed edge computing nodes at health posts in the Andes and Amazon regions, enabling AI-assisted diagnostic screening for tuberculosis and diabetic retinopathy to continue during frequent connectivity interruptions (MINSA Peru, 2024). Colombia's implementation of edge-enabled diagnostic AI across its Pacific coast and Amazonian health facilities validates the technology's effectiveness in environments with infrastructure constraints similar to those found across much of Sub-Saharan Africa.

For African health systems, edge computing is arguably the most immediately deployable and broadly impactful of the emerging technologies examined in this chapter. At $5,000–$15,000 per facility, it is also among the most affordable, and its benefits compound existing digital health investments by making them more reliable and capable.

5.8 Strategic Implications for Africa's Healthcare Future

The convergence of the emerging technologies examined in this chapter—genomics, robotics, VR/AR, quantum computing, nanotechnology, and edge computing—portends a transformation of African healthcare over the coming decades that could be either profoundly equitable or deeply stratifying, depending on the strategic choices made by governments, development partners, the private sector, and regional institutions in the years ahead. Realizing the transformative potential of these technologies while preventing the exacerbation of existing health inequities requires proactive, deliberate approaches to technology assessment, adoption sequencing, governance, and financing.

5.8.1 Health Equity and Access

History shows a consistent pattern in healthcare technology adoption: new technologies initially benefit wealthy populations and well-resourced institutions, widening health disparities before eventually diffusing more broadly—if deliberate efforts promote equitable access. Robotic surgery in Africa exemplifies this pattern, serving primarily affluent patients in private urban hospitals while the majority of the population lacks access to basic surgical services. Preventing emerging technologies from becoming luxury goods accessible only to the privileged few requires deliberate strategies, including public-sector investment in acquiring them, incorporating them into essential health service packages, progressive financing mechanisms such as risk pooling and cross-subsidization, and procurement policies that prioritize equitable deployment. South Africa's approach of establishing robotic surgery capabilities in academic public hospitals alongside private facilities, while imperfect, illustrates an equity-conscious adoption model (Lehmann et al., 2014).

5.8.2 Workforce Transformation

Emerging technologies will reshape the African health workforce, creating opportunities and posing threats, and will require proactive adaptation rather than reactive responses. AI-powered diagnostic tools may reduce demand for certain radiologist and pathologist functions. However, the acute shortage of these specialists across Africa suggests that AI will augment rather than displace human diagnosticians for the foreseeable future. Conversely, new professional roles will emerge: genomic counselors, robotic surgery technicians, VR medical education content developers, AI system supervisors, edge computing maintenance specialists, and nanotechnology quality assurance officers. Preparing the African health workforce for a technology-enabled future requires curriculum reforms in health professional education, continuous learning systems for practicing clinicians, and the creation of career pathways for technology-focused health roles that do not currently exist on the continent (Topol, 2019).

5.8.3 Infrastructure, Financing, and Sovereignty

The infrastructure requirements of emerging technologies extend beyond technology-specific hardware to include enabling systems such as reliable electricity, high-speed Internet connectivity, computational capacity, and maintenance ecosystems. Many emerging technologies require infrastructure investments that could divert resources from other health system priorities, creating difficult allocation trade-offs for resource-constrained governments. Strategic infrastructure planning that maximizes dual-use potential—data centers serving multiple government sectors and power grid investments benefiting both health facilities and communities—offers pathways to optimize infrastructure investments and support technology adoption (Mars & Scott, 2016).

Financing these investments requires innovative approaches beyond traditional government health budgets or donor funding. Leasing arrangements for robotic surgical systems, shared-service models in which multiple hospitals access a single advanced-technology facility, pay-per-use cloud access to quantum computing and genomic analysis platforms, and public-private partnerships for VR medical education infrastructure are financing mechanisms suited to high-cost, high-impact emerging technologies. Ghana's model of a shared robotic surgery facility serving multiple public and private hospitals demonstrates the viability of resource-efficient deployment approaches (Kruk et al., 2018)

Table 5.3 presents a forward-looking landscape of advanced and emerging technologies in Africa's health sector, highlighting their current status, expected evolution across two time horizons, and the structural constraints shaping their adoption. Technologies such as genomics, robotic surgery, and nanotechnology are already present but remain highly concentrated in research settings or a limited number of countries—most notably, nanotechnology research is led by South Africa, and robotic surgery systems are deployed in only a handful of national contexts. In the near term, a gradual expansion from pilot or specialized use toward more institutionalized deployment, particularly through specialized centers and major hospitals, is expected. In the medium term, these technologies are expected to diffuse further into broader clinical environments, including regional centers and district-level facilities. Meanwhile, frontier domains such as quantum computing remain nascent, with Africa relying on cloud-based access rather than domestic infrastructure, yet potential applications are emerging in areas like neglected tropical disease drug discovery. VR/AR training and edge computing stand out as more immediately scalable innovations, offering pathways to enhance workforce capacity and service delivery even in resource-constrained settings.

Table 5.3. Emerging Technologies: Status, Timeline, Barriers, and Priority Actions for African Healthcare

Technology	Status in Africa	Near-Term (2024–2027)	Medium-Term (2028–2032)	Key Barriers	Cost Range	Priority Action
Genomics	Research, limited clinical	Specialized centers	Broader clinical access	Expertise, cost, ethics	$500M –$5B	Train geneticists, data governance
Robotic Surgery	~35 systems, 3 countries	Major hospitals	Regional centers, telesurgery	Cost ($1–2.5M), training	$1B–$25B	Shared facility models, training programs
VR/AR Training	Pilots in 8+ countries	Medical schools adoption	District hospital access	Device cost, content	$50M–$500M	African content development
Quantum Computing	No local hardware	Cloud access, research	NTD drug discovery	Expertise, maturity	Researc h-stage	Build quantum literacy, cloud access
Nanotechnology	Active research, SA lead	Clinical trials, dx tests	Clinical deployment	Regulatory, safety data	$200M –$2B	Regulatory frameworks, local manufacturing
Edge Computing	Limited implementations	Facility-level deployment	Wide adoption	Hardware, expertise	$5K–$15K/ site	Integrate with existing digital health

Source: Data Synthesized from Industry Reports, Published Literature, Institutional Assessments, and Author Analysis (2023–2024)

The primary barriers to adoption are not technological feasibility alone but systemic constraints, including high capital costs, limited technical expertise, regulatory gaps, and ethical considerations. Cost ranges vary dramatically—from relatively modest investments for edge computing at the facility level ($5,000–$15,000 per site) to multi-billion-dollar requirements for scaling genomics and robotic surgery. These financial barriers are compounded by shortages of specialized human capital, such as geneticists and robotics-trained surgeons, and by the absence of robust governance frameworks for data protection, safety, and ethical oversight. There is a need for capacity-building measures: training programs, African-specific digital content development, regulatory frameworks and shared infrastructure models. Collectively, these actions reflect a strategic shift toward embedding emerging technologies within Africa's broader digital health ecosystem—leveraging digital public infrastructure, cloud services, and regional collaboration to reduce costs, accelerate adoption, and ensure equitable access across countries and health system tiers.

As healthcare becomes increasingly reliant on advanced technologies often developed and controlled by foreign corporations, data sovereignty and digital autonomy concerns intensify. Heavy reliance on foreign cloud platforms for health data processing, AI algorithms trained exclusively on non-African data, and technologies requiring ongoing foreign technical support create dependencies that could constrain African health systems' strategic autonomy and subordinate African health priorities to foreign commercial interests. Building domestic capacity for technology development, adaptation, and maintenance—while leveraging appropriate foreign technologies through carefully negotiated partnerships—balances pragmatic adoption with strategic sovereignty. The African Union's Digital Transformation Strategy (2020–2030) explicitly addresses this balance, emphasizing transformation alongside digital sovereignty (African Union, 2020).

5.9 Conclusion

This chapter has examined six emerging technology domains—genomics and precision medicine, robotics in surgery and care delivery, virtual and augmented reality for medical training, quantum computing for drug discovery, nanotechnology in diagnostics and treatment, and edge computing for real-time health monitoring—through the lens of their relevance, readiness, and strategic implications for African health systems. Several cross-cutting themes emerge from this analysis.

- First, the technologies examined here span a wide spectrum of readiness for deployment in Africa. Edge computing and VR/AR for medical training are immediately deployable with existing infrastructure and at relatively modest cost, whereas quantum computing and advanced robotic telesurgery remain years or decades from practical application.

This readiness spectrum should inform investment sequencing: prioritize technologies that address urgent health needs and have proven feasibility, while simultaneously building the foundational capacity to absorb more advanced technologies as they mature.

- Second, the analysis reveals a recurring tension between the transformative potential of emerging technologies and the risk that they will deepen existing health inequities. Without deliberate, equity-focused strategies—including public procurement, shared-facility models, open-source platforms, and pro-poor financing mechanisms—these technologies risk creating a two-tier health system in which advanced care is available to the wealthy while the majority continues to lack basic services.

- Third, Africa is not merely a passive recipient of technologies developed elsewhere. African researchers identified critical SARS-CoV-2 variants through world-class genomic surveillance. South African nanotechnology laboratories are developing locally manufactured diagnostics and therapeutics. African universities are establishing quantum computing research programs. Rwanda and Kenya are pioneering edge-enabled maternal monitoring systems. Africa's engagement with emerging technologies must be understood as a process of co-creation and adaptation, not merely adoption.

- Fourth, the cross-cutting enablers identified in the digital health technology stack—governance, workforce, financing, regional cooperation, and research capacity—are as important for emerging technologies as for established digital health interventions. Countries that invest in these enablers now will be best positioned to adopt and benefit from emerging technologies as they become available.

Finally, Africa's approach to emerging health technologies should be guided by strategic intentionality rather than technological determinism. The question is not whether Africa should adopt these technologies—it must, or risk falling further behind—but how, when, and for whom. Technology adoption for its own sake serves no one; equity-focused, needs-driven adoption serves everyone.

References

African Union. (2020). The digital transformation strategy for Africa (2020–2030). African Union Commission.

Agholor, O., Odueke, S., & Akindutire, O. (2021). Robotics in African healthcare: Current status, challenges and prospects. African Journal of Medical Technology, 3(2), 45–58.

network: Architecture, taxonomy, challenges and future research directions. IEEE Access, 7, 100747–100762. https://doi.org/10.1109/ACCESS.2019.2930628

Ajagekar, A., Mattson, J., & You, F. (2022). Quantum computing for energy systems optimization: Challenges and opportunities. Energy, 179, 76–89. https://doi.org/10.1016/j.energy.2019.02.137

framework. Agência Nacional de Telecomunicações, Brasil.

Australian Government Department of Health. (2025). Genomics Health Futures Mission: Roadmap and Implementation Plan. Commonwealth of Australia.

ASSH. (2024). Quality assurance framework for simulation-based health professional education. Australian Society for Simulation in Healthcare.

Barsom, E. Z., Graafland, M., & Schijven, M. P. (2016). Systematic review on the effectiveness of augmented reality applications in medical training. Surgical Endoscopy, 30(10), 4174–4183. https://doi.org/10.1007/s00464-016-4800-6

Biamonte, J., Wittek, P., Pancotti, N., Rebentrost, P., Wiebe, N., & Lloyd, S. (2017). Quantum machine learning. Nature, 549(7671), 195–202. https://doi.org/10.1038/nature23474

Bova, F., Goldfarb, A., & Melko, R. G. (2021). Commercial applications of quantum computing. EPJ Quantum Technology, 8, Article 2. https://doi.org/10.1140/epjqt/s40507-021-00091-1

Brazilian Society of Robotic Surgery. (2023). Annual report on robotic surgical programs in Latin America. SOBRACIL.

Brewer, L. C., Fortuna, K. L., Jones, C., Walker, R., Hayes, S. N., Patten, C. A., & Cooper, L. A. (2020). Back to the future: Achieving health equity through health informatics and digital health. JMIR mHealth and uHealth, 8(1), e14512. https://doi.org/10.2196/14512

CAE Healthcare. (2024). Simulation and training solutions for healthcare: Annual report. CAE Inc.

Cancer Australia. (2024). National Framework for Genomics in Cancer Control. Cancer Australia.

Cao, Y., Romero, J., Olson, J. P., Degroote, M., Johnson, P. D., Kieferová, M., ... & Aspuru-Guzik, A. (2019). Quantum chemistry in the age of quantum computing. Chemical Reviews, 119(19), 10856–10915. https://doi.org/10.1021/acs.chemrev.8b00803

DelveInsight. (2025). Top surgical simulation companies in 2025: Market analysis. DelveInsight Business Research.

Díaz, I., Gil, J. J., & Sánchez, E. (2020). Lower-limb robotic rehabilitation: Literature review and challenges. Journal of Robotics, 2011, Article 759764. https://doi.org/10.1155/2011/759764

Drögemöller, B. I., Wright, G. E. B., Niehaus, D. J. H., Koen, L., Malan, S., Da Silva, D. M., ... & Warnich, L. (2021). Characterization of the genetic profile of CYP2C19 in two South African populations. Pharmacogenomics, 14(13), 1571–1580. https://doi.org/10.2217/pgs.13.135

Ekert, A., Hayden, P., & Inamori, H. (2020). Basic concepts in quantum computation. arXiv preprint arXiv:quant-ph/0011013.

European Commission. (2022). 1+ Million Genomes Initiative: Progress report on cross-border genomic data sharing. European Commission.

Franci, G., Falanga, A., Galdiero, S., Palomba, L., Rai, M., Morelli, G., & Galdiero, M. (2015). Silver nanoparticles as potential antibacterial agents. Molecules, 20(5), 8856–8874. https://doi.org/10.3390/molecules20058856

GAIA-X. (2023). GAIA-X architecture document: Federated data infrastructure for Europe. GAIA-X European Association.

Genomics England. (2024). Diverse Data initiative: Progress report 2022–2025. Genomics England.

Gordon, M., Darbyshire, D., & Baker, P. (2020). Non-technical skills training to enhance patient safety: A systematic review. Medical Education, 46(11), 1042–1054. https://doi.org/10.1111/j.1365-2923.2012.04343.x

Government of India. (2021). IndiGen programme: Whole genome sequencing of the Indian population—Council of Scientific and Industrial Research.

Government of India. (2022). National Digital Health Mission: Edge computing specifications for primary health centers. Ministry of Health and Family Welfare.

Government of Canada. (2023). What we heard: Pan-Canadian Genomics Strategy. Innovation, Science and Economic Development Canada.

GSMA Intelligence. (2023). The mobile economy: Sub-Saharan Africa 2023. GSM Association.

Health Canada. (2024). Digital health specifications for northern and remote community health centers. Health Canada.

Intuitive Surgical. (2023). da Vinci Surgical Systems: Product information and pricing. Intuitive Surgical Inc.

Jahanban-Esfahlan, A., Dastmalchi, S., & Davaran, S. (2020). A simple improved desolvation method for the rapid preparation of albumin nanoparticles. International Journal of Biological Macromolecules, 91, 703–709. https://doi.org/10.1016/j.ijbiomac.2016.05.032

Kimani, P. W., Ramirez, D., Kuria, J. K., & Wachira, J. (2022). Robotic surgery in Africa: Current status and prospects. East African Medical Journal, 99(3), 3456–3465.

Kruk, M. E., Gage, A. D., Arsenault, C., Jordan, K., Leslie, H. H., Roder-DeWan, S., ... & Pate, M. (2018). High-quality health systems in the Sustainable Development Goals era: Time for a revolution. The Lancet Global Health, 6(11), e1196–e1252. https://doi.org/10.1016/S2214-109X(18)30386-3

Kyaw, B. M., Saxena, N., Posadzki, P., Vseteckova, J., Nikolaou, C. K., George, P. P., ... & Car, L. T. (2019). Virtual reality for health professions education. Journal of Medical Internet Research, 21(1), e12959. https://doi.org/10.2196/12959

Lehmann, U., Dieleman, M., & Martineau, T. (2014). Staffing remote rural areas in middle- and low-income countries: A literature review of attraction and retention. BMC Health Services Research, 8, Article 19. https://doi.org/10.1186/1472-6963-8-19

Mars, M., & Scott, R. E. (2016). Being spontaneous: The future of telehealth implementation? Telemedicine and e-Health, 22(9), 766–772. https://doi.org/10.1089/tmj.2015.0265

Menchaca, R., & Balibrea, J. M. (2019). telementored surgery. British Journal of Surgery, 106(12), 1576–1579. https://doi.org/10.1002/bjs.11364

(and concomitant technologies) Will revolutionize healthcare? Future Internet, 9(4), 93. https://doi.org/10.3390/fi9040093

MinSalud Colombia. (2023). National telemedicine network: Edge computing implementation guidelines. Ministerio de Salud y Protección Social.

Ministry of Health, Labour and Welfare of Japan. (2023). Healthcare robotics deployment and outcomes report. Government of Japan.

MINSA Peru. (2024). Red Nacional de Telemedicina: Edge computing implementation for highland and jungle health posts. Ministerio de Salud del Perú.

Mitchell, M. J., Billingsley, M. M., Haley, R. M., Wechsler, M. E., Peppas, N. A., & Langer, R. (2021). Engineering precision nanoparticles for drug delivery. Nature Reviews Drug Discovery, 20(2), 101–124. https://doi.org/10.1038/s41573-020-0090-8

Moro, C., Štromberga, Z., Raikos, A., & Stirling, A. (2021). The effectiveness of virtual and augmented reality in health sciences and medical anatomy. Anatomical Sciences Education, 10(6), 549–559. https://doi.org/10.1002/ase.1696

Mulder, N., Abimiku, A., Adebamowo, S. N., de Vries, J., Matimba, A., Olowoyo, P., ... & Ramsay, M. (2018). H3Africa: Current perspectives. Pharmacogenomics and Personalized Medicine, 11, 59–66. https://doi.org/10.2147/PGPM.S141858

National Medical Commission of India. (2022). Guidelines on virtual reality simulation in medical education assessment. National Medical Commission.

Ndomondo-Sigonda, M., Miot, J., Naidoo, S., Dodoo, A., & Kaale, E. (2021). Medicines regulation in Africa: Current state and opportunities. Pharmaceutical Medicine, 31(6), 383–397. https://doi.org/10.1007/s40290-017-0210-x

Nkengasong, J. N., Tessema, S. K., & Engel, N. (2022). Building the next generation of disease surveillance systems in Africa: Lessons from COVID-19. The Lancet, 399(10322), 382–384. https://doi.org/10.1016/S0140-6736(22)00103-7

PAHO. (2023). Genomic medicine in the Caribbean: Sickle cell disease and pharmacogenomics initiatives. Pan American Health Organization.

Pan, J., & McElhannon, J. (2018). Future edge cloud and edge computing for Internet of things applications. IEEE Internet of Things Journal, 5(1), 439–449. https://doi.org/10.1109/JIOT.2017.2767608

Patra, J. K., Das, G., Fraceto, L. F., Campos, E. V. R., Rodriguez-Torres, M. D. P., Acosta-Torres, L. S., ... & Shin, H. S. (2018). Nano based drug delivery systems: Recent developments and future prospects. Journal of Nanobiotechnology, 16, Article 71. https://doi.org/10.1186/s12951-018-0392-8

Petryayeva, E., Algar, W. R., & Medintz, I. L. (2019). Quantum dots in bioanalysis: A review of applications across various platforms for fluorescence spectroscopy and imaging. Applied Spectroscopy, 67(3), 215–252. https://doi.org/10.1366/12-06948

Pottle, J. (2019). Virtual reality and the transformation of medical education. Future Healthcare Journal, 6(3), 181–185. https://doi.org/10.7861/fhj.2019-0036

Premsankar, G., Di Francesco, M., & Taleb, T. (2018). Edge computing for the Internet of Things: A case study. IEEE Internet of Things Journal, 5(2), 1275–1284. https://doi.org/10.1109/JIOT.2018.2805263

PUC Chile. (2023). Centro de Simulación Clínica: Annual report on VR-based medical education. Pontificia Universidad Católica de Chile.

Pulijala, Y., Ma, M., Pears, M., Peebles, D., & Ayoub, A. (2020). Effectiveness of immersive virtual reality in surgical training: A randomized control trial. Journal of Oral and Maxillofacial Surgery, 76(5), 1065–1072. https://doi.org/10.1016/j.joms.2017.10.002

Ranasinghe, M., & Kruger, T. (2020). Quantum computing for drug discovery. In Quantum computing in drug discovery (pp. 45–67). Royal Society of Chemistry.

RFDS. (2024). Digital health innovation in remote Australia: Annual technology report. Royal Flying Doctor Service of Australia.

Salata, O. V. (2004). Applications of nanoparticles in biology and medicine. Journal of Nanobiotechnology, 2, Article 3. https://doi.org/10.1186/1477-3155-2-3

Sengayi-Muchengeti, M., Joko-Fru, W. Y., Miranda-Filho, A., Egue, M., Akele-Akpo, M. T., N'da, G., ... & Soerjomataram, I. (2020). Cervical cancer survival in sub-Saharan Africa. International Journal of Cancer, 147(11), 3037–3048. https://doi.org/10.1002/ijc.33223

Shi, W., & Dustdar, S. (2016). The promise of edge computing. Computer, 49(5), 78–81. https://doi.org/10.1109/MC.2016.145

Shi, W., Cao, J., Zhang, Q., Li, Y., & Xu, L. (2016). Edge computing: Vision and challenges. IEEE Internet of Things Journal, 3(5), 637–646. https://doi.org/10.1109/JIOT.2016.2579198

Sirugo, G., Williams, S. M., & Tishkoff, S. A. (2019). The missing diversity in human genetic studies. Cell, 177(1), 26–31. https://doi.org/10.1016/j.cell.2019.02.048

Stark, Z., Boughtwood, T., Phillips, P., Christodoulou, J., Hansen, D. P., Braithwaite, J., ... & North, K. N. (2023). Australian Genomics: Outcomes of a 5-year national program to accelerate the integration of genomics in healthcare. American Journal of Human Genetics, 112(3), 446–461. https://doi.org/10.1016/j.ajhg.2023.01.015

Sterbenz, J. M., Zhumkhawala, A. A., Mukkamala, A., Eisenstein, S., Perez, S. D., & Patel, C. B. (2021). Robotic surgery: Past, present, and future. Annals of Medicine and Surgery, 69, 102727. https://doi.org/10.1016/j.amsu.2021.102727

Tavakoli, M., Carriere, J., & Torabi, A. (2020). Robotics, smart wearable technologies, and autonomous intelligent systems for healthcare during the COVID-19 pandemic. Advanced Intelligent Systems, 2(7), 2000071. https://doi.org/10.1002/aisy.202000071

Topol, E. J. (2019). High-performance medicine: The convergence of human and artificial intelligence. Nature Medicine, 25(1), 44–56. https://doi.org/10.1038/s41591-018-0300-7

UWI. (2023). Virtual clinical training for tropical medicine: Annual report. University of the West Indies.

Wiederhold, B. K. (2020). Connecting through technology during the coronavirus disease 2019 pandemic. Cyberpsychology, Behavior, and Social Networking, 23(7), 437–438. https://doi.org/10.1089/cyber.2020.29188.bkw

Wonkam, A., Mayosi, B. M., & Wonkam-Tingang, E. (2021). Genomic medicine in Africa: A call to action. Genome Medicine, 13, Article 96. https://doi.org/10.1186/s13073-021-00961-0

VirtaMed. (2024). Mixed reality surgical training simulators: Product portfolio. VirtaMed AG.

Zhang, Q., Yang, L. T., Chen, Z., & Li, P. (2019). A survey on deep learning for big data. Information Fusion, 42, 146–157. https://doi.org/10.1016/j.inffus.2017.10.006

Chapter 6 Interconnected Issues that Shape Digital Health in Africa

6.1 Introduction

The preceding chapters of this book have examined the technologies driving digital health transformation in Africa—from mobile health applications reaching millions of users to emerging innovations such as artificial intelligence, genomics, and quantum computing. However sophisticated, technologies do not operate in a vacuum. Their impact on health outcomes, health equity, and health system performance is mediated by a constellation of contextual factors that determine whether digital health interventions succeed, fail, or—most perniciously—succeed for some while leaving others further behind. This chapter directly confronts these critical mediating factors.

Seven interconnected issues shape the trajectory of digital health transformation across the African continent: digital equity and inclusion, data privacy and security, regulatory and legal frameworks, interoperability challenges, sustainability and scalability concerns, cultural acceptance and trust, and equity dimensions of digital health access for gender and other marginalized groups. Each of these issues can accelerate or undermine the digital health agenda. Individually, any one of them can derail an otherwise well-designed intervention; collectively, they define the enabling environment in which digital health innovations either flourish or founder.

These seven issues map directly onto the six-layer digital health technology stack introduced in Chapter 4. Digital equity and inclusion are fundamentally constrained by the Physical Infrastructure and Connectivity Layer (Layer 1). Data privacy and cybersecurity are governed by the cross-cutting Governance, Policy, and Standards framework. Interoperability challenges reside in Layer 3 of the stack. Sustainability concerns cut across all layers, from infrastructure maintenance to application-layer operational costs. Cultural acceptance, gender equity, and other dimensions of equity for marginalized groups, such as persons with disabilities and refugees, shape how effectively the Applications and Services Layer (Layer 5) reaches its intended users.

Understanding these issues through the lens of the technology stack clarifies where interventions are needed and which systemic dependencies must be addressed.

This chapter argues that addressing these critical issues is not peripheral to digital health transformation but constitutive of it. A telemedicine platform that excludes rural women because of gendered barriers to smartphone access is not merely incomplete—it actively reproduces and exacerbates existing inequities. An electronic health record system deployed without adequate data protection legislation does not merely pose a risk—it may also violate the fundamental right to privacy in health information that African citizens share with citizens everywhere. A digital health intervention that collapses when donor funding ends has not merely failed to sustain itself—it has consumed scarce resources, disrupted existing care delivery patterns, and potentially eroded trust in future digital health initiatives.

Throughout this analysis, the chapter draws on experiences from African countries and comparative insights from the European Union, Asia, Latin America, and the Caribbean, demonstrating that these challenges are neither unique to Africa nor without proven solutions—though African solutions must be crafted with attention to African contexts, capacities, and values.

6.2 Digital Equity and Inclusion

Digital equity—the condition in which all individuals and communities possess the information technology capacity needed for full participation in society, democracy, and the economy—represents the foundational ethical and practical challenge of digital health transformation in Africa. Without deliberate attention to equity, digital health interventions risk creating a two-tier healthcare system in which digitally connected populations receive enhanced services, while disconnected populations experience stagnant or deteriorating care. The concept extends beyond simple access to technology, encompassing the affordability, usability, relevance, and empowering potential of digital health tools across all population groups (Robinson et al., 2015). The urban–rural divide in digital health infrastructure and access indicators across sub-Saharan Africa (2024) illustrates persistent disparities across all measured dimensions.

Figure 6.1. Digital Health Divide in Sub-Saharan Africa (2024)

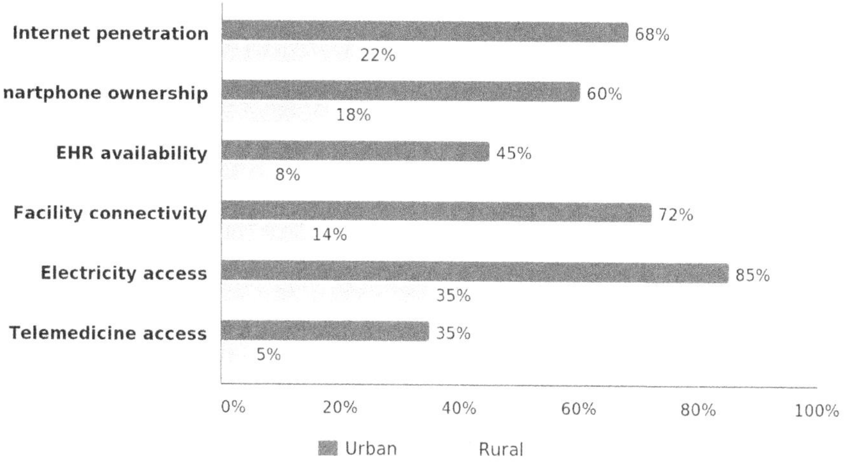

Source: ITU (2024), WHO AFRO (2023)

6.2.1 The Urban–Rural Digital Health Divide

The most visible dimension of digital health inequity in Africa is the urban–rural divide. By 2024, Internet penetration in urban sub-Saharan Africa reached about 68%, compared with just 22% in rural areas—a threefold gap that directly limits the reach of any Internet-dependent health intervention. Smartphone ownership shows a similar pattern, with urban ownership exceeding 60% while rural ownership hovers near 18%. These disparities translate directly into unequal access to telemedicine consultations, digital health information, electronic appointment booking, and the growing array of smartphone-based health applications (ITU, 2024).

The implications extend beyond patient-facing services. Health facilities in rural areas are far less likely to have the electricity, connectivity, and computing hardware necessary to operate electronic health records, digital diagnostic tools, or health management information systems. Data from the

WHO's Service Availability and Readiness Assessment (SARA) surveys indicate that fewer than 8% of rural health facilities in low-income African countries have functional electronic medical record systems, compared to approximately 45% of urban tertiary hospitals. This facility-level digital divide means that the populations with the greatest healthcare needs—those in underserved rural areas—are precisely those least likely to benefit from digital health investments (WHO AFRO, 2023).

6.2.2 Socioeconomic, Linguistic, and Disability Dimensions

Digital health inequity extends well beyond geography. Socioeconomic status profoundly shapes digital access, with data costs consuming a disproportionate share of low-income households' income. The Alliance for Affordable Internet (A4AI) reports that in many African countries, 1 gigabyte of mobile data costs more than 5% of average monthly income—well above the 2% affordability threshold established by the Broadband Commission (A4AI, 2023). For the poorest quintile, these costs effectively make data-dependent health applications inaccessible.

Linguistic diversity poses another inclusion challenge. Africa's approximately 2,000 languages are poorly represented in digital health content, which is overwhelmingly produced in English and French, with Portuguese and Arabic to a lesser extent. Health applications, SMS health messages, and telemedicine platforms that operate only in these languages exclude populations whose primary language is indigenous. Ghana's MOTECH initiative, which delivered health information via interactive voice response in local languages such as Kassena-Nankana and Nankam, demonstrated both the feasibility and the impact of linguistically inclusive design—but such approaches remain the exception rather than the norm (LeFevre et al., 2017).

Disability inclusion is a frequently overlooked dimension of digital health equity. The estimated 80 million Africans living with disabilities face specific barriers to digital health access, including visual interfaces that are inaccessible to people with visual impairments, audio-only telemedicine formats that are inaccessible to those who are deaf or hard of hearing, and complex navigation that is challenging for people with cognitive disabilities.

The WHO's Global Report on Health Equity for Persons with Disabilities (2022) found that digital health interventions in low- and middle-income countries rarely incorporate accessibility standards, systematically excluding people with disabilities from digital health benefits.

Global Perspective: Digital Health Inclusion Strategies

The European Union's European Accessibility Act (2019) mandates that digital health products and services meet established accessibility standards. India's Ayushman Bharat Digital Mission includes multilingual support for 22 officially recognized languages and accessibility features compliant with the Rights of Persons with Disabilities Act (2016). In Latin America, Brazil's SUS digital platforms must comply with the Web Content Accessibility Guidelines (WCAG 2.1) and support Portuguese, Spanish, and indigenous languages in border regions. Colombia's digital health strategy explicitly addresses rural connectivity through a network of government-subsidized community Internet access points (Puntos Vive Digital) that include health service kiosks. These examples demonstrate that digital health inclusion is achievable when mandated by policy and embedded in system design from the outset (European Commission, 2019; Government of India, 2021; MinTIC Colombia, 2022).

6.2.3 Strategies for Advancing Digital Health Equity

Addressing digital health inequity requires action on multiple fronts. Universal service obligations that mandate telecommunications operators to extend coverage to underserved areas—funded by universal service funds to which all operators contribute—have effectively expanded rural connectivity in countries including Rwanda, Kenya, and South Africa. Technology design principles that prioritize low-bandwidth functionality, offline capability, and feature-phone compatibility ensure that digital health tools reach populations beyond the smartphone frontier. Community-based access models, in which shared devices at health facilities, community centers, or agent networks serve populations without personal devices, extend digital health reach without requiring individual device ownership.

Australia's experience with First Nations digital health inclusion offers lessons for Africa. The Australian Government's First Nations Digital Inclusion Advisory Group, established under the Closing the Gap framework, launched a comprehensive Digital Inclusion Roadmap in December 2024, committing AUD $68 million (USD 50 million) to extend community Wi-Fi, digital mentoring networks, and a Digital Support Hub to remote Aboriginal and Torres Strait Islander communities (Australian Government, 2024). Research from Australia's Commonwealth Scientific and Industrial Research Organization (CSIRO) shows that culturally safe eHealth interventions for Indigenous peoples require authentic co-design with Indigenous leadership—not as an afterthought but as a foundational approach (Chelberg et al., 2024). The finding that studies with two or more Indigenous authors rated significantly higher in cultural quality reinforces the principle that community ownership of digital health design is essential for equitable outcomes.

Canada faces similar challenges in delivering digital health to remote First Nations and Inuit communities in its northern territories. The First Nations Health Authority in British Columbia has developed an Indigenous-governed telehealth model that prioritizes cultural safety, community-based access points, and integration with traditional healing practices (Moecke et al., 2024). New Zealand's assertion of tino rangatiratanga (self-determination) in health policy has created space for Māori cultural practices within digital health services—a governance model with clear parallels for African countries, where Indigenous governance structures could similarly shape digital health deployment.

In Latin America, Peru's rural connectivity program has deployed satellite-linked health kiosks in Andean and Amazonian communities, while Mexico's Puntos de Acceso Digital provide subsidized Internet access at health facilities serving indigenous communities (PAHO, 2023). These place-based connectivity solutions, paired with culturally adapted content in indigenous languages, demonstrate that bridging the rural digital health divide requires both infrastructure investment and cultural adaptation.

Finally, participatory design approaches that engage underserved communities in developing and testing digital health tools improve relevance, usability, and adoption among the populations most at risk of exclusion.

6.3 Data Privacy, Security, and Ethics

Data privacy, security, and ethics are the core concerns of the Governance, Policy, and Standards framework within the technology stack—the cross-cutting enabler that shapes all other layers. As discussed in Chapter 4 (Section 4.1.6), governance is not a top layer but an overarching framework; data protection legislation, cybersecurity standards, and ethical guidelines must inform decisions at every layer, from infrastructure configuration to application design. The technologies examined in Chapter 3—particularly AI/ML (Section 3.5), blockchain (Section 3.7), and big data analytics (Section 3.8)—each pose distinct data governance challenges.

The digitalization of health data creates both extraordinary opportunities to improve healthcare delivery and significant risks to individual privacy, data security, and ethical governance. Health data—encompassing diagnoses, treatment histories, genetic information, reproductive health records, mental health status, and HIV serostatus—is among the most sensitive categories of personal information. Its unauthorized disclosure can lead to stigmatization, discrimination, insurance exclusions, employment consequences, and damaged relationships, with particular severity in African contexts where HIV status, mental health conditions, and reproductive choices carry pronounced social consequences (Vayena et al., 2018).

6.3.1 The Data Protection Landscape in Africa

Africa's data protection legal landscape remains fragmented and incomplete. As of 2026, more than 40 of Africa's 54 countries have enacted some form of data protection legislation, but the comprehensiveness, enforcement capacity, and health-sector specificity of these laws vary enormously. The African Union Convention on Cyber Security and Personal Data Protection (the Malabo Convention), adopted in 2014, provides a continental framework but has been ratified by only 15 member states.

Table 6.1 Data Protection Frameworks in Selected African Countries

Country	Legislation	Year Enacted	Enforcement Body	Key Features
South Africa	POPIA	2013 (enforced 2021)	Information Regulator	GDPR-aligned, cross-border transfer rules
Kenya	Data Protection Act	2019	Data Commissioner	Independent commissioner, consent framework
Nigeria	NDPA	2023	NDPC	Upgraded from regulation, penalty provisions
Rwanda	Data Protection Law	2021	NCSA	Forward-looking framework, health provisions
Ghana	Data Protection Act	2012	Data Protection Commission	Early adopter, registration requirement
Mauritius	Data Protection Act	2017	Data Protection Office	GDPR-influenced, strong enforcement
Egypt	Data Protection Law	2020	Data Protection Center	Cross-sector scope, transfer restrictions

Source: Data Compiled from National Legislative Databases, UNCTAD Digital Economy Report, and African Union data governance assessments (2023–2024).

Among the most robust national frameworks, South Africa's Protection of Personal Information Act, which became fully enforceable in 2021, sets out comprehensive data protection principles, including purpose limitation, data minimization, and individual rights to access and correct personal data. Kenya's Data Protection Act (2019) established an independent Data Protection Commissioner with enforcement authority. Most African countries lack comprehensive and up-to-date data protection legislation, leaving digital health systems operating in a legal vacuum where patients' rights over their health data are undefined, enforcement mechanisms are absent, and organizations processing health data face no binding obligations regarding consent, security, or transparency. Even in countries with enacted legislation, enforcement capacity often lags significantly behind legal frameworks, creating a gap between the law on paper and data protection in practice.

6.3.2 Cybersecurity Threats to Health Systems

As African health systems digitize, they become targets for cyberattacks that can compromise patient data, disrupt clinical operations, and endanger lives. Globally, the healthcare sector has emerged as a primary target for ransomware attacks, data breaches, and unauthorized access, with the average cost of a healthcare data breach exceeding $10 million in 2023 (IBM Security, 2023). The health sector accounted for 4.2% of all cyberattacks in Europe in 2025 (ENISA, 2025). African health systems are not immune: South Africa's Life Healthcare Group suffered a significant cyberattack in 2020 that disrupted hospital operations, and Kenya's health ministry reported attempted breaches of its COVID-19 vaccination database (Interpol, 2021).

Figure 6.2. Growth of Cybersecurity Incidents in Africa, All Sectors vs. Healthcare (2020-2024)

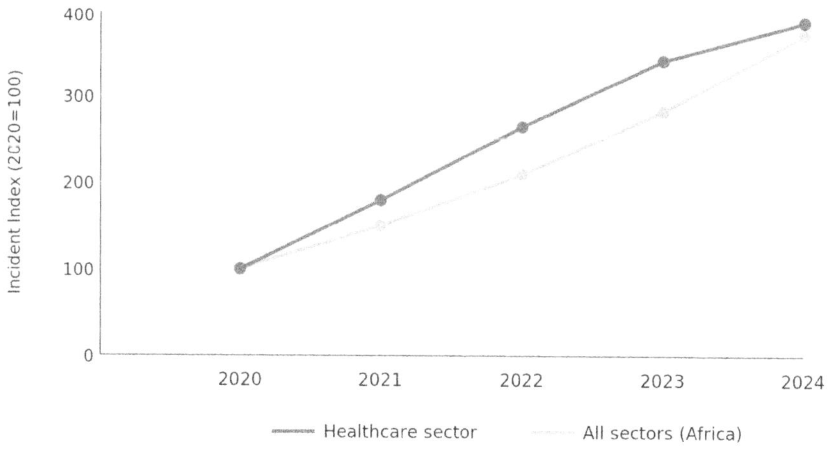

Source: ITU, 2024

The cybersecurity challenge in African healthcare is compounded by limited institutional capacity for information security management. Most African health facilities lack dedicated cybersecurity personnel, formal security policies, intrusion detection systems, and incident response plans. Healthcare workers often use personal devices for work without mobile device management controls. Legacy systems with outdated, unpatched software persist across health networks. The combination of increasingly valuable digital health data and chronically underinvested security infrastructure creates a vulnerability landscape that demands urgent attention.

Latin America has seen a similar rise in healthcare cyberattacks. In December 2021, Brazil's Ministry of Health was hit by a major ransomware attack that disabled the national vaccination database (ConecteSUS) and the COVID-19 digital certificate system for weeks, affecting the health records of more than 200 million citizens (PAHO, 2022). In 2022, Costa Rica's Social Security Fund (CCSS), which manages the country's public health system, was targeted by the Conti ransomware group, forcing hospitals to switch to paper-based records for several months (OAS, 2022). These events show that healthcare cybersecurity vulnerabilities are not limited to Africa but are a global challenge for health systems undergoing rapid digitalization. The lessons for African health systems are clear: cybersecurity investment must accompany digitalization from the outset, not be added after a breach.

In the Asia-Pacific region, Australia's 2022 Medibank data breach—during which the personal health data of 9.7 million current and former customers was stolen—prompted a comprehensive government response, including stricter penalties under the Privacy Act and a national Cyber Security Strategy with specific provisions for the health sector (Australian Government, 2023). Singapore's 2018 SingHealth breach, which compromised 1.5 million patient records, including the Prime Minister's, led to the creation of the Cybersecurity Agency's healthcare-specific security framework—a proactive regulatory response to healthcare cyber threats (CSA Singapore, 2019).

6.3.3 Ethical Dimensions of Health Data Governance

Beyond legal compliance and technical security, health data governance raises fundamental ethical questions about consent, ownership, purpose limitation, and benefit sharing—questions that resonate especially in African contexts shaped by historical experiences of extractive research and data exploitation. Providing meaningful informed consent for health data processing requires that patients understand how their data will be used, who will access it, how long it will be retained, and what risks disclosure might pose—information that is difficult to communicate in any setting and particularly challenging in environments with low digital literacy, linguistic diversity, and power imbalances between patients and providers (Tindana et al., 2015).

The question of data sovereignty—who controls, governs, and benefits from African health data—has grown more prominent as international tech companies, research organizations, and development agencies increasingly collect, process, and store African health data on servers outside the continent. The African Union's Data Policy Framework (2022) states that African data is a strategic resource that should be governed in accordance with African values and priorities, benefiting African populations rather than primarily serving foreign commercial or research interests. This principle challenges prevailing practices in which African health data flows to foreign cloud platforms, is analyzed by foreign algorithms, and generates intellectual property and commercial value captured primarily outside the continent (African Union, 2022).

Comparative Data Governance Frameworks

The European Union's General Data Protection Regulation (GDPR) has set the global benchmark for data protection, and its principles of lawful processing, purpose limitation, data minimization, and individual rights have influenced legislation worldwide—including several African data protection laws explicitly modeled after the GDPR. Brazil's Lei Geral de Proteção de Dados (LGPD) provides a Latin American model with specific provisions governing the processing of health data. India's Digital Personal Data Protection Act (2023) addresses the challenge of governing data at a massive scale while accommodating both individual rights and public health imperatives.

In the Caribbean, CARICOM's Harmonized Data Protection Legislation framework offers a model for regional harmonization among small states—a concept potentially applicable to African Regional Economic Communities seeking to establish interoperable data governance across member states (European Commission, 2016; Government of India, 2023; CARICOM, 2022).

6.4 Regulatory and Legal Frameworks

Regulatory and legal frameworks are the operational expression of Layer 6 (Governance, Policy, and Standards) in the technology stack. As Chapter 4 demonstrates, governance is not an abstract consideration but the framework that determines whether technologies deployed at other layers can operate legally, safely, and sustainably. The regulatory gaps examined in this section—in telemedicine, AI governance, and regional harmonization—directly constrain the scalability of the application-layer technologies discussed in Chapter 3.

The regulatory and legal environment for digital health in Africa remains a major barrier to sustainable digital health transformation. Digital health innovations—from telemedicine platforms to AI-powered diagnostic algorithms to blockchain-based health records—operate at the intersection of multiple regulatory domains, including healthcare regulation, telecommunications law, data protection legislation, consumer protection, professional licensing, and emerging technology governance. The absence, inadequacy, or fragmentation of regulatory frameworks across these domains creates legal uncertainty that discourages investment, limits scalability, exposes patients to unregulated services, and constrains the cross-border collaboration essential to continental digital health integration.

6.4.1 Telemedicine Regulatory Gaps

Telemedicine regulation exemplifies the regulatory deficit. Despite the COVID-19 pandemic's dramatic acceleration of telemedicine adoption across Africa, fewer than 15 African countries had developed comprehensive telemedicine-specific regulations by 2024. This lack of regulation creates uncertainty about key questions, including: under what conditions can a clinician offer remote care? What licensing requirements apply to telemedicine providers? Is a clinician licensed in Kenya legally permitted to provide telemedicine consultations to patients in Tanzania? What liability framework governs adverse outcomes from telemedicine encounters? How should telemedicine services be reimbursed by insurance schemes? (WHO AFRO, 2023).

The lack of clear answers to these questions has not prevented telemedicine from expanding—the COVID-19 pandemic demonstrated that when the alternative is no care at all, regulatory ambiguity becomes a secondary concern. However, as telemedicine shifts from an emergency response to a standard method of service delivery, clear regulations are crucial to ensure quality, patient safety, provider accountability, and insurance coverage. South Africa's Health Professions Council guidelines on telehealth, Kenya's draft telemedicine regulations, and Nigeria's National Telemedicine Policy represent progress, but harmonized regional frameworks—enabling cross-border telemedicine within Regional Economic Communities—remain missing.

6.4.2 AI and Algorithm Governance

The governance of artificial intelligence in healthcare poses a particularly acute regulatory challenge because AI-powered clinical tools operate in ways that defy traditional regulatory frameworks. Standard medical device regulation assumes that a product's behavior remains fixed once certified—it performs consistently over time. However, machine learning algorithms may continuously evolve as they are exposed to new data, potentially altering their diagnostic accuracy, bias profiles, and clinical recommendations after initial deployment. No African country has yet established comprehensive regulatory frameworks specifically for AI-based medical devices, resulting in a governance gap in which AI diagnostic tools are deployed without formal evaluation of their safety, efficacy, or suitability for African patient populations (WHO, 2021).

Algorithmic bias is particularly salient in Africa. AI diagnostic algorithms trained predominantly on data from European, North American, or East

Asian populations may perform poorly when applied to African patients, whose disease presentations, genetic profiles, skin pigmentation, and clinical contexts differ from those in the training data. Dermatology AI tools, for example, have shown significantly lower diagnostic accuracy for darker skin tones when trained primarily on images of lighter-skinned patients. Regulatory frameworks for health AI in Africa must therefore address not only safety and efficacy in general but also representational adequacy—whether an algorithm has been validated on data that reflect the diversity of African populations it will serve (Adamson & Smith, 2018).

International Regulatory Approaches to Health AI

The European Union's AI Act (2024), which classifies medical AI systems as "high-risk" and mandates conformity assessments, transparency obligations, and human oversight, offers the most comprehensive regulatory framework globally. The United States Food and Drug Administration's predetermined change control plan for AI/ML-based software as a medical device offers a model for regulating continuously learning algorithms. Singapore's AI Governance Framework for Healthcare, developed in collaboration with the WHO, provides practical guidance tailored to Asian healthcare contexts. The Brazilian Health Regulatory Agency (ANVISA) has issued specific guidance on software as a medical device, including AI-based diagnostic tools (European Commission, 2024; FDA, 2023; Singapore IMDA, 2020). Developing continental guidelines for health AI regulation that draw on international precedents while addressing Africa-specific concerns about algorithmic representativeness and data sovereignty is essential.

Overall, comparisons of regional regulatory frameworks across four domains—data protection, cybersecurity, telemedicine regulation, and AI governance—highlight clear regional disparities. The European Union leads consistently across all categories, with near-universal coverage in data protection (around 100%) and very high adoption in cybersecurity, telemedicine, and AI governance. Asia follows with a moderately strong performance, particularly in data protection and cybersecurity, though with noticeable gaps in telemedicine and AI governance. Latin America shows a similar but slightly lower trend, with relatively solid adoption in data protection but weaker coverage in more advanced or emerging regulatory areas such as AI governance.

Figure 6.3. Digital Health Regulatory Framework Maturity: Africa vs. Global Regions

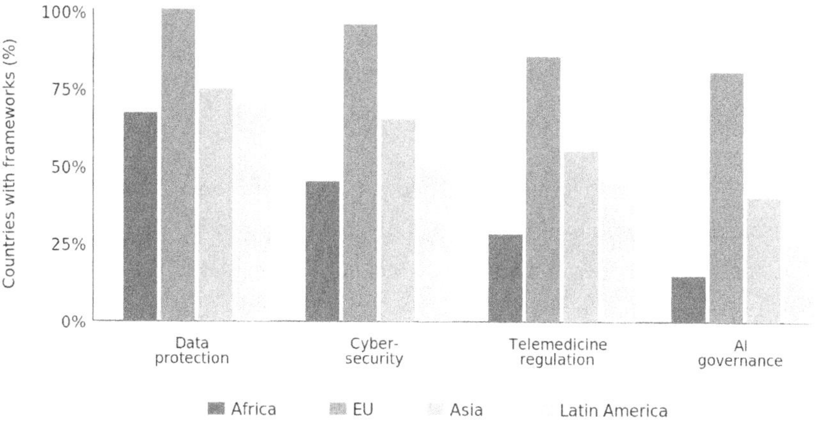

Source: Author's Elaboration

Africa, by contrast, lags significantly across all four domains, with the gap widening as the regulatory complexity increases. While about two-thirds of African countries have data protection frameworks, this drops sharply for cybersecurity, telemedicine regulation, and especially AI governance, where only a small minority of countries have established frameworks. The figure therefore illustrates a gradient of regulatory maturity: foundational areas like data protection are more widely adopted, while newer and more complex domains—particularly AI governance—remain underdeveloped. This pattern underscores the need for accelerated policy development, institutional capacity building, and regional harmonization efforts to support Africa's digital transformation and ensure safe, scalable deployment of emerging technologies in sectors such as health.

6.4.3 Regional Regulatory Harmonization

The fragmentation of regulatory frameworks across African countries creates a patchwork of regulations that imposes heavy compliance burdens on digital health innovators, limits economies of scale, and hinders cross-border health data exchange and telemedicine, both essential to continental health security. A digital health startup developing an AI diagnostic tool must navigate potentially 54 regulatory pathways to achieve continental coverage—a challenge that favors large multinational corporations with regulatory affairs capacity over African startups and social enterprises.

Regional regulatory harmonization, modeled on the African Medicines Agency's approach to pharmaceutical regulation and inspired by the EU's single digital market, provides a pathway to consistent regulation without requiring full continental uniformity. The East African Community, ECOWAS, and SADC could establish mutual recognition frameworks for digital health products, harmonized telemedicine standards, and interoperable data protection rules, enabling digital health innovations to expand regionally while preserving national sovereignty over health policy. The African Continental Free Trade Area protocol on digital trade will also provide a framework for aligning digital health regulations across the continent (African Union, 2023).

6.5 Interoperability Challenges

Interoperability—the ability of different information systems, devices, and applications to access, exchange, integrate, and cooperatively use data in a coordinated way—remains one of the most technically complex and organizationally challenging issues in digital health. In Africa, where digital health systems have often been built in an ad hoc, project-driven manner with limited coordination, the resulting environment is marked by fragmented, siloed systems that cannot communicate with one another. A patient's health records may be stored in separate, disconnected systems across different health facilities, each using different data formats, coding systems, and patient identifiers. This fragmentation undermines care continuity, wastes resources through duplicated tests and procedures, and restricts population-level data analytics essential for evidence-based health policy (Lehne et al., 2019).

6.5.1 Dimensions of Interoperability

Interoperability operates at multiple levels, each with distinct challenges. Technical interoperability—the ability of systems to exchange data using standardized communication protocols—is the most foundational layer and requires agreement on data transport mechanisms, messaging formats, and security protocols. Africa's adoption of HL7 Fast Healthcare Interoperability Resources (FHIR) as a health data exchange standard is progressing, with Kenya, South Africa, and Rwanda among the early implementers. However, most African health information systems still rely on proprietary data formats or earlier-generation standards.

Semantic interoperability—the ability of exchanged data to be understood and meaningfully interpreted by receiving systems—requires adopting common terminologies, coding systems, and data models. The use of the International Classification of Diseases (ICD-10) for disease classification, Systematized Nomenclature of Medicine—Clinical Terms (SNOMED CT) for clinical terminology, and Logical Observation Identifiers, Names and Codes (LOINC) for laboratory data remains limited across Africa, as many systems rely on locally developed coding schemes that cannot be mapped to international standards. Without semantic interoperability, even successful data exchange yields information that receiving systems cannot interpret accurately.

Organizational interoperability—the alignment of governance structures, policies, and workflows to support data exchange across institutional and jurisdictional boundaries—is arguably the most challenging dimension. Technical and semantic interoperability can be addressed by adopting standards; organizational interoperability requires changes to institutional culture, governance arrangements, legal frameworks, and incentive structures. Data-sharing agreements among health facilities, clear governance of health information exchanges, and policies that define who may access which data and under what conditions are prerequisites for functional interoperability, which remains largely undeveloped across the continent (WHO, 2020).

Table 6.2. Key Health Data Standards and their Adoption Status in Africa

Standard	Purpose	Global Status	African Adoption	Key Challenges
HL7 FHIR	Health data exchange protocol	Widely adopted	Early adoption (Kenya, SA, Rwanda)	Technical capacity, implementation cost
ICD-10/11	Disease and condition classification	Near-universal	Variable; ICD-10 moderate, ICD-11 minimal	Training, local adaptation
SNOMED CT	Clinical terminology	Growing adoption	Very limited; SA exploring	Licensing cost, complexity
LOINC	Laboratory observation codes	Established	Minimal adoption	Lab system fragmentation
OpenHIE	Health information exchange architecture	Growing	Rwanda, South Africa implementations	Governance, sustainability
DICOM	Medical imaging data exchange	Universal in imaging	Limited to major hospitals	Equipment cost, connectivity

Source: Adoption Status Based on Published Implementation Reports, WHO Digital Health Atlas data, and expert assessments (2023–2024).

Interoperability Models from Other Regions

The European Union's eHealth Digital Service Infrastructure (eHDSI) enables cross-border exchange of patient summaries and electronic prescriptions among 25+ member states and is built on agreed standards, including HL7 FHIR and Integrating the Healthcare Enterprise (IHE) profiles—demonstrating that interoperability is achievable even across sovereign nations with diverse health systems. IHE profiles provide standardized implementation frameworks that define how health information systems should communicate and exchange data to achieve interoperability in real-world healthcare settings. Rather than creating new standards, IHE profiles operationalize existing ones—such as HL7, DICOM, and ISO standards—by specifying precise workflows, data formats, and transaction sequences that ensure systems such as electronic health records, laboratory systems, imaging platforms, and health information exchanges can work together seamlessly.

India's Ayushman Bharat Digital Mission establishes a national Health Information Exchange using the ABDM architecture, featuring standardized APIs, unique health IDs, and a federated data model that connects public and private providers. In the Caribbean, PAHO's Information Systems for Health (IS4H) initiative has advanced interoperability across small island developing states by promoting shared standards and regional health information exchange protocols. These examples demonstrate that interoperability requires sustained institutional commitment and governance—not merely technical solutions (European Commission, 2023; Government of India, 2022; PAHO, 2023).

6.6 Sustainability and Scalability Concerns

Sustainability and scalability are cross-cutting concerns that affect every layer of the technology stack. Infrastructure (Layer 1) requires ongoing electricity and connectivity costs. Identity systems (Layer 2) require continuous maintenance and enrollment. Interoperability standards (Layer 3) require institutional commitment and technical capacity. Analytics platforms (Layer 4) require skilled personnel and computational resources. Applications (Layer 5) incur licensing, hosting, and user support costs. Governance frameworks (Layer 6) require institutional capacity for enforcement and evolution. A digital health system is only as sustainable as its least-funded layer.

The history of digital health in Africa is marked by pilot projects that showed promising results on a small scale but failed to continue after initial funding or to expand beyond their original sites. A systematic review by Tomlinson et al. (2013) described the "pilotitis" phenomenon—the proliferation of small-scale, donor-funded digital health pilots that rarely progress to sustainable, large-scale implementation.

Figure 6.4 Top Sustainability and Scalability Challenges for Digital Health in Africa

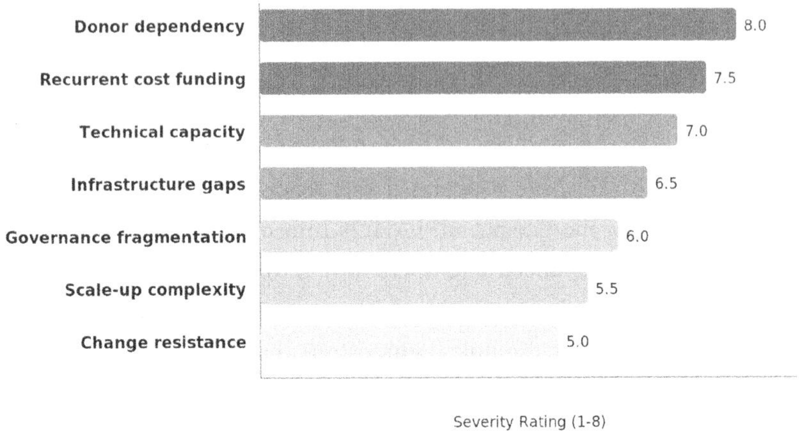

Source: Severity Ratings of Sustainability and Scalability Challenges as Reported by Digital Health Implementers across Africa.

The pilotitis pattern persists: one estimate suggests that fewer than 5% of digital health pilot projects in sub-Saharan Africa have achieved national-scale deployment and sustained operations for more than 5 years (WHO, 2019). The challenge of sustainability and scalability is not a secondary concern to be addressed after successful piloting; it is a fundamental design element that must inform digital health planning from the earliest stages.

6.6.1 The Donor Dependency Trap

The most common sustainability challenge is reliance on external donor funding. An estimated 70–80% of digital health initiatives in low-income African countries depend primarily on international development partners, creating a structural vulnerability: when donor priorities shift, project timelines expire, or global health funding contracts end, digital health systems embedded in service delivery face sudden funding gaps. Transitioning from donor-funded projects to government-supported programs requires deliberate planning for domestic resource mobilization, integration into national health budgets, and the development of revenue models that reduce donor dependency (Labrique et al., 2018).

Latin America provides valuable sustainability models. Argentina's national health information system (SISA) has been sustained through dedicated budget allocations within the Ministry of Health since its inception, avoiding the donor dependence that many African digital health programs face (PAHO, 2023). Chile's national EHR platform is financed through a mix of health ministry budgets and efficiency savings from reduced duplication of diagnostic tests—a model that demonstrates how digital health investments can generate measurable returns that justify continued public funding (MinSal Chile, 2023). Costa Rica's Caja Costarricense de Seguro Social (CCSS) has integrated its digital health systems into the country's social security financing structure, ensuring that digital health operational costs are treated as routine health system expenses rather than project-specific costs (CCSS, 2023).

The financial sustainability challenge is compounded by the total cost of ownership (TCO) of digital health systems, which is often underestimated during planning. Initial technology acquisition costs typically account for only 20–30% of a digital health system's total lifetime cost; the majority of expenditure occurs in ongoing operations, maintenance, software updates, user support, connectivity costs, hardware replacement, and continuous staff training due to turnover. African health budgets rarely include line items for digital health operations and maintenance, so even systems initially funded through capital grants often face unfunded recurrent costs (Khoja et al., 2013).

6.6.2 Scalability Barriers

Scalability—the ability to expand a digital health intervention from its initial implementation site to broader geographic or population coverage without proportional increases in cost or loss of effectiveness—is constrained by multiple factors in African contexts. Infrastructure differences mean that solutions designed for well-connected urban facilities might not work in rural areas with intermittent electricity and connectivity. Human capacity limitations mean that scaling requires training new users while supporting existing ones. Political and institutional fragmentation mean that scaling across administrative boundaries requires navigating different governance structures, procurement systems, and institutional cultures.

Successful scaling typically requires deliberate architectural choices: modular designs that enable incremental deployment; cloud-based or edge-computing architectures that accommodate variable infrastructure; open-source platforms that avoid vendor lock-in; and interoperable systems that integrate with existing health information infrastructure rather than creating parallel systems. The DHIS2 platform's successful scaling across 40+ African countries offers instructive lessons: its open-source model, web-based architecture, configurability to local reporting requirements, and strong community of practice have enabled continental adoption in a domain where most proprietary alternatives failed to achieve national scale (Braa & Sahay, 2017).

Lessons in Sustainability from Global Experiences

Thailand's universal health coverage system demonstrates that digital health sustainability is achievable when digital tools are embedded within—rather than bolted onto—health financing and service delivery systems. Brazil's e-SUS primary care information system, sustained entirely by the Ministry of Health budget after initial World Bank support, illustrates the transition from a donor-funded project to a government-owned program. In the Caribbean, Jamaica's electronic health record system has been maintained through a dedicated government health IT budget line, ensuring recurrent funding for operations and maintenance. Estonia's X-Road health information exchange, often cited as a global exemplar, has been sustained for over two decades through a national digital infrastructure strategy that treats health IT as core government infrastructure rather than a project—a mindset shift essential to African sustainability (Thai Ministry of Public Health, 2022; Estonian Ministry of Social Affairs, 2023; World Bank, 2022).

6.7 Cultural Acceptance and Trust

Cultural acceptance and trust primarily operate at the interface between the Applications and Services Layer (Layer 5) and the communities those applications are designed to serve. Even when infrastructure (Layer 1), identity (Layer 2), and interoperability (Layer 3) function well, applications that ignore cultural context will not be adopted. Trust is also shaped by the Governance Layer (Layer 6)—communities that view data governance as transparent and protective are more likely to engage with digital health tools than those that fear surveillance or data exploitation.

Technology adoption in healthcare is fundamentally mediated by cultural factors—the values, beliefs, social norms, and lived experiences that shape how individuals and communities perceive, evaluate, and decide whether to engage with digital health tools. In Africa, where healthcare-seeking behavior is shaped by diverse cultural traditions, pluralistic medical systems that include traditional and faith-based healing, community decision-making structures, and historical experiences with both colonial and postcolonial health systems, cultural acceptance cannot be assumed; it must be actively cultivated through approaches that respect local contexts, address legitimate concerns, and demonstrate tangible benefits (Olu et al., 2019).

6.7.1 Trust Deficits and Their Origins

Trust—or its absence—is the single most consequential determinant of digital health acceptance at the community level. Multiple sources of distrust complicate digital health adoption in African settings. Historical experiences of exploitative medical research, exemplified by the Pfizer meningitis trial controversy in Kano, Nigeria, and broader legacies of extractive biomedical research, have created deep reservoirs of skepticism about health data collection and sharing in some communities. Concerns about government surveillance, particularly in countries with histories of authoritarian governance or political repression, generate resistance to health information systems perceived as potential surveillance tools. Misinformation about digital health technologies—such as conspiracy theories about COVID-19 contact tracing applications—has undermined acceptance of digital health interventions (Okello et al., 2015).

Religious and spiritual beliefs shape how communities view health, illness, and the role of technology in healing. In contexts where illness is seen as caused by spiritual factors, purely biomedical digital health solutions may be perceived as irrelevant or even threatening to existing beliefs. Rather than dismissing these perspectives, culturally sensitive digital health approaches aim for complementarity—recognizing the role of faith and spiritual practices in health while providing digital tools that support evidence-based care within culturally acceptable frameworks.

Figure 6.5 Dimension of Cultural Trust and Acceptance in Digital Health

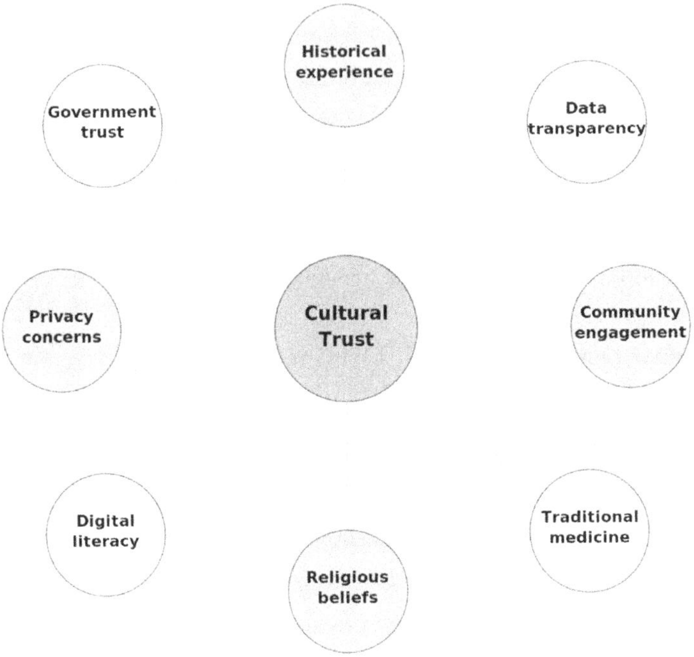

Source: Author's Elaboration

6.7.2 The Role of Traditional Medicine

According to WHO (2019), an estimated 80% of Africans use traditional medicine as their first point of contact for healthcare. The relationship between digital health and traditional medicine practice is complex yet significant. Digital health strategies that overlook traditional medicine practitioners risk excluding the healthcare providers most trusted by large segments of the population. Conversely, approaches that involve traditional healers as partners in digital health—for example, through community health information systems that include traditional practitioners in referral networks or through pharmacovigilance systems that document the use of traditional medicine alongside biomedical treatments—can improve both acceptance and clinical safety.

South Africa's Traditional Health Practitioners Act (2007) establishes a regulatory framework for traditional medicine that could be expanded to include digital health engagement. Ghana's Center for Plant Medicine Research has explored digital platforms to document and standardize herbal medicine formulations, thereby bridging traditional knowledge and digital health infrastructure. However, these efforts remain isolated, and a systematic approach to integrating traditional medicine practitioners into digital health ecosystems would enhance cultural acceptance and make the health system more comprehensive.

6.7.3 Building Trust Through Design and Engagement

Building cultural trust in digital health requires more than communication campaigns or awareness-raising activities; it demands fundamental shifts in how digital health interventions are designed, deployed, and governed. Community-centered design approaches that engage intended users and community leaders in defining problems, designing solutions, and conducting iterative testing create interventions that reflect local values, address locally prioritized health concerns, and incorporate culturally appropriate interaction patterns. Community health workers—who typically share cultural backgrounds with the populations they serve—act as critical bridges between digital health systems and community trust, translating technological capabilities into locally meaningful health benefits (Mehl & Labrique, 2014).

Transparency in data practices is crucial for building trust. Communities that clearly understand what health data is collected, how it is stored, who can access it, and what protections are in place are far more likely to engage with digital health tools than those who view data practices as opaque or exploitative. Rwanda's community-based health insurance scheme (Mutuelles de Santé) demonstrated that transparent governance structures and community involvement in decision-making promote high levels of trust and enrollment—principles that can be applied to digital health governance.

6.8 Gender Dimensions in Digital Health Access

Gender—the socially constructed roles, behaviors, activities, and attributes that a given society considers appropriate for women, men, and other gender identities—profoundly shapes access to, use of, and benefits from digital health technologies. In Africa, gender-based disparities in digital access intersect with pre-existing gender inequalities in healthcare access, economic resources, education, and decision-making power, creating compounded disadvantages that digital health interventions can either ameliorate or exacerbate. Without gender-intentional design and implementation, digital health risks can reproduce and magnify offline gender inequalities in digital forms (Tyers, 2020).

Figure 6.6 Gender Gap in Digital Health Access in Sub-Saharan Africa

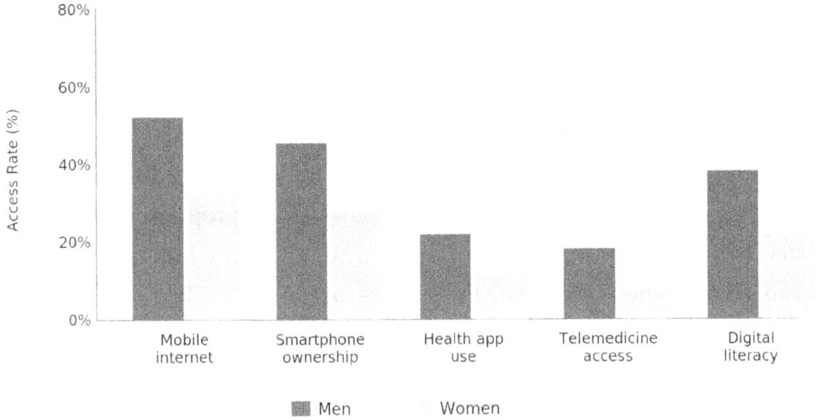

Source: GSMA (2024), WHO (2023)

6.8.1 The Gender Digital Divide

The gender digital divide in Africa remains significant and persistent. According to the GSMA's Connected Women report (2023), women in sub-

Saharan Africa are 37% less likely than men to use mobile Internet. This gap stems from intersecting barriers: lower rates of formal education and digital literacy among women, lower household incomes and reduced ability to afford devices and data, social norms in some communities that restrict women's access to and use of mobile phones, and gender-based violence and harassment in online spaces that discourage women's digital engagement. The mobile phone gender gap directly contributes to a gap in access to health information and services: women without mobile Internet cannot use telemedicine services, health information apps, or digital appointment systems (GSMA, 2023).

The health implications of the gender digital divide are especially severe because women shoulder a disproportionate share of healthcare needs—including maternal health services, reproductive health information, and child healthcare decision-making—while also facing greater barriers to accessing the digital tools designed to address them. Digital maternal health programs such as MomConnect in South Africa and mTrac in Uganda have shown that women actively engage with digital health tools when access barriers are addressed, content is relevant and culturally appropriate, and services deliver tangible value. However, programs that rely on smartphone ownership or mobile Internet access, without addressing the gender access gap, inevitably reach men more effectively than women.

6.8.2 Gender-Based Barriers to Digital Health Engagement

Beyond access to devices and connectivity, gender-based barriers to digital health engagement operate at multiple levels. At the household level, women in some communities require permission from male family members to own or use mobile phones, creating gatekeeping dynamics that limit women's autonomous access to health information and services. At the community level, social norms may stigmatize women who use technology in ways perceived as crossing gender roles, especially when that use involves accessing reproductive or sexual health information. At the institutional level, digital health systems designed without gender analysis may inadvertently exclude women through interface designs, content choices, or service delivery modalities that assume male patterns of technology use (Jennings & Gagliardi, 2013).

Safety and privacy concerns are especially important gender dimensions of digital health. Women who use digital platforms for reproductive health information, family planning, or support for gender-based violence face risks if controlling partners monitor their online activity. Digital health services that cover sensitive women's health topics must incorporate privacy-by-design features, such as discreet application interfaces, automatic history clearing, emergency exit options, and PIN-protected access, to ensure that digital health engagement does not increase women's vulnerability to surveillance or violence.

6.8.3 Gender-Responsive Digital Health Strategies

Advancing gender equity in digital health requires deliberate, multi-layered strategies. At the design level, gender-responsive digital health tools must be developed with women's input through participatory design processes, run on low-cost devices with minimal bandwidth, support voice- and visually based interfaces accessible to women with limited literacy, and address health topics prioritized by women. At the implementation level, gender-responsive deployment involves training female community health workers as digital health champions, placing digital health access points in spaces where women feel safe and comfortable, and scheduling digital health services at times that align with women's caregiving and livelihood responsibilities.

At the policy level, gender-responsive digital health governance should integrate gender analysis into national digital health strategies, establish gender-disaggregated monitoring indicators for digital health programs, and allocate dedicated resources to address gender-based barriers to digital health access. Kenya's Digital Health Act (2023) requires gender analysis in digital health program design, serving as a legislative model that other African countries could adapt. The African Union's Strategy for Gender Equality and Women's Empowerment (2018–2028) provides a continental framework for gender-responsive digital health policies (African Union, 2018).

Gender-Responsive Digital Health: International Examples

India's Accredited Social Health Activist (ASHA) program has trained nearly one million women community health workers to use digital tools for maternal and child health tracking, demonstrating that investing in women's digital capacity yields multiplier effects for community health outcomes. In Latin America, Mexico's digital health strategy includes a gender equity component that funds women's digital literacy programs linked to health service access. Bangladesh's Aponjon mobile health platform, delivered via feature phones and Bengali voice messages, reaches women with low literacy through a delivery modality designed to overcome gendered barriers to accessing text-based health information. In the Caribbean, the CARICOM Gender Equality Strategy explicitly addresses digital health access as a gender equity priority. These examples reinforce the principle that gender-responsive digital health is not an add-on but a core design requirement (WHO, 2023; CARICOM, 2021; Government of Bangladesh, 2022).

6.9 Conclusion

The analysis in this chapter underscores a central insight: digital health transformation in Africa is not fundamentally a technological challenge but a systemic one, shaped by interdependent social, institutional, and governance factors. The seven critical issues—digital equity, data governance, regulatory frameworks, interoperability, sustainability, cultural acceptance, and gender inclusion—are not peripheral constraints but core determinants of success. When viewed through the lens of the digital health technology stack, these issues are deeply embedded across all layers, from infrastructure to applications and governance. Addressing them in isolation is insufficient; progress requires coordinated, system-wide interventions that align technology deployment with broader health system strengthening and socioeconomic realities.

A recurring theme throughout the chapter is the risk of uneven progress—digital health innovations advance rapidly for connected, urban, and affluent populations while leaving rural, low-income, and marginalized groups even further behind. Evidence on urban–rural divides, affordability constraints, linguistic exclusion, disability access, and gender disparities shows that without intentional design, digital health can inadvertently reproduce and amplify existing inequities. Equity, therefore, must be treated not as a downstream outcome but as a foundational design principle, embedded in infrastructure investment, platform architecture, service delivery models, and policy frameworks from the outset.

Equally critical is governance—in its legal, regulatory, ethical, and institutional dimensions—as the enabling environment for digital health systems. Weak or fragmented data protection regimes, underdeveloped cybersecurity capacity, and regulatory gaps in areas such as telemedicine and artificial intelligence pose risks that can undermine trust, deter investment, and harm patients. At the same time, the lack of interoperability standards and sustainable financing models limits the scalability of otherwise promising innovations. The persistence of "pilotitis" and donor dependency underscores the need to transition from project-based approaches to nationally owned, institutionally embedded digital health systems that are financed, regulated, and maintained as core public infrastructure.

Finally, the chapter emphasizes that trust—rooted in cultural alignment, community engagement, and inclusive governance—is the ultimate currency for digital health adoption. Technologies that fail to resonate with local beliefs, exclude traditional health systems, or neglect gendered realities will struggle to achieve meaningful uptake, regardless of their technical sophistication. Conversely, approaches grounded in co-design, transparency, and community ownership show that digital health can be both innovative and inclusive. The path forward for Africa lies not in wholesale replication of external models but in adapting global lessons to African contexts—building digital health ecosystems that are equitable, trusted, interoperable, and sustainable, thereby strengthening health systems in ways that leave no one behind.

References

Australian Government. (2023). National Cyber Security Strategy 2023–2030. Commonwealth of Australia.

Australian Government. (2024). Measures for the First Nations Digital Inclusion Roadmap and Budget 2024–25. Department of Infrastructure, Transport, Regional Development, Communications, Sport and the Arts.

CCSS. (2023). Digitalización de servicios de salud: Informe anual. Caja Costarricense de Seguro Social.

Chelberg, G. R., Butten, K., Mahoney, R., & eHealth Research Collaboration. (2024). Towards a best practice framework for eHealth with Aboriginal and Torres Strait Islander peoples. Medical Journal of Australia, 221(6), 312–318.

CSA Singapore. (2019). Healthcare Cybersecurity Essentials. Cyber Security Agency of Singapore.

MinSal Chile. (2023). Estrategia Nacional de Salud Digital: Informe de implementación. Ministerio de Salud de Chile.

MinSalud Bolivia. (2023). Safci: Salud Familiar Comunitaria Intercultural—Marco de digitalización. Ministerio de Salud y Deportes.

MINSA Peru. (2024). Sistema Nacional de Información en Salud: Integración de medicina tradicional. Ministerio de Salud del Perú.

Moecke, D. P., Holyk, T., Beckett, M., et al. (2024). Scoping review of telehealth use by Indigenous populations from Australia, Canada, New Zealand, and the United States. Journal of Telemedicine and Telecare, 30(9), 1398–1416. https://doi.org/10.1177/1357633X231158835

OAS. (2022). Cybersecurity incident analysis: Costa Rica healthcare system attack. Organization of American States.

PAHO. (2022). Ciberseguridad en salud: Lecciones del ataque al Ministerio de Salud de Brasil. Organización Panamericana de la Salud.

Thai Ministry of Public Health. (2022). Digital health and traditional medicine integration: National framework. Ministry of Public Health, Kingdom of Thailand.

A4AI. (2023). Affordability report 2023: The Crisis of Internet Affordability in Africa. Alliance for Affordable Internet.

Adamson, A. S., & Smith, A. (2018). Machine learning and health care disparities in dermatology. JAMA Dermatology, 154(11), 1247–1248. https://doi.org/10.1001/jamadermatol.2018.2348

African Union. (2014). African Union Convention on Cyber Security and Personal Data Protection (Malabo Convention). African Union Commission.

African Union. (2018). Strategy for gender equality and women's empowerment (2018–2028). African Union Commission.

African Union. (2022). AU Data Policy Framework. African Union Commission.

African Union. (2023). Protocol on digital trade under the African Continental Free Trade Area: Negotiating framework. African Union Commission.

Braa, J., & Sahay, S. (2017). The DHIS2 open source software platform: Evolution over time and space. In Global health informatics (pp. 451–474). MIT Press.

CARICOM. (2021). CARICOM Gender Equality Strategy. Caribbean Community Secretariat.

CARICOM. (2022). Model harmonized data protection legislation for CARICOM member states. Caribbean Community Secretariat.

Estonian Ministry of Social Affairs. (2023). X-Road health information exchange: Two decades of sustainable operation. Republic of Estonia.

European Commission. (2016). Regulation (EU) 2016/679: General Data Protection Regulation. Official Journal of the European Union.

European Commission. (2019). Directive (EU) 2019/882: European Accessibility Act. Official Journal of the European Union.

European Commission. (2023). eHealth Digital Service Infrastructure: Cross-border health data exchange progress report. European Commission.

European Commission. (2024). Regulation (EU) 2024/1689 laying down harmonized rules on artificial intelligence (AI Act). Official Journal of the European Union.

FDA. (2023). Predetermined change control plans for machine learning-enabled medical devices: Guidance for industry. U.S. Food and Drug Administration.

Government of Bangladesh. (2022). Aponjon (MAMA Bangladesh) mobile health platform: National evaluation report. Ministry of Health and Family Welfare.

Government of India. (2021). Ayushman Bharat Digital Mission: Architecture and implementation framework. Ministry of Health and Family Welfare.

Government of India. (2022). National Digital Health Mission: Health information exchange specifications. Ministry of Health and Family Welfare.

Government of India. (2023). Digital Personal Data Protection Act, 2023. Ministry of Electronics and Information Technology.

GSMA. (2023). Connected Women: The mobile gender gap report 2023. GSM Association.

IBM Security. (2023). Cost of a data breach report 2023. IBM Corporation.

Interpol. (2021). African cyberthreat assessment report 2021. INTERPOL.

ITU. (2024). Measuring digital development: Facts and figures 2024. International Telecommunication Union.

Jennings, L., & Gagliardi, L. (2013). Influence of mHealth interventions on gender relations in developing countries: A systematic review. International Journal for Equity in Health, 12, Article 85. https://doi.org/10.1186/1475-9276-12-85

Khoja, S., Durrani, H., Scott, R. E., Sajwani, A., & Piryani, U. (2013). Conceptual framework for the development of a comprehensive e-health evaluation tool. Telemedicine and e-Health, 19(1), 48–53. https://doi.org/10.1089/tmj.2012.0073

Labrique, A. B., Vasudevan, L., Kottke, E., Tollefson, D., Breiman, R. F., & Mehl, G. (2018). mHealth innovations as health system strengthening tools: 12 common applications and a visual framework. Global Health: Science and Practice, 6(Supplement 1), S23–S35. https://doi.org/10.9745/GHSP-D-17-00069

LeFevre, A. E., Mohan, D., Hutchful, D., Jennings, L., Mehl, G., Labrique, A., ... & Moorthy, A. (2017). Mobile Technology for Community Health in Ghana: What happens when technical functionality meets standard operating procedures? Learning from mPedigree's GoldKeys. BMC Medical Informatics and Decision Making, 17, Article 174. https://doi.org/10.1186/s12911-017-0568-x

Lehne, M., Sass, J., Essenwanger, A., Schepers, J., & Thun, S. (2019). Why digital medicine depends on interoperability. NPJ Digital Medicine, 2, Article 79. https://doi.org/10.1038/s41746-019-0158-1

Makulilo, A. B. (2016). African data privacy laws. Springer International Publishing.

Mehl, G., & Labrique, A. (2014). Prioritizing integrated mHealth strategies for universal health coverage. Science, 345(6202), 1284–1287. https://doi.org/10.1126/science.1258926

MinTIC Colombia. (2022). Puntos Vive Digital: Impact evaluation and digital health access assessment. Ministry of Information Technologies and Communications.

Okello, G., Molyneux, S., Mwatasa, B., Muturi, C., & Marsh, V. (2015). Challenges to consent and community engagement in the conduct of a cluster randomised trial among schoolchildren in low-income settings. Trials, 16, Article 548. https://doi.org/10.1186/s13063-015-1064-7

Olu, O., Muneene, D., Bataringaya, J. E., Nahimana, M. R., Ba, H.,";"; Fergus, C., ... & Alemu, W. (2019). How can digital health technologies contribute to the sustainable attainment of universal health coverage in Africa? Frontiers in Public Health, 7, Article 341. https://doi.org/10.3389/fpubh.2019.00341

PAHO. (2023). Information systems for health (IS4H) in the Caribbean: Regional interoperability assessment. Pan American Health Organization.

Robinson, L., Cotten, S. R., Ono, H., Quan-Haase, A., Mesch, G., Chen, W., ... & Stern, M. J. (2015). Digital inequalities and why they matter. Information, Communication & Society, 18(5), 569–582. https://doi.org/10.1080/1369118X.2015.1012532

Singapore IMDA. (2020). Model AI governance framework for healthcare. Infocomm Media Development Authority, Singapore.

Thai Ministry of Public Health. (2022). Digital health sustainability within universal health coverage: Lessons from Thailand. Ministry of Public Health, Kingdom of Thailand.

Tindana, P., de Vries, J., Campbell, M., van Niekerk, M., & Parker, M. (2015). Community engagement strategies for genomic studies in Africa: A review of the literature. BMC Medical Ethics, 16, Article 24. https://doi.org/10.1186/s12910-015-0014-z

Tomlinson, M., Rotheram-Borus, M. J., Swartz, L., & Tsai, A. C. (2013). Scaling up mHealth: Where is the evidence? PLoS Medicine, 10(2), e1001382. https://doi.org/10.1371/journal.pmed.1001382

Tyers, A. (2020). Gender and digital health: From design to impact. Digital Health, 6, 1–12. https://doi.org/10.1177/2055207620918350

Vayena, E., Blasimme, A., & Cohen, I. G. (2018). Machine learning in medicine: Addressing ethical challenges. PLoS Medicine, 15(11), e1002689. https://doi.org/10.1371/journal.pmed.1002689

WHO. (2019). WHO guideline: Recommendations on digital interventions for health system strengthening. WHO Press.

WHO. (2020). Global strategy on digital health 2020–2025. WHO Press.

WHO. (2021). Ethics and governance of artificial intelligence for health: WHO guidance. WHO Press.

WHO. (2022). Global report on health equity for persons with disabilities. WHO Press.

WHO. (2023). Gender and health: Overview and analysis. WHO Press.

WHO AFRO. (2023). Digital health in the WHO African Region: Policy, regulatory, and implementation landscape assessment. WHO Regional Office for Africa.

World Bank. (2022). Digital health in the Caribbean: Sustainability and governance assessment. World Bank Group.

PART 2

Foundations of Digital Health in Africa

Chapter 7 Digital Infrastructure for the Health Sector

7.1. Overview

Digital infrastructure—Internet connectivity, reliable electricity, cloud and data center capacity, and end-user devices—constitutes Layer 1 (Physical Infrastructure and Connectivity) of the digital health technology stack introduced in Chapter 4. As the foundational layer on which every other layer depends, deficiencies in Layer 1 infrastructure cascade upward, undermining interoperability platforms (Layer 3), analytics capabilities (Layer 4), and end-user applications (Layer 5) that the health system relies on. This chapter examines Layer 1 in depth, providing a detailed analysis of Africa's physical infrastructure that complements the architectural overview in Chapter 4.

This chapter examines Africa's digital infrastructure landscape through a health-sector lens, quantifies critical gaps that constrain progress, analyzes the urban–rural divide, and benchmarks Africa against other regions, including the European Union, Asia, and Latin America. It explores investment needs and outlines strategies for leveraging broader infrastructure development to improve health outcomes.

7.2 Internet Connectivity and Broadband Access

As the most fundamental component of Layer 1 of the digital health technology stack, Internet connectivity is the circulatory system of digital health, enabling data transmission between health facilities, supporting telemedicine consultations, powering cloud-based applications, and facilitating real-time disease surveillance reporting. Africa's connectivity landscape has improved dramatically over the past decade—driven by the deployment of submarine cables along both coasts, the rapid expansion of mobile networks, and emerging satellite solutions—yet significant gaps persist, particularly in rural and peri-urban areas (GSMA, 2023; ITU, 2023).

Mobile networks are the primary means of connectivity across the continent, covering approximately 85% of Africa's population. In 2024, 4G Long Term Evolution (LTE) reached roughly 65% of urban populations and only 28% of rural populations. Mobile broadband underpins the vast majority of telemedicine encounters, health data reporting via platforms such as DHIS2, and mobile health (mHealth) applications for community health workers, expectant mothers, and patients managing chronic conditions. However, affordability remains a persistent barrier: in many low-income African countries, one gigabyte of mobile data can consume between 5% and 10% of average monthly household income, far exceeding the 2% threshold recommended by the Broadband Commission for Sustainable Development (Alliance for Affordable Internet, 2023).

Fixed broadband penetration remains extremely low at approximately 12% continent-wide, concentrated almost exclusively in capital cities and major commercial centers, with average download speeds frequently below 5 megabits per second (Mbps). While fixed broadband offers greater bandwidth reliability for hospital-based systems, electronic health record platforms, and picture archiving and communication systems (PACS), its limited geographic footprint renders it impractical as the primary connectivity solution for most African health systems. Satellite Internet, particularly the emerging generation of Low Earth Orbit (LEO) constellations such as Starlink and OneWeb, promises to expand coverage to the most remote and underserved areas, though current costs and the technical expertise required for installation and maintenance limit widespread adoption in health settings (ITU, 2023).

Global and Regional Comparisons

Africa's connectivity challenges become clearer when benchmarked against other developing regions. In the European Union, broadband penetration exceeds 90%, and virtually every health facility is connected to high-speed Internet, enabling the widespread adoption of interoperable electronic health records and telemedicine as standard practice. In Southeast Asia, countries such as Thailand and Vietnam have achieved 70–80% mobile broadband penetration through deliberate government policies that combine universal service obligations with competitive licensing frameworks. India's Digital India program, which subsidized data costs and aggressively expanded 4G infrastructure, drove mobile broadband costs to among the lowest globally, directly enabling the Ayushman Bharat Digital Mission to reach hundreds of millions of citizens (Mehl & Labrique, 2014; WHO, 2021).

Figure 7.1. Internet Connectivity by Technology: Africa vs. Global Average

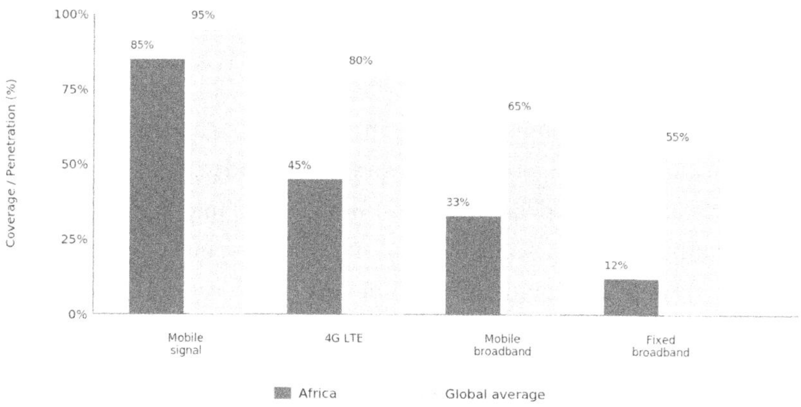

Sources: GSMA (2023), ITU (2023), World Bank (2022)

In Latin America and the Caribbean, Brazil's Programa Conecta SUS has invested in connecting all primary health care units to broadband Internet, demonstrating that national political commitment can rapidly close connectivity gaps for health facilities, even where general population coverage remains uneven. Similarly, Colombia's Vive Digital program prioritized health and education institutions in its national broadband deployment, reducing time-to-connectivity for rural clinics from years to months (OECD, 2020).

Australia's National Broadband Network (NBN) provides a particularly instructive model for large, geographically dispersed countries. The Australian government invested AUD 51 billion (USD 37 billion) in a publicly owned wholesale broadband network designed to reach 100% of the population using a mix of fiber-to-the-premises, fixed wireless, and satellite technologies. By 2025, over 8.6 million premises were connected, and the government committed an additional AUD 2.4 billion (USD 1.7 billion) to extend full-fiber access to an additional 1.5 million premises, including 660,000 in regional and rural communities (Australian Government, 2024). The NBN's cross-subsidization model—where metropolitan revenues subsidize rural deployment at uniform wholesale prices—demonstrates how public ownership can ensure equitable geographic access. Australia's Better Connectivity Plan, which provides over AUD 1.1 billion (USD 800 million) to rural and regional communities, and its Regional Connectivity Program (AUD 368 million, equivalent to USD 263 million across 297 place-based projects), show how targeted complementary programs can address remaining gaps (Australian Department of Infrastructure, 2025).

Canada faces challenges similar to those in Africa in connecting remote and Indigenous communities. The Canadian Radio-television and Telecommunications Commission (CRTC) Broadband Fund, funded by levies on telecommunications providers rather than tax revenues, has improved connectivity in over 290 communities, including health care centers, schools, and community centers. A landmark 2024 investment of CAD 271.9 million (USD 200 million) for fiber to four Inuit communities in Nunavut illustrates the scale of investment required for the most remote populations (CRTC, 2024). Canada's Universal Broadband Fund (CAD 3.225 billion, equivalent to USD 2.35 billion) explicitly targets 50/10 Mbps speeds for all Canadians, with dedicated provisions for Indigenous communities—only 35% of First Nations households on reserves currently have access to these speeds, compared with 99% in urban areas (ISED Canada, 2024). The transferable lesson for Africa is that universal service mechanisms funded by industry levies, combined with dedicated programs anchored in national broadband strategies for all communities, can systematically close connectivity gaps.

Several African countries have made noteworthy progress in expanding broadband access for all. Kenya's National Broadband Strategy has progressively connected county hospitals and major health facilities to fiber-optic networks. Rwanda, leveraging its small geographic size and strong governance structures, has achieved near-universal 4G coverage and connected most district hospitals via a national fiber backbone. Nevertheless, across sub-Saharan Africa, the continental average for health facility Internet connectivity remains about 30%, compared with 55% in Latin America, 48%

in Southeast Asia, and 88% in the European Union (WHO, 2023; GSMA, 2023).

Table 7.1.Benchmarking Africa's Digital Health Infrastructure with Other Regions

Region	Broadband Penetration	Facilities Digitized	Grid Electricity in Facilities	EHR Adoption	Data Center Capacity
Sub-Saharan Africa	38%	22%	52%	15%	2.5%
South Asia	45%	38%	70%	25%	5%
Latin America & Caribbean	62%	55%	82%	42%	8%
Southeast Asia	58%	48%	78%	35%	10%
European Union	92%	88%	99%	82%	28%
East Asia	88%	82%	98%	78%	32%

Sources: WHO (2023); ITU (2023); World Bank (2022); European Commission (2022); OECD (2020)

7.3 The Urban-Rural Digital Divide

Within Layer 1 of the technology stack, the most consequential infrastructure challenge for digital health in Africa is not aggregate connectivity or electrification rates, but the stark divide between urban and rural areas. Across the continent, urban areas achieve approximately 78% Internet coverage, 85% electricity access, and 65% of health facilities connected to some form of Internet service. Rural areas, where the majority of Africa's population resides and where health needs are often most acute, lag substantially: 28% Internet coverage, 35% electricity access, and only 18% of health facilities connected in 2023. This average gap of 50 percentage points across key infrastructure indicators directly constrains rural digital health implementation and perpetuates health outcome disparities (World Bank, 2022; GSMA, 2023).

The urban-rural divide in digital health infrastructure mirrors and reinforces existing health inequities. Rural facilities, which typically serve larger geographic catchment areas with higher disease burdens and fewer health workers, are precisely the facilities that could benefit most from telemedicine, digital decision-support tools, and electronic supply chain management—yet they are the least likely to have the infrastructure to support these interventions. This creates a paradox: the communities most in need of digital health solutions are the least able to access them.

Figure 7.2. The Urban-Rural Digital Divide in Health Infrastructure

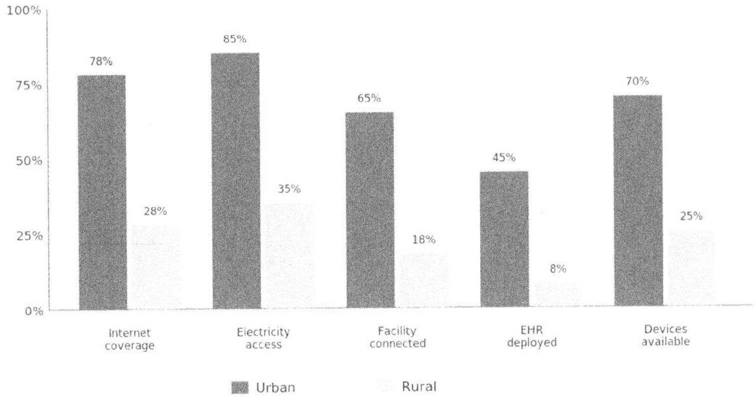

Source: World Bank (2022), WHO (2023), GSMA (2023)

Comparative experience from other regions offers valuable lessons. India's BharatNet project, which aims to connect all 250,000 gram panchayats (village councils) to fiber-optic broadband, has shown that large-scale rural connectivity is both technically and financially feasible with sustained political commitment and phased deployment. In Latin America, Mexico's Red Compartida wholesale shared-network model is designed to incentivize private operators to extend coverage to underserved rural communities by providing access to shared infrastructure at regulated prices. In the European Union, the Recovery and Resilience Facility has allocated billions of euros for rural broadband expansion and explicitly includes healthcare connectivity targets in member states' recovery plans (European Commission, 2021; World Bank, 2022).

Australia's experience with the urban–rural digital divide is especially relevant, despite its much higher income level. The 2024 Regional Telecommunications Review found that many regional and remote communities still lack high-speed Internet access, despite decades of investment. The government is exploring low Earth orbit (LEO) satellite solutions and has established a LEO Satellite Working Group (Australian Government, 2024). The Royal Flying Doctor Service, which provides healthcare across Australia's vast interior, has adopted Starlink satellite connectivity to support telemedicine and edge computing in areas where terrestrial networks are unavailable—a model directly applicable to African flying doctor services and remote clinics (RFDS, 2024).

Strategies for Bridging the Divide

Within Africa, several promising strategies have emerged to narrow the urban–rural digital health infrastructure gap. Universal Service and Access Funds (USAFs), financed by telecommunications operator levies, have been deployed in countries such as Ghana, Uganda, and Nigeria to subsidize extending infrastructure to underserved areas, though challenges with fund governance and disbursement have limited their effectiveness in some contexts. Community network models, in which local organizations own and operate small-scale cellular or Wi-Fi networks, have proven successful in countries such as South Africa, where the Zenzeleni Community Network in the Eastern Cape provides affordable Internet access to rural health facilities and households. Mobile first design strategies, which optimize digital health applications for smartphones and feature phones over low-bandwidth connections, acknowledge that mobile devices are far more ubiquitous than fixed Internet connections in rural Africa (GSMA, 2023; ITU, 2023).

7.4 Electricity and Power Supply Reliability

Reliable electricity—the most critical component of Layer 1 of the technology stack—is essential to digital health systems. Computers, servers, networking equipment, medical devices with digital components, cold-chain refrigerators, and mobile phones used by community health workers all require a reliable power supply. However, Africa's electricity landscape presents formidable challenges for health system digitization: only 52% of health facilities in sub-Saharan Africa have access to grid electricity in 2023, and among those connected, 68% face frequent outages—defined as unplanned power interruptions lasting more than one hour—with some areas experiencing an average of 4.6 hours of daily downtime. Voltage fluctuations, common in many grid-connected areas, can damage sensitive computing equipment and medical devices, necessitating investments in uninterruptible power supply (UPS) systems and voltage stabilizers, thereby increasing the total cost of ownership (WHO, 2023; IEA, 2022).

Figure 7.3 Power Sources in African Health Facilities

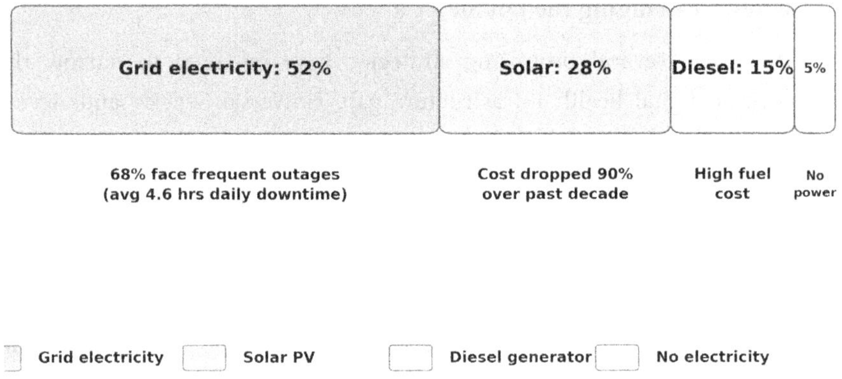

Source: WHO (2023), IEA (2022)

Solar photovoltaic systems, now installed at an estimated 28% of health facilities, are an increasingly viable and reliable alternative, especially for rural and off-grid facilities. The significant drop in solar panel costs—around 90% over the past decade—along with advances in battery storage technology, has made solar-plus-battery systems cost-competitive with diesel generators for many health facility applications, offering benefits such as lower operating costs, less maintenance, and no fuel dependence. Organizations such as the United Nations Foundation's Sustainable Energy for All initiative and Power Africa have supported the deployment of solar energy systems in health facilities across several African countries, demonstrating that solar power can reliably sustain digital health equipment, vaccine cold chains, and facility lighting simultaneously (IEA, 2022; IRENA, 2023).

Diesel generators, which serve roughly 15% of facilities, remain crucial for backup power in areas with unreliable grid connections, but their high fuel costs, maintenance requirements, noise, and environmental impact make them suboptimal as primary power sources. An estimated 5% of African health facilities—mainly small primary care posts in remote locations—have no electricity, making digital health interventions fundamentally impossible without concurrent energy investments.

Lessons from Other Regions

In Latin America, Chile's Programa Energías Renovables para Centros de Salud has installed solar systems at rural health posts across the Atacama and Andes regions, demonstrating that solar energy is effective for health facilities in high-altitude, extreme-temperature environments. Costa Rica, which generates over 99% of its electricity from renewable sources, has achieved near-universal electrification of health facilities through its integrated national grid—an aspiration that African countries with significant hydroelectric and geothermal potential (such as Ethiopia, Kenya, and the Democratic Republic of Congo) could eventually emulate (IEA, 2022).

India's Saubhagya scheme, which aimed to achieve universal household electrification, designated health facilities as priority connection sites and paired grid extension with off-grid solar solutions for the most remote locations. In Southeast Asia, Myanmar's National Electrification Plan included health facilities in its village-level electrification prioritization criteria, ensuring that clinic power preceded or accompanied household connections. In Latin America, Peru's National Photovoltaic Household Electrification Program has demonstrated that solar energy can reliably power digital health systems in high-altitude and jungle communities where grid extension is neither economically nor technically feasible (IEA, 2022; World Bank, 2022).

7.5 Data Centers and Cloud Infrastructure

Data centers and cloud computing infrastructure—the third component of Layer 1 that directly enables Layers 3 and 4 of the technology stack—form the backbone of scalable digital health systems, providing the storage, processing, and hosting capabilities needed for electronic health records, health information exchanges, disease surveillance dashboards, and analytics platforms. Africa's data center capacity has grown rapidly in recent years, yet it remains modest by global standards: the continent hosts approximately 2.5% of the world's hyperscale data center capacity, concentrated primarily in South Africa, Kenya, Nigeria, and Egypt. The majority of digitally stored African health data is hosted on servers outside the continent—in Europe, North America, or the Middle East—raising concerns about data sovereignty, latency, regulatory compliance, and dependence on international connectivity (Africa Data Centers Association, 2023).

Cloud computing offers compelling advantages for health systems in resource-constrained settings: it reduces the need for large capital investments in on-premises server infrastructure, provides elastic scalability to handle growing data volumes, enables automated software updates and security patching, and supports centralized management of distributed health information systems. Several African countries have begun adopting cloud-based health information platforms. Rwanda's health information exchange runs on cloud infrastructure, and Kenya's DHIS2 national instance uses cloud hosting for reliability and disaster recovery. However, cloud adoption for health data is complicated by regulatory uncertainty over data residency requirements, limited local cloud infrastructure, concerns about vendor lock-in, and the need for reliable Internet connectivity to access cloud-hosted applications (Kiberu et al., 2014; WHO, 2023).

The European Union's approach to health data infrastructure, embodied in its European Health Data Space initiative, offers a governance model that Africa could adapt. The EHDS sets clear rules for health data storage, sharing, and secondary use while promoting interoperability across member states. Canada's Shared Services Canada provides government-wide cloud infrastructure that hosts health data for federal health programs, while provinces maintain their own health data hosting arrangements—a federated model that mirrors the distributed governance of African health systems across national and subnational levels (Government of Canada, 2024). Brazil's national health data cloud, operated by DATASUS, demonstrates how a centralized yet distributed cloud infrastructure can serve a large, geographically diverse health system while maintaining national data sovereignty (European Commission, 2022; OECD, 2020).

Data Sovereignty Considerations

As African countries digitize health data, the question of where that data is stored and processed has profound implications for privacy, security, and sovereignty. The African Union's Convention on Cyber Security and Personal Data Protection (Malabo Convention) provides a continental framework, but ratification remains incomplete. The African Union Data Policy Framework (2022) adopts a balanced approach to data sovereignty, defining it as the right of African states to govern data generated within their jurisdictions while avoiding overly restrictive measures, such as blanket data localization, that could hinder innovation and regional integration. Instead, it promotes "controlled openness," enabling trusted cross-border data flows through harmonized legal and regulatory frameworks, common data protection standards, and a continental mechanism for data exchange to support the African Digital Single Market.

The Framework also affirms that countries may safeguard national security and the public interest, but such measures should be proportionate and not undermine continental interoperability. Crucially, it extends sovereignty beyond regulation to include economic and technological dimensions, emphasizing the need for African investment in data infrastructure, local ecosystems, and skills to ensure that data value remains within the continent, thereby advancing a model of "smart data sovereignty" that combines national control, regional coordination, and openness.

The implication is that countries must balance the practical advantages of cloud providers with the imperative to maintain control over citizens' health data. Investing in local and regional data center capacity, skills, and local enterprise ecosystems, while developing clear data residency regulations, is a strategic priority for Africa's digital health future.

7.6 Hardware and Device Availability

The availability and distribution of digital devices—the fourth and most visible component of Layer 1 of the technology stack—smartphones, tablets, desktop computers, and digitally enabled medical equipment—directly shape the feasible scope of digital health interventions at each level of the health system. Device availability in Africa varies significantly by facility level, creating distinct digital health opportunity and challenge landscapes across primary, secondary, and tertiary care settings (PATH, 2021; WHO, 2023).

Figure 7.4. Digital Device Availability by Health Facility Level

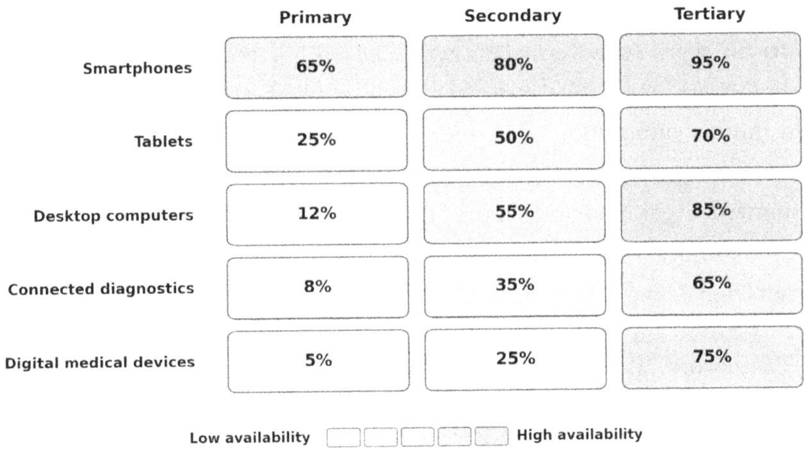

Source: PATH (2021), WHO Service Availability and Readiness Assessment (2022)

The heat map of digital device availability across primary, secondary, and tertiary health care levels shows a concentration of equipment in tertiary hospitals and a relative scarcity at the primary care level. Smartphones are the most widely available digital device across all facility levels: 95% penetration in tertiary hospitals, 80% in secondary facilities, and 65% in primary care settings. This near-ubiquity of smartphones, many of which are personal devices owned by health workers rather than facility assets, has driven the global shift toward mobile-first digital health strategies and underpins the success of community health worker platforms, mHealth applications, and mobile data collection tools. The declining cost of functional Android devices, now available for under $50 in many African markets, further accelerates this trend (GSMA, 2023).

Desktop computers, which remain essential for data-intensive tasks such as electronic health record management, laboratory information systems, and radiology reporting, present a different picture. While tertiary hospitals achieve 85% desktop availability, secondary facilities reach only 55%, and primary care facilities just 12%. This scarcity at the primary care level, where most patient encounters occur, represents a significant bottleneck to deploying health information systems. Tablets, positioned between smartphones and desktops in both capability and cost, offer a promising middle ground: their larger screens facilitate clinical data entry and the use of decision-support tools, while their portability suits the mobile work patterns of community health workers and outreach teams.

Digital medical devices—including connected diagnostic equipment, digital blood pressure monitors, Bluetooth-enabled pulse oximeters, and point-of-care ultrasound devices—are heavily concentrated in tertiary facilities (75% availability) and have minimal presence in primary care (5%). This concentration limits the potential for digital diagnostics and remote monitoring at the community level, where early detection and triage would have the greatest impact on health outcomes. Investment in affordable, rugged, and connected point-of-care devices designed for primary care and community settings is a critical frontier for digital health infrastructure development in Africa (PATH, 2021).

Comparative Insights

Australia's approach to health facility device provisioning integrates device procurement into broader digital health infrastructure programs. The Australian Digital Health Agency includes device specifications and lifecycle management guidance in its My Health Record implementation toolkit, ensuring that health facilities have the hardware needed to participate in the national health information exchange. The government's AUD 1.7 billion (USD 1.2 billion) digital health budget includes dedicated funding for device procurement at Aboriginal and Torres Strait Islander health services, recognizing that digital inclusion requires targeted investment in underserved communities (Australian Digital Health Agency, 2024).

India's Common Service Centers scheme has shown that shared device infrastructure at the village level can enable digital health services without requiring every facility to own dedicated equipment. Thailand's Universal Coverage Scheme includes device provisioning and maintenance as a standard component of health facility operating budgets, ensuring that digital infrastructure is treated as essential equipment alongside clinical supplies. These experiences underscore the importance of device procurement strategies that address the full spectrum of care levels, not merely tertiary hospitals (WHO, 2021; World Bank, 2022).

7.7 Infrastructure Investment Needs and Funding Mechanisms

Achieving a comprehensive digital health infrastructure across Africa requires substantial, sustained investment. Current estimates indicate a total investment need of approximately $6.3 billion USD over five years, distributed across four major categories: connectivity infrastructure ($2.5 billion for fiber-optic deployment, mobile network expansion, and satellite terminal installation at health facilities); power systems ($1.8 billion for solar installations, grid connections, battery storage, and backup power); data centers and cloud infrastructure ($0.8 billion for local data center development, cloud migration, and hosting services); and end-user devices ($1.2 billion for computers, tablets, smartphones, medical devices, and networking equipment). These estimates encompass both initial capital expenditure and the operational expenditure necessary to sustain infrastructure over a five-year horizon (World Bank, 2022; AfDB, 2021).

Funding mechanisms for digital health infrastructure investment can draw on multiple sources. Government capital budgets are the most sustainable long-term funding source, but competition with other development priorities and fiscal constraints limit allocations in many countries. Development partners, including the World Bank, the African Development Bank, the Global Fund, and bilateral donors, have increasingly integrated digital health infrastructure into their health system-strengthening portfolios.

Figure 7.5 Digital Health Infrastructure Investment Needs for 5 years

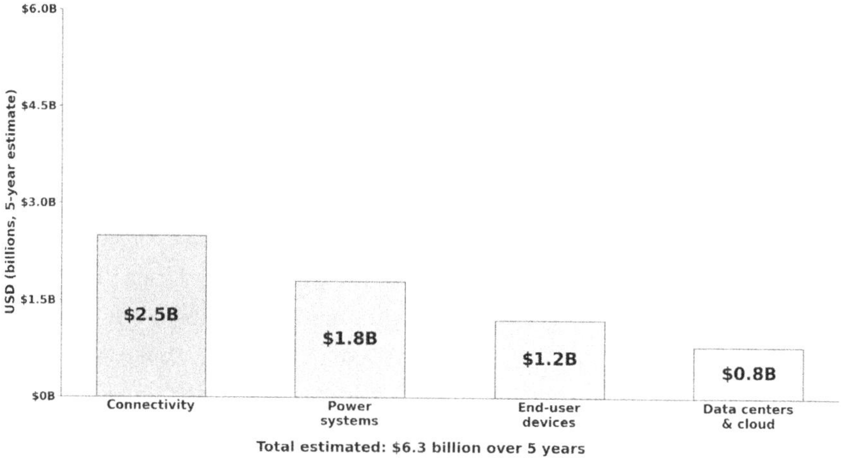

Source: World Bank (2022), AfDB (2021).

The private sector contributes through direct investment in commercial infrastructure that health systems can leverage (particularly broadband networks) and through targeted health-sector investments via corporate social responsibility programs and social enterprise models. Philanthropic organizations, including the Bill and Melinda Gates Foundation, the Rockefeller Foundation, and the Patrick J. McGovern Foundation, have funded innovative digital health infrastructure pilots and scaling initiatives (AfDB, 2021; WHO, 2023).

Innovative Financing Approaches

Beyond traditional funding channels, several innovative financing mechanisms show promise for digital health infrastructure. Social impact bonds and development impact bonds, which link financial returns to measurable health outcomes, have been piloted in several African countries for health service delivery and could be adapted for infrastructure investments. Blended finance structures, which combine concessional public or philanthropic capital with commercial investment to de-risk projects, have proven effective for energy infrastructure and could be similarly applied to health facility connectivity and electrification. Domestic resource mobilization through earmarked taxes or telecommunications levies directed to Universal Service and Access Funds offers a pathway to sustainable national funding, provided governance and disbursement mechanisms are strengthened (World Bank, 2022; Broadband Commission, 2021).

7.8 Public–Private Partnerships in Infrastructure Development

Public–private partnerships (PPPs) are a critical mechanism for accelerating the deployment of digital health infrastructure across Africa, leveraging private-sector capital, technical expertise, and operational efficiency to complement public-sector resources and policy authority. The rationale for PPPs in digital health infrastructure is compelling: governments possess the mandate to ensure universal health coverage and the regulatory authority to shape market conditions, while private-sector actors possess the technical capabilities, financial resources, and implementation capacity to deploy infrastructure rapidly at scale (World Bank, 2022; GSMA, 2023).

Partnership Models in Practice

Telecommunications companies are the most established PPP partners for digital health infrastructure. In Kenya, Safaricom has partnered with the Ministry of Health to provide preferential data rates for health facilities and health workers. In Nigeria, MTN's partnership with state governments has extended mobile network coverage to underserved health zones. Across the continent, the GSMA's Mobile for Development Health program has facilitated partnerships between mobile operators and health ministries, demonstrating the commercial viability of health-sector connectivity when structured appropriately (GSMA, 2023).

Technology companies increasingly provide cloud infrastructure and technical support. Microsoft's AI for Health program has provided cloud computing credits and technical assistance to African health organizations. Google's partnership with Africa CDC has supported the development of cloud-based disease surveillance and genomic sequencing platforms. Amazon Web Services has established an African cloud region in Cape Town, enabling health data to be hosted on the continent while still benefiting from global cloud infrastructure. These technology PPPs typically combine in-kind contributions (cloud credits, technical expertise) with capacity-building components that develop local technical talent (Africa CDC, 2022; World Bank, 2022).

Solar energy companies have become key PPP partners for electrifying health facilities. Companies such as d.light, M-KOPA, and Greenlight Planet, operating under long-term service agreements, finance, install, and maintain solar-plus-battery systems at health facilities, with governments paying a monthly service fee rather than the full upfront capital cost. This model, deployed in Uganda, Tanzania, Sierra Leone, and other countries, aligns private profit incentives with public health objectives by tying payments to system performance and uptime. The World Bank's Lighting Africa program has supported the development of quality standards and market infrastructure for off-grid solar products, including those designed for health facility applications (IEA, 2022; IRENA, 2023).

Ensuring Effective Partnerships

Successful PPPs require clear contractual frameworks specifying performance standards, accountability mechanisms, and dispute-resolution procedures. They demand transparent governance structures that prevent conflicts of interest and enable efficient decision-making. PPPs require capacity within government agencies to negotiate, manage, and monitor complex partnership agreements. Moreover, they must align private profit incentives with public health objectives through carefully designed incentive structures, performance metrics, and risk-sharing arrangements. Countries such as Kenya, Rwanda, and South Africa, which have established dedicated PPP units within their finance or health ministries, have generally achieved better outcomes from public–private health infrastructure partnerships than countries without such institutional frameworks (World Bank, 2022).

7.9 Global Benchmarking and Lessons for Africa

Benchmarking Africa's Layer 1 infrastructure against other regions provides both a measure of the gap to be closed and actionable strategies for closing it. While direct comparisons must account for differences in economic development, population distribution, governance capacity, and historical investment levels, the experiences of other regions offer concrete lessons for African policymakers and implementers (WHO, 2021; World Bank, 2022).

Figure 7.6 Global Benchmarking: Health Facility Digitization Rates

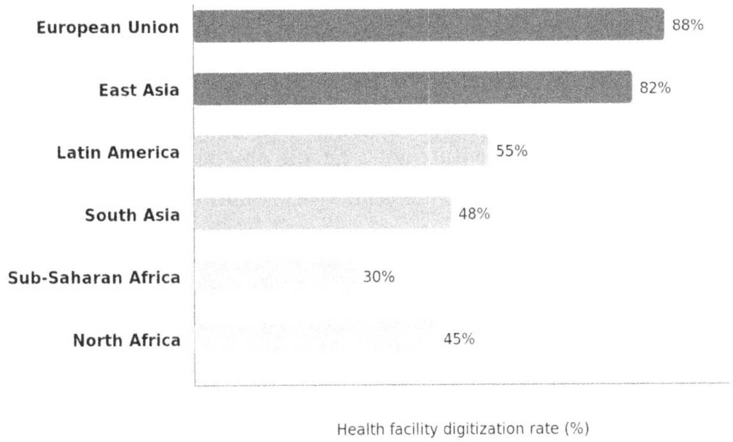

Sources: WHO (2023), World Bank (221), EU Digital Health Network (2023)

The European Union's experience demonstrates the transformative impact of political commitment backed by sustained investment. The EU's Digital Single Market strategy and the European Health Data Space initiative have created an enabling environment for digital health infrastructure by establishing clear regulatory standards, investing in cross-border interoperability, and dedicating substantial funding through mechanisms such as the Connecting Europe Facility and Horizon Europe. EU Member States have achieved near-universal health facility digitization, with the remaining gaps concentrated in rural areas of newer member states—a challenge that mirrors Africa's own urban–rural divide (European Commission, 2022).

East Asian economies, particularly South Korea and Taiwan, offer models of rapid digital health infrastructure development driven by industrial policy and technology investment. South Korea's nationwide health information network, built over two decades of sustained government investment, connects nearly all hospitals and clinics to a unified electronic health record system, supported by universal broadband connectivity and advanced data center infrastructure. The key lesson for Africa is the importance of long-term strategic planning paired with phased implementation that builds incrementally on each successive investment (WHO, 2021).

South Asia, and India in particular, offers perhaps the most directly relevant comparisons for Africa, given similarities in scale, diversity, resource constraints, and the coexistence of advanced tertiary facilities with underserved rural primary care. India's approach—combining ambitious national digital identity (Aadhaar) and payment (UPI) infrastructure with progressive health-specific digitization through the Ayushman Bharat Digital Mission—demonstrates how general-purpose digital public infrastructure can accelerate health-sector digitization. Africa's growing digital public infrastructure ecosystem, including mobile money systems, national identification programs, and open-source health platforms such as DHIS2 and OpenMRS, provides analogous foundations for a similar trajectory (Mehl & Labrique, 2014; WHO, 2021).

Latin America and the Caribbean offer instructive examples of health-sector infrastructure development in middle-income contexts: Brazil's SUS digital transformation, Uruguay's Salud (the national health information system), and Costa Rica's EDUS electronic health record system all demonstrate that sustained political commitment, phased implementation, and effective use of open-source software can achieve significant digitization of health facilities even in constrained fiscal environments. These experiences are particularly relevant for Africa's upper-middle-income countries and for demonstrating proof-of-concept approaches that can be adapted across different economic contexts (OECD, 2020; WHO, 2021).

7.10 Conclusion

This chapter has demonstrated that digital infrastructure is not merely a technical prerequisite for digital health transformation but its foundational determinant. Connectivity, reliable electricity, data center capacity, and device availability—collectively forming Layer 1 of the digital health technology stack—shape what is feasible across all higher layers, from interoperability and analytics to service delivery. Persistent infrastructure gaps across Africa, particularly in rural and underserved areas, continue to constrain the reach, quality, and equity of digital health systems. As such, investments in digital health that do not simultaneously address foundational infrastructure risk underperformance, fragmentation, or outright failure.

A central insight from the chapter is that Africa's digital divide is structural, especially between urban and rural contexts. Evidence shows that while urban centers increasingly benefit from expanding broadband, reliable electricity, and device availability, rural areas—where health needs are often greatest—remain systematically excluded. This divide is not only technological but also deeply intertwined with broader development inequalities, reinforcing disparities in health access and outcomes. Bridging this gap requires deliberate policy choices, including universal service obligations, targeted rural connectivity programs, decentralized energy solutions such as solar systems, and mobile-first design approaches tailored to low-resource environments.

The chapter also highlights that infrastructure development at scale is fundamentally a challenge of financing and governance. The estimated multi-billion-dollar investment needs cannot be met by public funding alone; instead, a blended approach combining government budgets, development finance, private-sector participation, and innovative financing instruments is essential. Public–private partnerships are a particularly powerful mechanism, aligning public health objectives with private-sector capabilities in telecommunications, energy, and cloud infrastructure. However, their effectiveness depends on robust institutional capacity, transparent governance, and well-designed incentive structures that ensure equitable access and long-term sustainability.

Finally, global benchmarking shows that Africa's infrastructure challenges, while significant, are not insurmountable. Experiences from the European Union, Asia, Latin America, and comparable regions demonstrate that rapid progress is achievable through sustained political commitment, strategic investment, and integrated sectoral planning. The key lesson is that digital health infrastructure must be treated as core national infrastructure—akin to roads, water, and electricity—rather than as a peripheral component of health projects. By embedding digital infrastructure within broader development strategies and aligning it with the continent's digital public infrastructure agenda, Africa can build a resilient foundation for inclusive, scalable, and transformative digital health systems that serve all populations.

References

ARENA. (2024). Hybrid renewable energy for remote communities: Health facility electrification outcomes. Australian Renewable Energy Agency.

Australian Department of Infrastructure. (2025). Better Connectivity Plan for Regional and Rural Australia: Implementation report. Australian Government.

Australian Digital Health Agency. (2024). Digital health implementation toolkit: Device specifications and lifecycle management. Australian Digital Health Agency.

Australian Government. (2024). National Broadband Network: Investment and upgrade program. Commonwealth of Australia.

Canada Health Infoway. (2024). Technology procurement support program: Annual report. Canada Health Infoway.

CARICOM. (2023). Regional data centre cooperation framework for the Caribbean Community. Caribbean Community Secretariat.

CRTC. (2024). Broadband Fund: Projects selected for funding and policy review (Telecom Regulatory Policy CRTC 2024-328). Canadian Radio-television and Telecommunications Commission.

CRTC. (2026). Indigenous stream of the Broadband Fund: Development process. Canadian Radio-television and Telecommunications Commission.

CTU. (2023). Caribbean telecommunications regulatory harmonization: Annual report. Caribbean Telecommunications Union.

Government of Canada. (2024). Shared Services Canada: Cloud infrastructure for government health programs. Government of Canada.

Health Canada. (2024). Digital health specifications for northern and remote community health centres. Health Canada.

ISED Canada. (2024). Universal Broadband Fund: Program update and coverage statistics. Innovation, Science and Economic Development Canada.

RFDS. (2024). Digital health innovation in remote Australia: Annual technology report. Royal Flying Doctor Service of Australia.

Africa CDC. (2022). Digital health strategy for Africa 2020–2030. Africa Centres for Disease Control and Prevention.

Africa Data Centres Association. (2023). Africa data centre market outlook 2023. ADCA.

African Development Bank. (2021). African economic outlook 2021: From debt resolution to growth—The road ahead for Africa. AfDB.

Alliance for Affordable Internet. (2023). Affordability report 2023. Web Foundation.

Broadband Commission for Sustainable Development. (2021). Connecting Africa through broadband: A strategy for doubling connectivity by 2021 and reaching universal access by 2030. ITU/UNESCO.

European Commission. (2021). Recovery and resilience facility: Factsheet on digital. European Commission.

European Commission. (2022). European health data space: Regulation proposal. European Commission.

GSMA. (2023). The mobile economy: Sub-Saharan Africa 2023. GSM Association.

International Energy Agency. (2022). Africa Energy Outlook 2022. IEA Publications.

International Renewable Energy Agency. (2023). Renewable energy statistics 2023. IRENA.

International Telecommunication Union. (2023). Measuring digital development: Facts and figures 2023. ITU.

Kiberu, V. M., Mars, M., & Scott, R. E. (2014). Barriers and opportunities to implementation of sustainable e-health programmes in Uganda: A literature review. African Journal of Primary Health Care & Family Medicine, 6(1), 1–8. https://doi.org/10.4102/phcfm.v6i1.727

Mehl, G., & Labrique, A. (2014). Prioritizing integrated mHealth strategies for universal health coverage. Science, 345(6202), 1284–1287. https://doi.org/10.1126/science.1258926

Organisation for Economic Co-operation and Development. (2020). Health at a glance: Latin America and the Caribbean 2020. OECD Publishing. https://doi.org/10.1787/6089164f-en

PATH. (2021). Digital health in low- and middle-income countries: A landscape assessment. PATH.

World Health Organization. (2021). Global strategy on digital health 2020–2025. WHO.

World Health Organization. (2023). Service availability and readiness assessment (SARA): An annual monitoring system for service delivery. WHO.

World Bank. (2022). Digital Africa: Technological transformation for jobs. World Bank Group.

Chapter 8 Digital Identity and Registries for Health

8.1 Introduction: Why Identity Is the Linchpin of Digital Health

Digital health systems are only as reliable as the identity infrastructure on which they are built. Every clinical encounter, laboratory result, prescription, insurance claim, and surveillance report must be linked to a correctly identified patient, delivered by a verified health worker, and associated with a known facility. When identity infrastructure fails—when a patient cannot be uniquely identified across facilities, when a health worker's credentials cannot be verified, or when a facility's services and location are unknown to the broader system—the entire digital health ecosystem breaks down. Duplicate records proliferate, care continuity is severed, surveillance data becomes unreliable, and the interoperability that Layers 3 through 5 of the technology stack depend on becomes impossible.

This chapter examines Layer 2 of the digital health technology stack introduced in Chapter 4 (Section 4.1.2): the Digital Identity and Registries Layer. This layer includes the master patient index (MPI), unique patient identifiers (UPIs), health worker and facility registries, and digital identity systems that authenticate users across platforms. As the chapter will demonstrate, Layer 2 serves as the critical bridge between Layer 1's physical infrastructure and the interoperability, analytics, and application layers above it. Without a reliable identity infrastructure, investments in electronic health records, telemedicine, and health information exchange cannot deliver their full value.

The chapter is organized into four parts. First, it examines the core conceptual and technical issues surrounding identity in the health sector. Second, it assesses how African countries are currently addressing universal patient identity. Third, it systematically reviews global experiences in Europe, Asia, Latin America, Australia, and Canada. Fourth, it identifies gaps in Africa's identity infrastructure and proposes actionable strategies to address them.

8.2 Core Issues of Identity in the Health Sector

8.2.1 The Problem of Patient Identification

The ability to uniquely and reliably identify a patient across encounters, facilities, and time is the foundational requirement for any digital health system. Without it, a patient's medical history is fragmented across disconnected records; a clinician cannot know which medications the patient is already taking, which allergies have been documented, or which diagnostic tests have already been performed. At the population level, disease surveillance cannot accurately count cases when the same individual presents at multiple facilities and is counted multiple times. Insurance systems cannot detect duplicate claims. Research datasets cannot build longitudinal cohorts.

The challenge of patient identification is compounded in low- and middle-income countries by several structural factors. Civil registration systems are incomplete: across Sub-Saharan Africa, only an estimated 46% of births are registered, leaving a significant proportion of the population without the foundational civil identity document on which health identification typically depends (UNICEF, 2023). Population mobility is high, with patients frequently crossing facility, district, and national boundaries for care, particularly in nomadic areas and in Southern and East Africa, where cross-border migration is substantial. Paper-based record systems—still the norm in most African primary care facilities—assign local medical record numbers that have no meaning outside the issuing facility. Where electronic systems exist, they often operate as isolated silos, each assigning its own identifiers without mechanisms for cross-referencing (Boulle et al., 2023; Katurura & Cilliers, 2018).

McFarlane et al. (2019) identified six attributes that an ideal patient identifier must possess: it must be unique (no two patients share the same identifier), unchanging (the identifier persists over the patient's lifetime), ubiquitous (available across all care settings), uncomplicated (easy to use in practice), inexpensive (affordable for resource-constrained systems), and uncontroversial (acceptable to patients and the public). No single identification strategy perfectly satisfies all six attributes simultaneously, which is why effective patient identity management requires a layered approach combining multiple strategies—unique identifiers, demographic matching, biometrics, and crosswalk services—rather than relying on any single mechanism.

8.2.2 The Architecture of Health Identity Infrastructure

The architecture of health identity infrastructure, illustrated in Figure 8.1, comprises several interconnected components. At the apex sits the national identity or civil registration system, which serves as the authoritative source for identity proofing—establishing that a person is who they claim to be. Below this is the master patient index (MPI) or health identity registry, which issues and maintains the health-sector unique patient identifier (UPI), creates a "golden record" for each individual by reconciling information from multiple sources, and provides crosswalk services that link the UPI to local medical record numbers used by individual facilities. The MPI interacts with three specialized registries: the patient registry (demographics, consent, longitudinal records), the health worker registry (credentials, licensure, deployment), and the facility registry (location, services, capacity). At the base, local electronic systems—hospital EMRs, clinic records, laboratory systems, pharmacy systems, and insurance platforms—each maintain their own identifiers but connect to the MPI through standardized identity services.

The WHO and Integrating the Healthcare Enterprise (IHE) recommend a set of FHIR-based interoperability profiles for managing patient identity across systems. The Patient Master Identity Registry (PMIR) profile supports the creation and management of patient identity data. The Patient Identifier Cross-Reference for Mobile (PIXm) profile enables cross-referencing of patient identifiers across systems. The Patient Demographics Query for Mobile (PDQm) profile supports querying patient demographics from a central registry. Together, these profiles provide the technical foundation for interoperable patient identity management (WHO, 2023; IHE, 2024).

8.2.3 Beyond Patients: Health Worker and Facility Registries

While patient identity receives the most attention, reliable identification of health workers and health facilities is equally important for the functioning of digital health systems. A health worker registry provides an authoritative, up-to-date listing of all health professionals authorized to practice, their qualifications, licensure status, facility assignments, and contact information. Without such a registry, clinical systems cannot verify that the person entering orders or prescribing medications is a legitimate, credentialed health worker. Telemedicine platforms cannot authenticate remote providers. Workforce planning cannot accurately assess the deployment and distribution of health personnel.

Figure 8.1. Architecture of the Digital Identity and Registries Layer

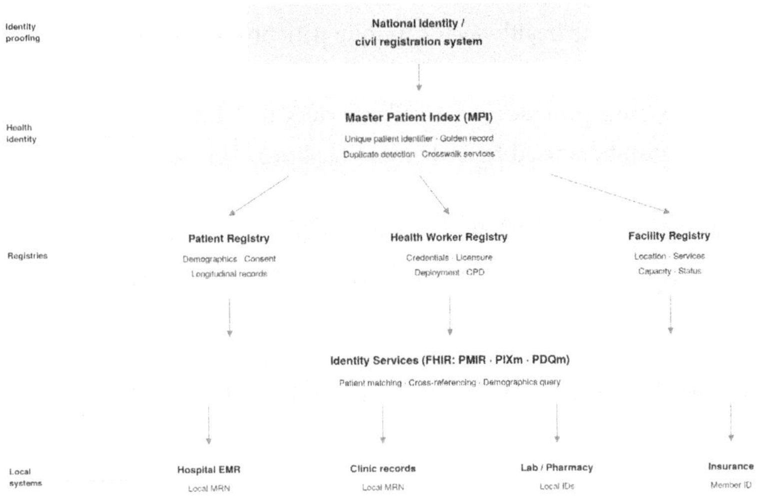

Source: Adopted from OpenHIE, IHE and Author's Elaboration

A facility registry provides an authoritative listing of all health facilities, including geographic coordinates, services offered, operational status, and administrative relationships. Facility registries are essential for referral systems (directing patients to facilities that offer the services they need), supply chain management (knowing where to deliver medicines and supplies), and health system performance monitoring (benchmarking facilities against their peers). The OpenHIE framework identifies the facility registry, health worker registry, and client (patient) registry as three core components of a functioning health information exchange (OpenHIE, 2024).

8.3 African Approaches to Health Identity

8.3.1 Current Landscape

Africa's approaches to health identity are diverse, fragmented, and at different stages of maturity. A 2023 landscape analysis of the Southern African Development Community (SADC) found that most countries were in the early to middle stages of implementing unique patient identifiers, and that existing identification methods often failed to support patient tracking across facilities and programs (Osler et al., 2023). The study also found that even where UPI systems were in place, identifiers were often not captured at the point of care, undermining their utility for care coordination and surveillance.

South Africa is among the continent's most advanced in implementing patient identity. The Health Patient Registration System (HPRS) aims to create a master patient index covering the entire public health sector, using the South African national identity number (RSA ID) as the primary linking variable. However, the Western Cape Provincial Health Data Centre—one of the most sophisticated health data linkage environments in Africa—has documented that fewer than 30% of patient records in its master patient index contain a valid RSA ID, with duplicate rates estimated at 10–20% (Boulle et al., 2023). This experience illustrates a critical lesson: even where a national identity number exists, its utility for health purposes depends on consistent capture at the point of care.

Rwanda has achieved relatively strong patient identification by integrating national identity numbers with the national EMR system, which is deployed across all 502 public health facilities. The country's small geographic size, strong governance structures, and comprehensive community-based health insurance (CBHI) scheme—which requires identification for enrollment—have collectively supported more complete patient identification than in most African countries (Rwanda Biomedical Center, 2022).

Ethiopia is pursuing an ambitious integration of health identity with the national digital ID system. The Fayda national digital identity, currently being rolled out, is intended to serve as the foundational identity layer across government services, including healthcare. Ethiopia's Ministry of Health has identified unique patient identification as a crucial component of its digital health blueprint, with plans to link health identifiers to the Fayda system (Melkamu, 2024).

Namibia offers a noteworthy example of an open-source approach. The Ministry of Health and Social Services, supported by the University of California, San Francisco (UCSF), deployed SanteMPI—an open-source master patient index recognized as a digital public good—that provides real-time validation of national identifiers against the Namibia National Population Registry (NPRS). The system generates a unique seven-character Health ID for each patient and provides a mobile application for health facility staff to query the MPI at the point of care (UCSF Global Health Informatics, 2024).

Nigeria illustrates the challenges of patient identification in a large, federated country with an incomplete national identity system. A 2022 study found that no current patient identification strategy in Nigeria simultaneously meets all six attributes of an ideal identifier (Oleribe et al., 2022). The National Identification Number (NIN), administered by the National Identity Management Commission (NIMC), serves as a potential linking variable, but coverage remains incomplete, and integration with health information systems is fragmented. The study proposed a decentralized, offline patient ID generation and matching algorithm that could operate without continuous connectivity to a central authority—an approach particularly relevant to resource-constrained settings.

8.3.2 Common Challenges Across Africa

Several challenges recur across African implementations of health identity infrastructure:

- First, incomplete civil registration limits the population available for health identity linkage.
- Second, multiple parallel identification systems—for HIV programs, immunization, insurance, and general clinical care—create fragmentation rather than a unified identity infrastructure.

- Third, infrastructure constraints, including intermittent connectivity and unreliable power, complicate the deployment of centralized identity verification systems.
- Fourth, data quality issues, including misspelled names, inconsistent date-of-birth recording, and missing demographic fields, reduce the accuracy of matching algorithms.
- Fifth, governance gaps, including the lack of clear data protection legislation in many countries, create uncertainty about how health identity data should be stored, shared, and protected.
- Sixth, the lack of unique identifiers for health workers and facilities in many countries compounds the challenge of patient identification by making it difficult to verify the provenance of clinical records.

The Smart Africa Alliance Digital Health Blueprint (2024), championed by the Government of Rwanda and Africa CDC, explicitly addresses these challenges. It recommends that African countries establish national health information systems with integrated access and identity management, set up national data gateways to manage terminology, and develop patient consent management systems integrated with the identity infrastructure (Smart Africa, 2024).

8.4 Global Experiences in Health Identity

8.4.1 Four Models for Connecting National IDs with Health Identifiers

Global experience reveals four principal models for integrating national civil identity with health-sector patient identification, as illustrated in Figure 8.2. Understanding these models is essential for African countries as they make strategic decisions about their identity architecture.

- **Model 1: Direct Civil ID Reuse.** In this model, the national civil identity number serves directly as the health identifier. This approach is common in the Nordic countries (Sweden, Denmark, Finland), South Korea, and Thailand. In Sweden, the personal identity number (personnummer) is used extensively across public services, including healthcare. In Denmark, the CPR number serves as the standard patient identifier in FHIR-based health information exchange. The advantage of direct reuse is simplicity and universal coverage in countries with complete civil registration. The disadvantage is that broadly exposing the national ID across the health ecosystem increases privacy and surveillance risks (WHO, 2023).

- **Model 2: Health-Specific UPI Linked to Civil ID.** In this model, the health sector issues its own identifier but links it to the national civil identity for verification and de-duplication. Australia's Individual Healthcare Identifier (IHI), issued through the Healthcare Identifiers Service, is one of the strongest examples globally. Persons with Medicare or Department of Veterans' Affairs records are automatically assigned an IHI, while others can obtain one after identity verification. The IHI is used within the My Health Record system, while the national identity remains a verified attribute rather than the visible clinical key (Australian Digital Health Agency, 2024). India's Ayushman Bharat Health Account (ABHA) follows a similar model: it is a 14-digit health-specific identifier that can be created using Aadhaar for identity proofing but functions as a distinct health identifier within the ABDM ecosystem (Sharma et al., 2023). The United Kingdom's NHS number and France's Identité Nationale de Santé (INS) are further examples of health-governed identifiers linked to state identity infrastructure.

- **Model 3: Federated Provincial or Institutional IDs.** In this model, provinces, insurers, or facilities maintain their own identifiers, linked via a client registry or master patient index. Canada exemplifies this approach: there is no single national health identifier, and each province issues its own health card number. Ontario's Provincial Client Registry stores demographic data and uniquely identifies patients using local or global identifiers, which are validated against the Registered Persons Database (Canada Health Infoway, 2024). This model is realistic for countries with decentralized governance or no universal national ID, though it requires robust registry infrastructure to achieve cross-jurisdictional interoperability.

Figure 8.2. Four Models for Connecting National IDs with Health Patient Identification.

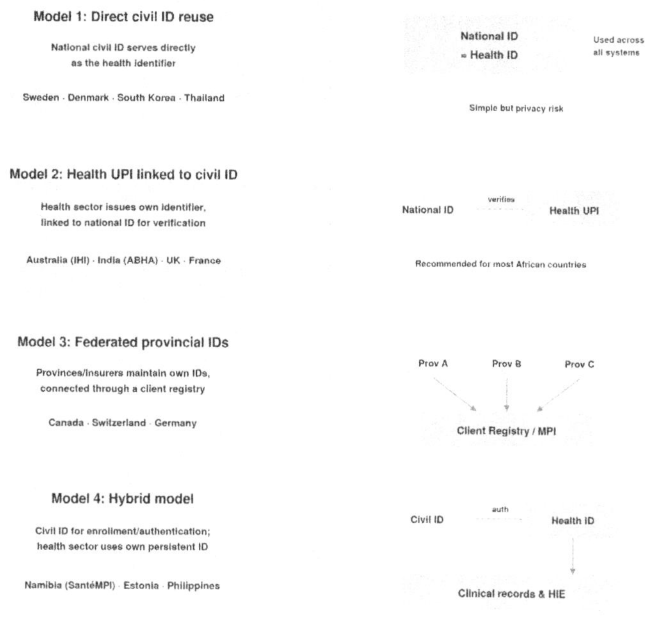

Source: Author's Synthesis based on WHO, IHE and Country Reports

- **Model 4: Hybrid Model.** In this model, the civil ID is used primarily for enrollment and authentication, while the health sector uses its own persistent identifier for information exchange and longitudinal records. Namibia's SanteMPI implementation, which validates against the National Population Registry but issues a distinct Health ID, exemplifies this approach. Estonia's digital health ecosystem uses a similar architecture: the national e-ID authenticates users, while the health information system maintains its own record structures. The

Philippines is emerging as another hybrid case, with the National ID integrated into the Department of Health systems for verification, while health applications maintain their own identifiers (Philippine Statistics Authority, 2026).

8.4.2 European Experiences

Europe spans both ends of the identity spectrum. The Nordic countries show that direct reuse of civil ID can be highly effective where civil registration is universal, trusted, and digitally mature. By contrast, the United Kingdom and France demonstrate the advantages of a health-governed identifier linked to state identity but operated within the health sector. France's INS, built on social security infrastructure, has been mandatory for referencing health data since 2021. At the EU level, cross-border exchange under MyHealth@EU and the European Health Data Space does not require a single EU-wide patient number; instead, member states must reliably identify patients within their own systems and exchange data interoperably across borders (European Commission, 2022).

The European lesson for Africa is that both approaches can work, but the more mature systems separate identity proofing from clinical interoperability. For most African countries, where civil registration coverage is incomplete and population mobility is high, the health-governed identifier linked to civil identity—the second model—offers a safer and more adaptable approach.

8.4.3 Asia-Pacific Experiences

India's ABHA system is the most directly relevant Asian model for Africa, given similarities in scale, diversity, and the coexistence of public and private health systems. By March 2024, over 568 million ABHA accounts had been created, demonstrating that health identity infrastructure can be deployed at a population scale in a resource-constrained setting when built on existing digital public infrastructure—in India's case, the Aadhaar biometric identity system (Balsari et al., 2024). Singapore's National Electronic Health Record relies on trusted state identity infrastructure for access and authentication, representing a tightly integrated model suited to a small, highly connected city-state. Thailand and South Korea use direct national ID linkage, with hospitals maintaining local identifiers mapped to the national number for insurance and record linkage (WHO, 2021).

8.4.4 Latin American and Caribbean Experiences

In Latin America, the dominant trend is to use robust civil registration and national identification numbers as the practical basis for health identification. Chile and Costa Rica, with near-universal birth registration, frequently use the national identification number (RUT/RUN in Chile) as the linking patient identifier. Uruguay's national electronic health record platform enables clinical information exchange across providers through high-assurance digital identity methods (PAHO, 2023). However, reliance on national IDs without a proper health interoperability layer creates risks: populations with incomplete civil registration—including newborns, migrants, refugees, and undocumented persons—may be excluded from digital health systems precisely when they need access most (PAHO, 2024).

PAHO's interoperability guidance explicitly recommends unique identifiers for patients, providers, and facilities, and its work on civil registration and vital statistics (CRVS) reinforces that health identification should not fail when civil identity is incomplete. The LACPASS initiative, using blockchain-enabled verifiable health credentials for cross-border exchange, demonstrates how regional identity interoperability can be achieved without requiring a single regional identifier (PAHO, 2023).

Canada's federated model offers perhaps the most directly applicable lessons for African countries with decentralized governance structures. The absence of a single national health identifier has not prevented Canada from building functional health information systems; rather, it has required investment in registries, standards, and patient identity management at the provincial level, with national-level interoperability frameworks linking them. For African countries where provinces, states, or counties operate semi-autonomous health systems, Canada's experience shows that functional identity infrastructure can be built incrementally from the subnational level upward (Canada Health Infoway, 2024; Bhatia et al., 2024).

8.5 Addressing Gaps: A Strategic Agenda for Africa

8.5.1 Master Patient Index and Unique Patient Identifier

The top priority for African health identity infrastructure is establishing functional master patient indices at the national or subnational level. Countries can begin by creating a national patient identity authority within the Ministry of Health, drawing on global models such as Australia's ADHA and India's NHA, and by deploying open-source MPI solutions like SanteMPI or OpenHIE to enable rapid, cost-effective implementation. Countries can then strengthen identity integrity and inclusivity by linking the MPI to national civil registration systems (as seen in Estonia and India's ABHA), issuing persistent health Unique Patient Identifiers(similar to Australia's IHI and the UK's NHS number), and incorporating exception pathways for underserved populations, such as newborns, migrants, and refugees, while enabling offline functionality to address connectivity constraints in low-resource settings. Finally, ongoing system optimization is needed through continuous duplicate resolution using probabilistic matching and the adoption of international interoperability standards—particularly FHIR-based identity profiles such as PMIR, PIXm, and PDQm.

Further, the experience suggests the following strategic approach.

- First, countries should adopt the hybrid model—using national ID or civil registration for identity proofing while issuing and maintaining a health-sector UPI to support clinical operations and interoperability.

- Second, the MPI should be implemented as an open-source digital public good, following Namibia's SanteMPI deployment, to reduce costs and avoid vendor lock-in.

- Third, the MPI must include robust capabilities for duplicate detection and resolution, recognizing that data quality in African settings will inevitably produce duplicate records that require systematic management.

- Fourth, exception pathways must be designed from the outset for newborns (who lack national IDs), migrants, refugees, and undocumented populations—groups that are often the most vulnerable and in greatest need of health services.

- Fifth, the MPI must operate in low-connectivity environments, supporting offline identity verification and batch synchronization upon restoration of connectivity.

Table 8.1 Strategic Priorities for MPI Implementation in Africa

Priority	Action	Global Model	Timeframe
Establish MPI governance	Create national patient identity authority within MoH	Australia (ADHA), India (NHA)	Year 1
Deploy open-source MPI	Implement SanteMPI or equivalent as digital public good	Namibia, OpenHIE	Year 1–2
Link to civil ID	Validate identities against national ID/ civil registry	Estonia, India (ABHA)	Year 1–3
Issue health UPI	Generate persistent health identifier for each individual	Australia (IHI), UK (NHS No.)	Year 2–3
Build exception pathways	Accommodate newborns, migrants, refugees, undocumented	PAHO guidance, UNHCR	Year 1–2
Enable offline operation	Support offline ID generation and batch sync	Nigeria algorithm model	Year 2–3
Resolve duplicates	Implement probabilistic matching and manual review	South Africa PHDC	Ongoing
Adopt FHIR identity profiles	Implement PMIR, PIXm, PDQm for interoperability	IHE, WHO SMART Guidelines	Year 2–4

Source: Author's Elaboration

8.5.2 Health Worker Registry

Africa faces a severe health workforce crisis: the continent bears 24% of the global disease burden yet accounts for only 3% of the global health workforce (WHO, 2022). Accurate tracking of the health workforce through a comprehensive registry is essential for workforce planning, equitable deployment, credential verification, and management of continuing professional development.

Ghana's Human Resource Information System, integrated with payroll systems, has improved workforce data quality and reduced ghost workers on government payrolls (Ghana Health Service, 2021). South Africa's Health Professions Council maintains a digital register of all licensed health professionals, providing a model for credential verification that could be adopted across the continent. The WHO National Health Workforce Accounts framework provides standardized indicators and reporting templates for health worker registries, offering a foundation for African countries to build on (WHO, 2022).

Key actions for health worker registries include establishing unique health worker identifiers linked to licensure and credentialing bodies, integrating registry data with payroll and deployment systems to eliminate ghost workers, linking registries to EMR systems to verify prescribing and ordering authority, and developing regional frameworks for cross-border credential recognition—essential for the growing number of health workers practicing across African borders.

8.5.3 Facility Registry

A comprehensive, up-to-date facility registry is essential for effective referral systems, supply chain management, and health system performance monitoring. Many African countries maintain facility lists, but these lists are often outdated, incomplete, and disconnected from the digital health systems that rely on them. The WHO Master Facility List (MFL) initiative provides guidance and tools for establishing and maintaining authoritative facility registries, and several African countries have made progress in developing digital facility registries aligned with this guidance (WHO, 2023).

Key actions include establishing a national master facility list as the single authoritative source, assigning unique facility identifiers that are used consistently across all health information systems, incorporating geospatial coordinates for every facility to support mapping and spatial analysis, regularly updating the registry to reflect new facilities, closures, and changes in services offered, and making the registry available as a shared service via APIs that other systems can query.

8.5.4 Biometrics and Digital Identity Integration

Biometric identification—using fingerprints, iris scans, facial recognition, or other measurable biological characteristics to verify identity—holds particular promise for African health settings where documentary identification may be incomplete. India's Aadhaar system demonstrated that biometric identity can be deployed at scale, with over 1.3 billion enrollments forming the identity-proofing foundation for the ABHA health identifier. Several African countries, including Kenya (Huduma Namba), Nigeria (NIN), and Ethiopia (Fayda), are developing or deploying national biometric identity systems that could underpin health identity infrastructure.

However, biometric approaches in health settings face specific challenges. Fingerprint quality can be compromised in populations engaged in manual labor. Infant biometrics remain technically challenging. Privacy and surveillance concerns are heightened when biometric data is linked across government systems. The cost of biometric capture devices at the point of care adds to facility-level infrastructure requirements. For these reasons, biometrics are best understood as a complement to other identity mechanisms rather than a standalone solution—they strengthen identity proofing at enrollment and can support re-identification of patients who have lost their identity documents, but they should be embedded within a broader identity governance framework that includes privacy protections, consent mechanisms, and oversight (Jain et al., 2016; Simprints, 2024).

8.5.5 An Eight-Point Agenda for Africa

Drawing on the global evidence reviewed in this chapter, the following eight-point strategic agenda is proposed for strengthening Layer 2 of the digital health technology stack across Africa:

1. Create an authoritative national patient identity registry or MPI with a "golden record." This should serve as the single source of truth for patient identity across all health programs and systems.

2. Keep the national ID as a verified attribute, not the sole operational key. Use the national ID for identity proofing and de-duplication, but issue and maintain a persistent health UPI for clinical operations.

3. Issue a persistent health-sector UPI for longitudinal care and interoperability. This identifier should follow the patient across facilities, programs, and time.

4. Support local identifiers and crosswalks. Allow facilities to retain their existing medical record numbers while linking them to the national UPI via crosswalk services, avoiding the need to renumber all legacy systems.

5. Adopt FHIR/IHE identity services. Implement the PMIR, PIXm, and PDQm profiles to standardize identity matching and synchronization across systems.

6. Require two-identifier verification at the point of care. Patient safety should depend on at least two identifiers (such as name and date of birth) rather than a single identifier.

7. Provide exception pathways for vulnerable populations. Design identity systems that accommodate newborns, migrants, refugees, visitors, and undocumented people from the outset.

8. Support pseudonymous or privacy-enhanced identities for sensitive use cases. Certain conditions (HIV, mental health, reproductive health) require additional privacy protections that the identity system must accommodate.

This combination is safer than raw national ID reuse and more interoperable than disconnected local medical record numbers. As this chapter has shown, drawing on global evidence, the best practice is not "national ID or UPI" but rather "national ID for trusted identity proofing, UPI for health operations, linked through a governed registry."

8.6 Conclusion

The Digital Identity and Registries Layer (Layer 2) is the critical enabler that transforms disconnected digital health tools into a coherent, interoperable health information ecosystem. Without reliable patient identification, the electronic health records examined in Chapter 3 become fragmented silos. Without health worker and facility registries, the interoperability infrastructure described in Chapter 4 cannot verify the provenance of clinical data. Without a governed identity architecture, the application-layer innovations described throughout this book—telemedicine, AI diagnostics, digital payments, and surveillance systems—cannot realize their full potential.

Africa's path forward requires a pragmatic, phased approach that builds on existing national identity infrastructure while establishing health-specific identity governance. Global evidence is clear: the most effective architecture uses national identity for proofing and deduplication, a health-sector UPI for clinical operations, and governed registries for patients, health workers, and facilities, all connected via standardized interoperability profiles. Countries that invest in this foundational layer will find that every subsequent digital health investment—from EMRs to analytics to telemedicine—delivers substantially greater value.

References

Australian Digital Health Agency. (2024). Healthcare Identifiers Service: Individual Healthcare Identifier (IHI) specifications. Australian Digital Health Agency.

Balsari, S., Sesia, P., & Patnaik, S. (2024). India's evolving digital health strategy. npj Digital Medicine, 7, Article 285. https://doi.org/10.1038/s41746-024-01279-2

Bhatia, R. S., Desveaux, L., & Bhyat, R. (2024). The Connected Care for Canadians Act: An important step toward interoperability of health data. Canadian Medical Association Journal, 196(48), E1383–E1388. https://doi.org/10.1503/cmaj.241161

Boulle, A., Heekes, A., Tiffin, N., Smith, M.,van de Merwe, L. & Fox, M. P. (2023). Record linkage for routinely collected health data in an African health information exchange. International Journal of Population Data Science, 8(1), 1771. https://doi.org/10.23889/ijpds.v8i1.1771

Canada Health Infoway. (2024). Interoperability: Shared Pan-Canadian Interoperability Roadmap. Canada Health Infoway.

European Commission. (2022). Proposal for a regulation on the European Health Data Space. COM(2022) 197 final.

Ghana Health Service. (2021). Human Resource Information System Implementation Report Ghana Health Service.

IHE. (2024). IT Infrastructure Technical Framework: Patient identity management profiles (PMIR, PIXm, PDQm). Integrating the Healthcare Enterprise.

Jain, A. K., Nandakumar, K., & Ross, A. (2016). 50 years of biometric research: Accomplishments, challenges, and opportunities. Pattern Recognition Letters, 79, 80–105. https://doi.org/10.1016/j.patrec.2015.12.013

Katurura, M. C., & Cilliers, L. (2018). Electronic health record system in the public health care sector of South Africa: A systematic literature review. African Journal of Primary Health Care & Family Medicine, 10(1), e1–e8. https://doi.org/10.4102/phcfm.v10i1.1746

McFarlane, T. D., Dixon, B. E., Grannis, S. J., & Gibson, P. J. (2019). Patient matching: Approaches and challenges. In Health Information Exchange (pp. 171–193). Academic Press.

Melkamu, G. (2024). Digital identity integration with Ethiopia's health system: Ministry of Health perspective. Presented at ID4Africa Livecast on Digital ID for Health. ID4Africa.

Oleribe, O. O., Okeibunor, J., & Osler, M. (2022). Scaling up a decentralized offline patient ID generation and matching algorithm: Insights from Nigeria. Frontiers in Digital Health, 4, 985337. https://doi.org/10.3389/fdgth.2022.985337

OpenHIE. (2024). OpenHIE architecture specification: Core components. Open Health Information Exchange.

Osler, M., Hildebrand, K., Goemaere, E., Ford, N., Smith, M.,";"; Boulle, A. (2023). Progress towards unique patient identification and case-based surveillance within the Southern African Development Community. Frontiers in Public Health, 11, 1197064. https://doi.org/10.3389/fpubh.2023.1197064

PAHO. (2023). Digital health in the Americas: Interoperability guidance and LACPASS verifiable credentials. Pan American Health Organization.

PAHO. (2024). Civil registration and vital statistics for health identification: Regional guidance. Pan American Health Organization.

Philippine Statistics Authority. (2026). National ID integration with Department of Health systems: Implementation report. Philippine Statistics Authority.

Rwanda Biomedical Center. (2022). National Health Information Exchange: Implementation and impact report. RBC.

Sharma, R. S., Rohatgi, A., Jain, S., & Singh, D. (2023). The Ayushman Bharat Digital Mission (ABDM): Making of India's digital health story. CSI Transactions on ICT, 11, 3–9. https://doi.org/10.1007/s40012-023-00375-0

Simprints. (2024). Biometrics for health: Lessons from field deployments in low-resource settings. Simprints Technology.

Smart Africa. (2024). Smart Africa Alliance Digital Health Blueprint. Smart Africa Secretariat / Africa CDC.

UCSF Global Health Informatics. (2024). SanteMPI deployment in Namibia: Master patient index for national health identity. University of California, San Francisco.

UNICEF. (2023). Birth registration: Global and regional estimates. United Nations Children's Fund.

WHO. (2021). Global strategy on digital health 2020–2025. World Health Organization.

WHO. (2022). Global strategy on human resources for health: Workforce 2030 progress report. World Health Organization.

WHO. (2023). Classification of digital interventions, services and applications in health (2nd ed.). World Health Organization.

Chapter 9 Interoperability and Health Information Exchange

9.1 Introduction: The Imperative of Interoperability

A health system in which every hospital, clinic, laboratory, pharmacy, and insurance platform operates its own digital system—each storing patient data in proprietary formats, assigning its own identifiers, and unable to share information with the others—is not a digital health system. It is a collection of digital silos that replicates the fragmentation of paper records in electronic form. Interoperability—the ability of different information systems, devices, and applications to access, exchange, integrate, and cooperatively use data in a coordinated manner—transforms isolated digital tools into a functioning digital health ecosystem (HIMSS, 2024).

This chapter examines Layer 3 of the digital health technology stack introduced in Chapter 4 (Section 4.1.3): the Interoperability and Data Exchange Layer—the third of five foundation layers in the stack model. This layer comprises health information exchange (HIE) platforms, application programming interfaces (APIs), messaging standards such as HL7 and FHIR, terminology services including SNOMED CT, ICD, and LOINC, and the governance frameworks that regulate data sharing. Layer 3 sits above Layer 2's identity infrastructure(Chapter 8), which provides patient, health worker, and facility identifiers that enable meaningful data exchange, and below Layer 4's analytics capabilities, which depend on interoperable data flows to generate actionable insights.

The chapter proceeds in four parts. First, it examines the core components of a national interoperability architecture. Second, it assesses Africa's current HIE landscape. Third, it systematically reviews global HIE models from Europe, Canada, Australia, Asia, and Latin America. Fourth, it proposes a strategic framework for building interoperability infrastructure across African health systems.

9.2 Components of a National Interoperability Architecture

Achieving interoperability is not a matter of deploying a single software product. As global experience shows, countries that have achieved meaningful health data exchange have done so by building a national interoperability stack comprising five interconnected components, as illustrated in Figure 9.1.

Figure 9.1. Five Components of National Interoperability Architecture

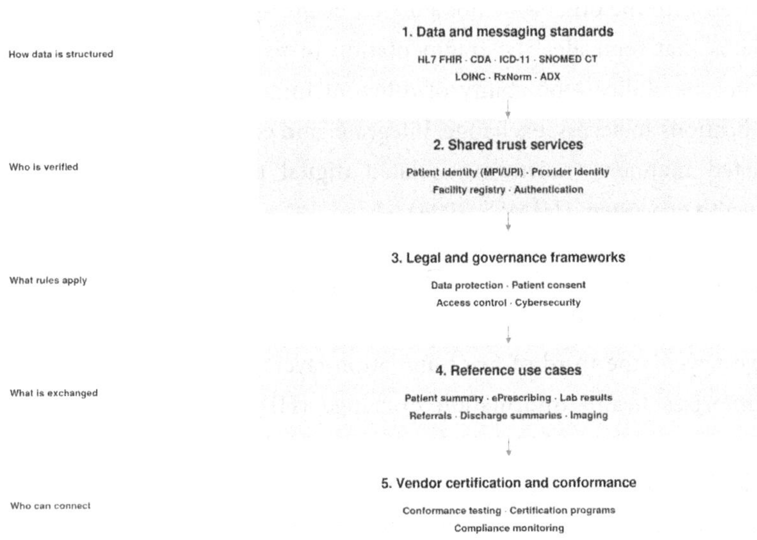

Source: Author's Synthesis Based on WHO, OpenHIE and Country Reports

Data and messaging standards define how health data is structured, coded, and transmitted across systems. HL7 Fast Healthcare Interoperability Resources (FHIR) has become the dominant global standard for health data exchange, offering a modular, API-based approach that is developer-friendly and well-suited to modern web architectures. Clinical document standards, such as HL7 Clinical Document Architecture (CDA), remain important for structured document exchange. Terminology standards—ICD for diagnoses,

LOINC for laboratory observations, SNOMED CT for clinical terms, and RxNorm for medications—ensure that the same concept is understood consistently across systems, enabling semantic interoperability (HL7 International, 2024; WHO, 2023).

Shared trust services provide the identity verification, authentication, and authorization infrastructure that enables secure data exchange. As detailed in Chapter 8, these services include patient identity services (master patient index, unique patient identifier), provider identity services (health worker registry, credential verification), and facility identity services (master facility list, service directory). Without these trust services, systems cannot reliably determine who the patient is, whether the requesting provider is authorized to access data, or which facility generated a given record (OpenHIE, 2024).

Legal and governance frameworks set the rules for collecting, storing, sharing, and using health data. These frameworks include data protection legislation (such as South Africa's POPIA, Kenya's Data Protection Act, and the EU's GDPR), patient consent mechanisms, access control policies, cybersecurity requirements, and institutional arrangements for overseeing data exchange. As discussed in Chapter 4 (Section 4.1.6), governance, policy, and standards are one of six cross-cutting enablers—alongside digital health strategy, digital health skills, research and development, the healthtech ecosystem, regional coordination and financing—that shape all five foundation layers of the technology stack.

Reference use cases define the specific clinical and administrative scenarios in which data exchange is implemented. Rather than attempting to exchange all data for all purposes at once, successful HIE implementations start with a small set of high-value use cases and expand incrementally. The most common initial use cases include patient summary exchange (a concise summary of a patient's key clinical information shared among providers), electronic prescribing and dispensing, laboratory result exchange, diagnostic imaging sharing, referral and counter-referral communication, and discharge summary exchange (WHO, 2023; European Commission, 2022).

Vendor certification and conformance ensure that electronic health record systems, laboratory information systems, and other point-of-service applications used by health facilities can connect to and exchange data through the national interoperability architecture. This component includes developing conformance testing tools, establishing certification programs for health IT products, and implementing compliance monitoring to ensure ongoing adherence to interoperability standards (IHE, 2024).

9.3 Africa's Health Information Exchange Landscape

9.3.1 Current State

Africa's HIE landscape is marked by significant policy ambition and substantial implementation gaps. A 2023 systematic review of HIE policy and standards across African digital health systems found that many countries had outlined HIE development initiatives in their strategic documents and proposed adopting interoperability architectures and standards, yet implementation remained fragmented and largely donor-driven (Abegaz et al., 2023). A 2025 scoping review confirmed persistent challenges, including limited technical capacity, fragmented infrastructure, and inadequate regulatory support, while noting encouraging developments, such as the use of OpenHIE, alignment with the African Union Digital Health Strategy, and growing public-private partnerships (Kgasi et al., 2025).

Rwanda is Africa's most mature HIE implementation. The national health information exchange links the OpenMRS-based EMR system, deployed across all 502 public health facilities, with laboratory, pharmacy, and community-based health insurance systems, enabling longitudinal patient records and cross-facility care coordination. Rwanda's success reflects a combination of strong governance, a small geographic scale, comprehensive EMR deployment, and sustained investment over more than a decade (Rwanda Biomedical Center, 2022).

South Africa's Western Cape Province operates one of the continent's most sophisticated health data linkage environments through the Provincial Health Data Center (PHDC), which integrates data from multiple health information systems using a stepwise, deterministic record-linkage approach. Although not a real-time HIE in the traditional sense, the PHDC demonstrates the analytical value of linked health data and offers a model for population-level health intelligence that other provinces and countries aim to replicate (Boulle et al., 2023).

Kenya is developing a national shared health record based on FHIR standards, with the Community Health Toolkit (CHT) serving as a major data source from community health workers. In 2024, Kenya's Ministry of Health adopted the CHT for national scale, enabling bidirectional data exchange between community-level systems and the national shared health record through the OpenHIE architecture and FHIR resources (Medic, 2024). Kenya is also developing a FHIR-based client registry as the single source of truth for patient identity, representing one of the most standards-aligned HIE implementations on the continent.

Ethiopia's eHealth architecture defines syntactic and semantic standards, including ICD-10, LOINC, RxNorm, and SNOMED, along with shared services such as a health worker registry, a master facility registry, and a national health data dictionary. The architecture provides a comprehensive blueprint, though implementation across the country's decentralized health system remains at different stages (Federal Ministry of Health, Ethiopia, 2018).

Nigeria's Digital Health Services Bill 2025 mandates that all digital health platforms be compatible with the country's EHR infrastructure, marking a legislative push for interoperability. The African Union's HIE Guidelines, which Nigeria is adopting, set technical standards for health data sharing that align with the Malabo Convention on Cybersecurity and Personal Data Protection (Tech in Africa, 2026).

At the continental level, two major initiatives are shaping the future of interoperability in Africa. The Smart Africa Alliance Digital Health Blueprint (2024), championed by Rwanda and Africa CDC, provides a roadmap for a "single digital health market" across Africa, with detailed specifications for patient identity, key registries, semantic interoperability, consent management, and data integration (Smart Africa, 2024). The HELINA-led "Africa on FHIR" initiative, in collaboration with Africa CDC, HL7 International, and WHO, aims to scale the adoption of HL7 FHIR across the continent through capacity building, conformance testing, and the establishment of the Africa Standards and Interoperability Lab (SIL-Africa), hosted in Rwanda (HELINA, 2025).

9.3.2 Common Challenges

Several structural challenges constrain HIE development across Africa.

- First, the proliferation of vertical, program-specific information systems—separate systems for HIV, tuberculosis, malaria, immunization, and maternal health—creates data silos that are difficult to integrate across programs.

- Second, the limited adoption of common data standards means that even when systems exist, they often cannot exchange data because they use incompatible formats and terminology.

- Third, the shortage of health informatics professionals with the technical skills to implement and maintain interoperability infrastructure is a critical human capacity constraint.

- Fourth, the lack of comprehensive data protection legislation in many countries creates legal uncertainty regarding health data sharing.

- Fifth, the donor-driven nature of many digital health investments has led to fragmented implementations optimized for specific programs rather than integrated into national architectures (Abegaz et al., 2023; Kgasi et al., 2025).

9.4 Global HIE Models and Their Transferability to Africa

Global experience identifies four principal platform models for health information exchange, as illustrated in Figure 9.2. Each model reflects distinct governance structures, infrastructure conditions, and historical trajectories and offers transferable lessons for African health systems.

Figure 9.2. Global Platform Models for Health Information Exchange

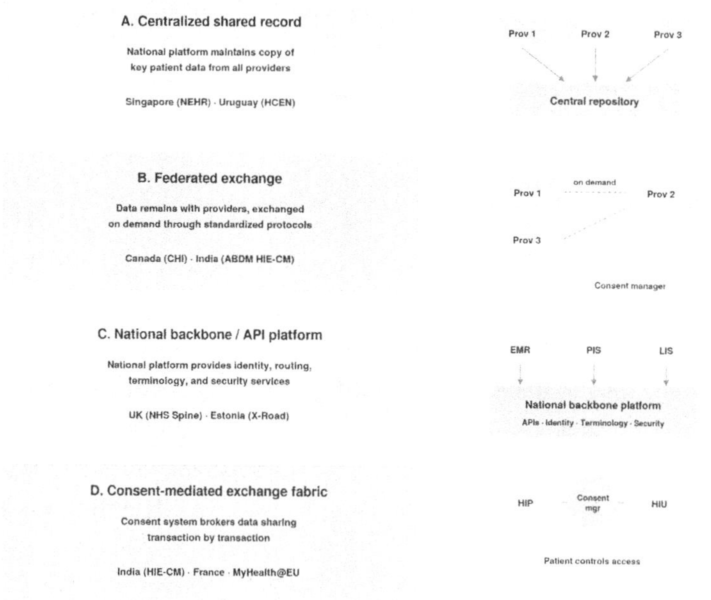

Source: Author's Synthesis based on Country Report and WHO/OpenHIE Frameworks

9.4.1 Centralized Shared Record Model

In this model, a national platform stores and provides access to key patient data contributed by providers. Singapore's National Electronic Health Record (NEHR) is the strongest example: it serves as a national repository for clinical information, and recent legislation under the Health Information Bill framework requires licensed providers to contribute data. Uruguay's Historia Clinica Electronica Nacional (HCEN) is the leading Latin American example: it enables secure access to clinical information across providers, and more than 90% of users have at least one clinical document on the platform. Uruguay also emphasizes terminology services for semantic interoperability, making it one of the clearest examples of a national exchange platform with strong interoperability governance (Government of Uruguay, 2023; Ministry of Health Singapore, 2024).

Transferability to Africa: The centralized model is feasible for countries with strong governance, compact geography, and high connectivity—conditions that Rwanda and potentially smaller African countries, such as Mauritius or Cabo Verde, may meet. For larger, more diverse countries, the infrastructure and governance requirements for maintaining a centralized repository may be prohibitive.

9.4.2 Federated Exchange Model

In this model, data remains with source providers and is exchanged on demand via standardized protocols. Canada exemplifies this approach: there is no single national HIE platform, and Canada Health Infoway has advanced common building blocks, including the pan-Canadian Patient Summary (PS-CA) and the pan-Canadian FHIR Exchange (CA: FeX). Provincial and territorial systems remain in place but are made interoperable through shared specifications, registries, and exchange patterns (Canada Health Infoway, 2024).

India's Ayushman Bharat Digital Mission (ABDM) has built one of the clearest consent-based federated HIE models through its Health Information Exchange and Consent Manager (HIE-CM). This is not a single national repository but a national exchange fabric composed of identities, registries, and consent-mediated data flows. The HIE-CM enables patients to control which providers can access their health records, with consent managed on a transaction-by-transaction basis (Sharma et al., 2023; Balsari et al., 2024).

Transferability to Africa: The federated model is particularly relevant for large, decentralized African countries such as Nigeria, South Africa, Ethiopia, and Kenya, where provincial or state-level health systems operate with considerable autonomy. Canada's experience shows that interoperability can advance without a single centralized national EHR—what matters is agreement on common content, FHIR exchange methods, and connected-care workflows across jurisdictions. India's consent-mediated model is relevant in contexts where patient trust in data sharing requires explicit, granular consent mechanisms.

9.4.3 National Backbone and API Platform Model

In this model, a national platform provides identity, routing, terminology, and security services that enable other systems to exchange data. England's NHS Spine is the clearest example: it is not just a record repository but a national platform for APIs, messaging, identity, and exchange services. Estonia's X-Road, discussed extensively in Chapters 4 and 8, provides similar backbone services for the entire digital government ecosystem, including health (NHS England, 2024; e-Estonia, 2025).

Transferability to Africa: The backbone model is attractive because it does not require replacing existing systems; instead, it provides the middleware and services that enable them to interoperate. Countries that have already deployed DHIS2, OpenMRS, and other systems could benefit from a backbone platform that connects these existing investments through shared identity, terminology, and routing services. The OpenHIM Platform, developed by Jembi in South Africa, provides exactly this kind of middleware for low- and middle-income country health systems, implementing the OpenHIE specification with FHIR-based exchange, patient matching, and data warehousing capabilities (Jembi, 2024).

9.4.4 Consent-Mediated Exchange Fabric

In this model, a consent management system brokers data-sharing transactions on a per-transaction basis, with patients controlling who can access their data and for what purpose. India's HIE-CM is the primary example. France's digital health approach integrates consent and identity services as core components of its national interoperability framework (PAHO, 2024).

Transferability to Africa: Consent-mediated exchange is increasingly important as African countries develop data protection legislation that requires explicit patient consent for health data sharing. The model aligns well with the African Union's emphasis on data sovereignty and individual rights, though implementation requires robust digital identity infrastructure (Layer 2) and connectivity (Layer 1) to manage consent transactions in real time.

9.4.5 Regional and Cross-Border Exchange

Beyond national HIEs, regional exchange mechanisms are emerging and offering models to meet Africa's cross-border health data needs. The EU's MyHealth@EU supports cross-border Patient Summary and ePrescription services, connecting national HIEs through common EU rules and services rather than requiring a single EU-wide system. In Latin America, PAHO's Pan-American Highway for Digital Health is positioned as a regional initiative to support connected health and continuity of care across more than 20 countries. Chile's 2024 law on clinical record interoperability illustrates how legal mandates can drive interoperability at the national level (European Commission, 2022; PAHO, 2024).

Australia is transitioning from its My Health Record (a national shared summary record) to Health Connect Australia, a broader national HIE program that enables secure information sharing among healthcare participants. This evolution from a centralized, document-oriented approach to a hybrid model that combines a national summary record with a broader API-based interoperability architecture is a path many countries, including those in Africa, are likely to follow (Australian Digital Health Agency, 2024).

Across Africa, the East African Community's Digital Regional East Africa Community Health Initiative has recommended shared digital health standards to enable cross-border healthcare, including regional principles for data sharing, system interoperability, and digital tool design. The African Union's HIE Guidelines and the Smart Africa Digital Health Blueprint provide the continental governance framework for developing such regional exchange (Smart Africa, 2024).

9.5 A Strategic Framework for African HIE Development

Drawing on the global evidence reviewed in this chapter, the following strategic framework is proposed for building Layer 3 of the digital health technology stack across African countries.

The model proposes a progressive, standards-based approach to building interoperable digital health ecosystems, moving from foundational readiness to scaled implementation and regional integration. In the early phase (Years 1–2), the focus should be on establishing foundational standards and governance frameworks. Countries should adopt HL7 FHIR as the national exchange standard, alongside globally recognized terminologies such as ICD-11, LOINC, and SNOMED CT to ensure semantic and syntactic interoperability. At the same time, enabling institutions should be established through data protection legislation, consent frameworks, and the creation of a national HIE governance body, drawing on global models such as the EU's European Health Data Space and India's HIE-CM. Parallel investments in trust services, including Master Patient Indexes (MPI) and health worker and facility registries, ensure reliable identity management—an essential prerequisite for secure data exchange.

In the intermediate phase (Years 2–4), attention should shift toward operationalization and service delivery. Countries are expected to deploy interoperability middleware platforms, such as OpenHIM, that align with the OpenHIE architecture to enable real-time data exchange across systems. This phase prioritizes high-impact use cases, starting with patient summaries, e-prescriptions, and laboratory results, and gradually expanding to referrals, imaging, and discharge summaries. These use cases are selected to demonstrate immediate value in clinical care and system efficiency while building confidence in digital health systems. The roadmap emphasizes learning from global and regional experiences—such as EU MyHealth@EU and Uruguay's national HIE—to ensure that implementation is practical and scalable.

In the advanced phase (Years 3–5 and beyond), the focus should shift toward system maturity, ecosystem alignment, and sustainability. This includes establishing vendor conformance frameworks and requiring compliance with interoperability standards (particularly FHIR) for all health IT procurement to prevent fragmentation and vendor lock-in. Countries are also encouraged to align with regional interoperability initiatives, such as the AU HIE Guidelines and the Smart Africa frameworks, enabling cross-border health data exchange through Regional Economic Communities. Finally, sustained capacity building—through training in FHIR, interoperability architecture, and governance—ensures that the health workforce and institutions can manage and evolve the system over time.

Table 9.1 Strategic Framework for Health Information Exchange Development in Africa

Component	Priority Actions	Global Models	Timeframe
Standards adoption	Adopt HL7 FHIR as national exchange standard; adopt ICD-11, LOINC, SNOMED CT for terminology	WHO SMART Africa Guidelines on FHIR	Year 1-2
HIE platform	Deploy OpenHIM or equivalent as national interoperability middleware	OpenHIE, Jembi, Kenya	Year 2-3
Trust services	Connect to MPI (Chapter 8), health worker and facility registries	OpenHIE, Australia IHI	Year 1-3
Governance	Enact data protection legislation; establish consent frameworks; create national HIE governance body	EU EHDS, India HIE-CM	Year 1-2
Use cases	Begin with patient summary, e-prescription, lab results; expand to referrals, imaging, discharge	EU MyHealth@EU, Uruguay HCEN	Year 2-4
Vendor conformance	Establish national conformance testing; require FHIR compliance for health IT procurement	SIL-Africa, HELINA	Year 3-5
Regional exchange	Align with AU HIE Guidelines and Smart Africa Blueprint; develop cross-border exchange with regional economic communities	EU MyHealth@EU, PAHO Pan-American Highway	Year 3-5
Capacity building	Train health informatics workforce in FHIR, interoperability architecture, and HIE governance	Africa on FHIR, HELINA DHALP	Ongoing

Note. Timeframes are indicative and will vary by country context.

Sequencing matters. The global evidence is consistent on one critical point: countries should build the national interoperability architecture first and deploy individual applications second. The temptation to deploy EMRs, telemedicine platforms, and surveillance dashboards without first establishing the identity services, data standards, and exchange infrastructure that connect them leads to the proliferation of digital silos that are expensive and difficult to integrate. As the broad best practice emerging from every region reviewed in this chapter confirms, the strongest HIE strategies combine common standards, shared identity and registry services, API-based exchange, legal mandates, and a few high-value exchange use cases. The exact platform may be centralized, federated, or hybrid, but the winning pattern is the same—national interoperability architecture first, individual applications second.

9.6 Conclusion

Layer 3 of the digital health technology stack—the Interoperability and Data Exchange Layer—transforms a collection of isolated digital health tools into a connected health information ecosystem. Without interoperability, the EMRs examined in Chapter 3, the applications categorized in Chapter 4, and the identity infrastructure built in Chapter 8 cannot deliver their full value. The clinical, surveillance, administrative, and financial data generated across the health system remain trapped in silos, inaccessible to the clinicians, managers, and policymakers who need them most.

The global evidence reviewed in this chapter demonstrates that interoperability is not a product to be purchased but an architecture to be built—comprising standards, trust services, governance frameworks, reference use cases, and vendor conformance, all developed incrementally and governed continuously. Africa's path forward requires embracing FHIR as the continental exchange standard, deploying open-source interoperability middleware such as OpenHIM, establishing governed registries for patients, health workers, and facilities, and starting with high-value exchange use cases that deliver immediate clinical benefit. The continental initiatives already underway—the Smart Africa Digital Health Blueprint, the Africa on FHIR initiative, and the AU HIE Guidelines—provide the policy and technical foundations for country-level implementation.

References

Abegaz, T. M., Berhie, A. Y., & Tilahun, B. C. (2023). Health information exchange policy and standards for digital health systems in Africa: A systematic review. PLOS Digital Health, 2(2), e0000118. https://doi.org/10.1371/journal.pdig.0000118

Australian Digital Health Agency. (2024). Health Connect Australia: National health information exchange program. Australian Digital Health Agency.

Balsari, S., Sesia, P., & Patnaik, S. (2024). India's evolving digital health strategy. npj Digital Medicine, 7, Article 285. https://doi.org/10.1038/s41746-024-01279-2

Boulle, A., Heekes, A., Tiffin, N., Smith, M., van de Merwe, L., & Fox, M. P. (2023). Record linkage for routinely collected health data in an African health information exchange. International Journal of Population Data Science, 8(1), 1771. https://doi.org/10.23889/ijpds.v8i1.1771

Canada Health Infoway. (2024). Interoperability: Shared Pan-Canadian Interoperability Roadmap. Canada Health Infoway.

e-Estonia. (2025). X-Road: Secure data exchange layer. e-Estonia.

European Commission. (2022). Proposal for a regulation on the European Health Data Space. COM(2022) 197 final.

Federal Ministry of Health Ethiopia. (2018). Information Revolution Strategic Plan (2018–2025). Federal Democratic Republic of Ethiopia.

Government of Uruguay. (2023). Historia Clinica Electronica Nacional: Platform report. Ministerio de Salud Publica.

HELINA. (2025). Africa on FHIR and SIL-Africa: Capacity building for interoperability across the continent. Health Informatics in Africa.

HIMSS. (2024). Interoperability in healthcare: Definition and framework. Healthcare Information and Management Systems Society.

HL7 International. (2024). FHIR Release 5: Fast Healthcare Interoperability Resources specification. Health Level Seven International.

IHE. (2024). IT Infrastructure Technical Framework: Interoperability profiles for health information exchange. Integrating the Healthcare Enterprise.

Jembi. (2024). OpenHIM Platform: Streamlining health information exchange for low- and middle-income countries. Jembi Health Systems.

Kgasi, M., Ochieng, B., & Katurura, M. (2025). Adoption, barriers and opportunities of interoperability and eHealth standards in Africa: A scoping review. BMJ Health and Care Informatics, 32(1), e101210.

Medic. (2024). Revolutionizing healthcare in Kenya and Nepal: Standardizing data exchange for optimal delivery. OpenHIE Impact Stories.

Ministry of Health Singapore. (2024). Health Information Bill: National Electronic Health Record contribution requirements. Ministry of Health, Republic of Singapore.

NHS England. (2024). NHS Spine: National platform for APIs, messaging, and identity services. National Health Service England.

OpenHIE. (2024). OpenHIE architecture specification: Core components. Open Health Information Exchange.

PAHO. (2024). Pan-American Highway for Digital Health: Regional interoperability initiative. Pan American Health Organization.

Rwanda Biomedical Center. (2022). National Health Information Exchange: Implementation and impact report. RBC.

Sharma, R. S., Rohatgi, A., Jain, S., & Singh, D. (2023). The Ayushman Bharat Digital Mission (ABDM): Making of India's digital health story. CSI Transactions on ICT, 11, 3–9. https://doi.org/10.1007/s40012-023-00375-0

Smart Africa. (2024). Smart Africa Alliance Digital Health Blueprint. Smart Africa Secretariat / Africa CDC.

Tech in Africa. (2026). Healthtech regulation 2025: AU HIE guidelines and Nigeria Digital Health Services Bill. Tech in Africa.

WHO. (2023). Classification of digital interventions, services and applications in health (2nd ed.). World Health Organization.

Chapter 10 Data Management, Quality, and Analytics

10.1 Introduction: Data as the Currency of Digital Health

Data is the essential foundation of a functioning health system. Without dependable, timely, and interoperable health data, the full potential of digital technologies cannot be realized. The connectivity infrastructure of Layer 1, the identity registries of Layer 2, and the interoperability platforms of Layer 3 all serve one main purpose: to generate, transmit, store, and make accessible data that enables better health decisions—at the bedside, in the district office, at the national planning table, and across continental surveillance networks.

This chapter examines Layer 4 of the digital health technology stack introduced in Chapter 4 (Section 4.1.4): the Data Management and Analytics Layer, one of the stack's five foundational layers. As shown in Figure 10.3, this layer includes data warehouses and data lakes for structured storage, analytics engines for business intelligence and performance monitoring, and AI/ML platforms for predictive modeling and clinical decision support. Layer 4 transforms raw data from the Interoperability Layer (Layer 3, Chapter 9) into actionable insights that inform the applications and services in Layer 5 (Chapters 3 and 4).

The chapter also explores Africa's health data landscape and situates African progress within the context of global best practices from Europe, Asia, Latin America, Australia, Canada, New Zealand, and the Caribbean. It analyzes data availability and collection systems, data quality across five dimensions, health data standards and their adoption, data governance frameworks, and financing for sustainable health data ecosystems.

Figure 10.1. Architecture of the Data Management and Analytics Layer

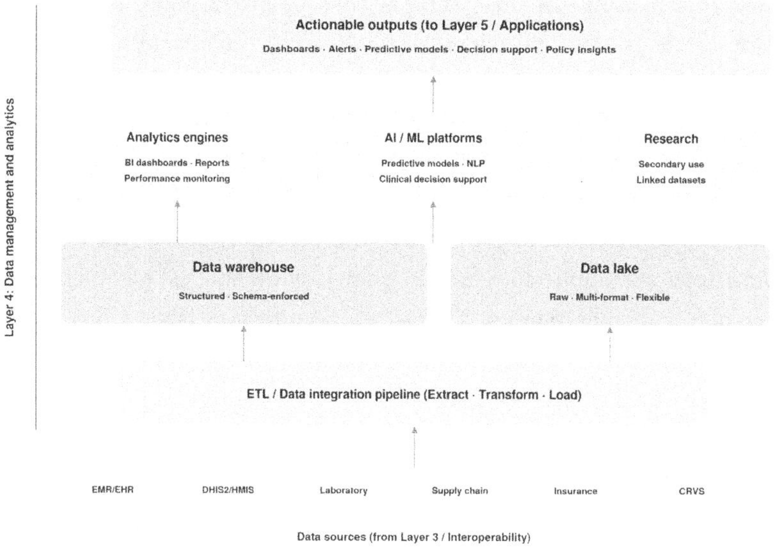

Source: Adapted from WHO (2023) and the Author's Elaboration

10.2 The Health Data Landscape in Africa

10.2.1 A Paradox of Innovation and Deficit

Africa's health data landscape is marked by a paradox. The continent has led the way in adopting open-source health information systems, particularly the District Health Information Software 2 (DHIS2), which is now used in more than 47 African countries, covering more than 1.4 billion people, making Africa the global leader in DHIS2 adoption (HISP, 2023). Community health information systems have grown significantly. Mobile data collection platforms—including ODK, KoBoToolbox, and CommCare—have enabled real-time data collection in settings that previously relied on paper-based registers.

At the same time, significant gaps remain. The WHO (2022) estimates that fewer than half of births and deaths in Africa are officially registered, creating a major gap in vital statistics. Only 31 of 54 African countries have civil registration systems capable of producing useful mortality statistics, and fewer than a third report cause-of-death data of sufficient quality for national planning. This lack of data has serious consequences: populations whose births are not registered and whose deaths leave no data trail are excluded from the health systems meant to serve them.

The fragmentation of data systems compounds these structural deficits. A single patient may have data recorded across multiple non-interoperable systems—such as an EMR for HIV treatment, a paper register for antenatal care, and a separate mobile app for community follow-up—all of which fail to communicate with one another. This siloed architecture creates duplication and inefficiency, undermining the longitudinal patient data essential for continuity of care (Vital Wave, 2021).

10.2.2 The Urban–Rural Data Divide

The urban–rural divide in health data availability reflects deeper inequalities in infrastructure and staffing. A 2021 survey across six sub-Saharan African countries found that 78% of urban health facilities had an electronic data system, compared with just 32% of rural facilities. Completeness of monthly facility reporting was about 40 percentage points higher in urban areas (PATH, 2021). These disparities cause national aggregate data to systematically underrepresent the health status of rural populations, leading to skewed resource allocation away from the communities most in need.

Comparative experience highlights both the challenges and opportunities. In the European Union, health data reporting completeness exceeds 90% in virtually all member states. Brazil's SUS health information system covers more than 85% of the population nationwide, supported by a constitutional mandate for health data transparency and the integration of community health agent reporting into the national HMIS. Thailand's Health Data Center (HDC) platform achieves 98% coverage across public-sector facilities. Australia's My Health Record system, with over 23 million registered individuals, demonstrates that near-universal participation in national health data systems is achievable when enrollment is opt-out rather than opt-in—a policy choice that increased coverage from under 20% to over 90% within two years of implementation (Australian Digital Health Agency, 2024). In New Zealand, the National Health Index assigns a unique identifier to every person who uses health and disability services, enabling near-complete longitudinal data linkage across a population of five million (Ministry of Health New Zealand, 2024).

10.3 Data Quality Across Five Dimensions

Data quality in health systems is conventionally assessed across five principal dimensions: completeness, accuracy, timeliness, consistency, and interoperability. Each presents distinct challenges in the African context, and deficits in one dimension frequently cascade into others.

Table 10.1 Core Dimensions of Health Data Quality and Their Status in African Health Systems

Dimension	Definition	African Status
Completeness	All required data fields populated	Low in Central/West Africa; higher in vertical programs with dedicated funding
Accuracy	Data correctly represents actual health events	Compromised by manual transcription errors; 13–55% discrepancy rates between registers and DHIS2
Timeliness	Data available when needed for decisions	Median 47-day lag from facility to national level; COVID-19 catalyzed innovation
Consistency	Data coherent across sources and time	Fragmented vertical programs create inconsistent denominators and double-counting
Interoperability	Data exchangeable across systems	Most challenging: fewer than 10% of countries have functional HIE platforms

Completeness remains a foundational challenge. At the facility level, incompleteness stems from high clinical workloads, insufficient training, poorly designed tools with an excessive number of data elements, and inadequate supervisory feedback. Ghana's experience illustrates a positive trajectory: automated validation rules in DHIS2 reduced the share of incomplete monthly reports from 35% to under 15% within two years (Bhattacharya et al., 2019). Canada's Canadian Institute for Health Information (CIHI) achieves near-complete hospital discharge data through mandatory reporting requirements tied to provincial funding—demonstrating that linking data reporting to health system financing can drive completeness (CIHI, 2024).

Manual transcription from paper to digital systems compromises accuracy. Studies across multiple African countries have documented discrepancy rates between source registers and DHIS2 entries for key indicators ranging from 13% to 55% (Wagenaar et al., 2016). India's ABDM incorporates more than 200 automated validation checks that flag anomalies before data is accepted, dramatically reducing downstream quality issues (National Health Authority India, 2022). New Zealand's National Minimum Dataset uses automated matching algorithms to compare data against the National Health Index, verifying and correcting demographic inconsistencies at the point of submission (Ministry of Health New Zealand, 2024).

Timeliness is critical for surveillance and outbreak response. In Africa, the median time from facility-level data collection to national availability is 47 days (WHO Africa, 2022). The EU's European Surveillance System (TESSy) requires near-real-time reporting of notifiable diseases across all 27 member states. The Caribbean Public Health Agency (CARPHA) operates a regional event-based surveillance system that provides 24-hour notification of priority conditions across 24 Caribbean states and territories, demonstrating that even small, resource-constrained health systems can achieve rapid reporting when regional infrastructure pools technical capacity (CARPHA, 2023).

Consistency is undermined by fragmented program architectures with different denominators and coding practices. Population denominator data pose specific challenges: many African countries conduct censuses infrequently and lack the capacity for intercensal projections. Australia manages this through the Australian Bureau of Statistics' Estimated Resident Population, updated quarterly with birth, death, and migration data, providing health systems with reliable, current denominators for coverage calculations (ABS, 2024).

Interoperability remains the most challenging dimension globally. As detailed in Chapter 9, fewer than 10% of African countries have operational health information exchange systems. The standards landscape is presented in Section 10.4 below.

10.4 Health Data Standards and Their Adoption in Africa

Health data standards are the common languages that enable different systems to exchange and interpret data consistently. Without shared standards, digital health systems become isolated silos incapable of generating the population-level insights that justify their development costs.

Table 10.2 Health Data Standards Adoption Across Africa

Standard	Description	Africa Adoption	Global Benchmark
ADX/DHIS2	Aggregate data exchange via DHIS2	~85% (45+ countries)	Africa leads globally
ICD-10/11	Diagnosis and mortality coding	~58%	EU ~95%; ICD-11 transition underway
OpenHIE	Open architecture for HIE	~42%	Africa leads globally
HL7 v2	Legacy hospital messaging	~35%	Widely deployed globally
HL7 FHIR	Modern API-based exchange	~8%	EU, US, Australia >60%
LOINC	Laboratory observation codes	~5%	US, EU, Brazil >70%
SNOMED CT	Clinical terminology	~3%	Mandatory in EU, US, Australia

Africa's standards landscape reveals a striking pattern: the continent leads globally in adopting standards for resource-constrained settings (ADX/DHIS2 at 85%, OpenHIE at 42%) but trails significantly in clinical interoperability standards (FHIR at 8%, SNOMED CT at 3%) that are increasingly required for patient-level data exchange (Kgasi et al., 2025). This pattern reflects both the success of aggregate reporting infrastructure and the gap in individual-level clinical data exchange capabilities.

Figure 10.2. Health Data Standards Adoption Rates Across Africa

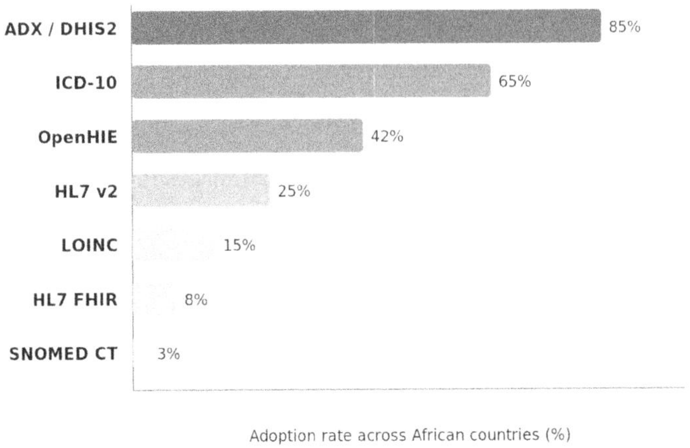

Source: Author's estimates based on WHO (2023) and Kgasi et al. (2025)

The HELINA-led "Africa on FHIR" initiative, in collaboration with Africa CDC, HL7 International, and WHO, aims to bridge this gap through continental capacity building, conformance testing, and the establishment of the Africa Standards and Interoperability Lab (SIL-Africa) in Rwanda (HELINA, 2025). Kenya's FHIR sandbox environment and South Africa's HAPI FHIR server pilot mark important country-level milestones.

The transition to ICD-11 presents both opportunities and challenges. ICD-11 features a digital-first architecture and expanded codes for conditions prevalent in low- and middle-income countries. However, fewer than 15% of African countries have begun formal transition planning, compared with over 60% in Europe. In 2023, Jamaica completed ICD-11 implementation across all public hospitals through a centralized task force and alignment with CARPHA's regional initiative, serving as a model for phased regional transition (WHO, 2022).

10.5 DHIS2 and Data Analytics

DHIS2 is one of the most significant achievements in Africa's digital health and data analytics movement. Originally piloted in South Africa in the mid-1990s, it has since become the standard HMIS for more than 47 African countries. DHIS2 enables aggregate data collection, supports dashboards and analytics, and increasingly provides tracker features for individual-level longitudinal data. During the COVID-19 pandemic, DHIS2 was adapted for contact tracing and case monitoring across more than 30 African countries, demonstrating both its flexibility and the institutional trust governments place in it (HISP, 2023).

Despite these achievements, reporting rates remain below 80% in many countries, and data accuracy relative to source registers ranges from 45% to 87%, closely tied to the intensity of data quality initiatives, the availability of trained data clerks, and the strength of supervisory feedback (Wagenaar et al., 2016). Closing the gap between DHIS2 deployment and reliable data production requires sustained investment in workforce capacity, connectivity, and quality improvement.

10.6 Global Experiences in Health Data Management

The European Health Data Space (EHDS), the most ambitious regional health data governance framework to date, provides a model for the structured secondary use of health data. Its core distinction between primary use (patients accessing their own records across borders) and secondary use (researchers accessing de-identified data through national data access bodies with ethical review) offers a governance architecture that African countries could adopt. The EHDS mandates HL7 FHIR R4 for cross-border exchange, promoting harmonization across 27 diverse national health systems (European Commission, 2022).

Brazil's Rede Nacional de Dados em Saude (RNDS), launched under the Lei Geral de Protecao de Dados (LGPD), establishes a federated health information exchange using HL7 FHIR R4. Patients access their electronic health summaries via the Meu DigiSUS application, and providers query records across facilities via the RNDS API. Brazil's experience shows that FHIR-based data management is feasible in a large, federated, resource-constrained system serving over 200 million people—a model directly applicable to Nigeria, Ethiopia, or the DRC (PAHO, 2021).

India's ABDM established a federated consent architecture through the Health Information User/Health Information Provider model, giving patients control over who can access their records via a personal data locker. By 2024, more than 568 million ABHA identifiers had been issued, and over 200,000 facilities had registered with the national health facility registry. The consent management framework is viewed as a model for low- and middle-income countries seeking to balance open data for public health with individual privacy (Sharma et al., 2023; Balsari et al., 2024).

Thailand's Health Data Center (HDC), integrated with the National Health Security Office claims database, has achieved near-universal coverage of public-sector facilities. The HDC aggregates data via HL7 messaging and provides near-real-time analytics for surveillance, quality monitoring, and resource allocation. South Korea's national health insurance claims database—covering virtually the entire population through mandatory universal coverage—enables population-scale analytics for utilization, quality, and cost management, a level few countries achieve (OECD, 2023). The ASEAN Digital Health Framework provides a regional architecture for health data exchange that balances national sovereignty with cross-border utility (WHO, 2021).

Australia's approach combines the My Health Record national shared summary with an increasingly sophisticated analytics infrastructure. The Australian Institute of Health and Welfare (AIHW) operates one of the world's most comprehensive health data linkage environments, connecting hospital records, primary care data, pharmaceutical benefits data, and mortality data through privacy-preserving linkage methods that enable population-level analytics without exposing individual records (AIHW, 2024).

New Zealand's health data system is based on the National Health Index (NHI), which assigns a unique identifier to each person using health services. The NHI enables linkage across primary care, hospital, pharmaceutical, and laboratory datasets, as well as mortality data, creating one of the most comprehensive longitudinal health data environments for the entire population. New Zealand's Integrated Data Infrastructure (IDI) expands health data linking to education, social services, and justice datasets, enabling whole-of-government analytics for health equity and research on social determinants (Statistics New Zealand, 2024).

The Caribbean Public Health Agency, which serves 24 Caribbean states and territories, has created a regional health information system that integrates national data into a unified surveillance and analytics platform. CARPHA's eHealth Caribbean Initiative has facilitated ICD-11 adoption, strengthened regional disease surveillance, and standardized health workforce data. The collaborative model—pooling technical capacity at the regional level to support national functions that individual small states cannot afford independently—offers a directly applicable model for Africa's smaller states in West and Central Africa (CARPHA, 2023).

10.7 Data Warehousing and Data Lakes for Health

Transforming raw health data into actionable intelligence requires purpose-built storage and processing infrastructure. While transactional systems such as DHIS2 and OpenMRS are optimized for data capture and operational reporting, they are not designed to support the complex, cross-system analytical queries required for population health management, epidemiological research, and health system performance monitoring. This is where data warehouses and data lakes play a critical role in Layer 4 of the technology stack.

A health data warehouse is a structured repository that consolidates data from multiple source systems—such as EMRs, HMIS, laboratory and pharmacy systems, insurance claims, and civil registration—into a unified, consistent schema optimized for analytical queries. Data warehouses ensure data quality through extract-transform-load (ETL) processes that clean, standardize, and validate data before it enters the repository. South Africa's Western Cape Provincial Health Data Center (PHDC) exemplifies this approach in Africa: it integrates data from more than 15 health information systems into a unified analytical environment that supports population-level epidemiological analysis, care cascade monitoring for HIV and tuberculosis, and health system performance benchmarking (Boulle et al., 2023).

A data lake, in contrast, stores raw data in its original format—structured, semi-structured, and unstructured—without requiring predefined schemas. Data lakes are particularly valuable for health systems that need to integrate diverse data types, including clinical text, medical images, genomic sequences, and sensor data from IoMT devices (see Chapter 3, Section 3.6). The flexibility of data lakes comes with increased analytical complexity: data must be transformed at query time rather than at the point of storage, which requires more advanced analytical tools and technical expertise.

In practice, most advanced health data architectures use a hybrid approach. Australia's AIHW operates a data linkage environment that combines the schema enforcement of a data warehouse for core administrative datasets (hospital separations, Medicare claims, and pharmaceutical benefits) with the flexibility of a data lake for research datasets integrating genomic, environmental, and social determinants data (AIHW, 2024). Canada's CIHI maintains standardized data holdings for hospital and primary care data while supporting linked research datasets that incorporate non-traditional data sources (CIHI, 2024). India's ABDM architecture envisions a federated data lake approach in which data remains with source providers but can be accessed through standardized APIs with patient consent, thereby avoiding the need for a centralized national data repository (Sharma et al., 2023).

In Africa, the OpenHIM Platform, developed by Jembi, provides an open-source solution for health data warehousing. The platform uses ClickHouse for data warehousing and Grafana for analytics dashboards, and it integrates with the HAPI FHIR server for standards-based data storage and exchange. This architecture enables countries to build analytical capabilities on top of their existing transactional systems without replacing them, offering a practical pathway from data collection to data intelligence (Jembi, 2024).

Key considerations for African health data warehousing include data sovereignty, which involves deciding whether data is stored on local servers or in international cloud environments; privacy-preserving linkage methods that enable population-level analysis without exposing individual records; the technical capacity to maintain ETL pipelines and ensure data quality; and governance structures to control data access for different user communities—from clinicians and program managers to researchers and policymakers.

10.8 Analytics Engines and Business Intelligence

Analytics engines transform stored data into insights through dashboards, statistical analysis, performance monitoring, and data visualization. In the health sector, analytics serves three primary functions: operational analytics for real-time monitoring of service delivery; tactical analytics for program management and resource allocation; and strategic analytics for policy formulation and health system planning.

DHIS2 is the most widely used health analytics platform in Africa, featuring built-in dashboards, pivot tables, data visualization tools, and GIS mapping capabilities. DHIS2 analytics support routine monitoring of health indicators at the facility, district, and national levels, and the platform has been adapted for specialized analytical applications, including vaccine coverage tracking, disease surveillance, and supply chain monitoring. The platform's accessibility—requiring only a web browser and an Internet connection—makes it a practical entry point for health analytics in most African settings (HISP, 2023).

Beyond DHIS2's built-in analytics, countries are increasingly adopting dedicated business intelligence (BI) platforms to address more sophisticated analytical needs. Rwanda's Health Information Exchange integrates DHIS2 data with EMR, insurance, and supply chain data to generate cross-system analytics that would not be possible from any single source system. Kenya's eCHIS (electronic Community Health Information System) creates dashboards that combine community health worker reporting data with facility-level indicators, enabling integrated analysis of community- and facility-based service delivery.

Globally, Thailand's Health Data Center (HDC) demonstrates the potential of an integrated analytics platform. The HDC collects data from hospital information systems nationwide via HL7 messaging, generating near-real-time analytics for disease surveillance, service quality monitoring, and resource allocation. The platform achieves 98% reporting completeness across public-sector facilities because analytics outputs are directly linked to facility performance management and insurance reimbursement, creating a feedback loop in which data quality directly influences institutional incentives (WHO, 2021).

South Korea's national health insurance claims database underscores the value of comprehensive administrative data for health analytics. Because nearly the entire population is covered by mandatory national health insurance and claims are processed centrally, South Korea can compile and analyze population-scale datasets on utilization patterns, quality measurement, cost management, and outcomes research with a level of completeness and timeliness that few countries can match (OECD, 2023).

10.9 Predictive Analytics, Machine Learning, and AI for Health

Predictive analytics and machine learning represent the most advanced analytical capabilities in Layer 4, enabling health systems to shift from retrospective reporting to proactive, anticipatory decision-making. Although these capabilities remain in the early stages across most of Africa, several promising developments signal a growing role for AI-powered analytics in African health systems.

10.9.1 DHIS2 Climate Health Analytics Platform (CHAP)

One of the most significant recent developments in African health analytics is the DHIS2 Climate Health Analytics Platform (CHAP), developed through the DHIS2 Climate and Health project, coordinated by the HISP Center at the University of Oslo and funded by the Wellcome Trust. CHAP integrates weather and environmental data with routine health data already captured in national DHIS2 systems, enabling ministries of health to train machine learning models on their own data to predict sub-seasonal malaria, dengue, and other climate-sensitive disease incidence.

Since the project's inception in 2024, more than 10 countries have used CHAP to develop customized predictive models. In Togo, the National Malaria

Control Program used CHAP to analyze precipitation and temperature alongside malaria incidence data, identifying districts that required expanded seasonal malaria chemoprevention (SMC) campaigns in response to shifting climate patterns. The analysis showed that increasing SMC from four to five monthly cycles in three northern regions would yield the greatest health impact given changing rainfall patterns. Togo's Ministry of Health used this analysis to advocate for updated budget allocations from the Global Fund (DHIS2, 2025).

The CHAP platform is significant for three reasons. First, it integrates machine learning into the existing national health information system, eliminating the need for separate, externally managed platforms. Second, it enables national health teams to train, validate, and improve models using their routine data, promoting local ownership and sustainability. Third, it provides actionable outputs—district-level disease forecasts linked to specific programmatic interventions—rather than abstract statistical outputs that require specialized interpretation (HISP, 2024).

10.9.2 AI for Disease Diagnosis and Clinical Decision Support

As detailed in Chapter 3, AI-powered diagnostic tools have shown promising results in African health settings. The CAD4TB algorithm for tuberculosis screening from chest X-rays has been deployed across South Africa, Kenya, Tanzania, and other countries. AI-based retinal imaging for diabetic retinopathy screening has been piloted in Kenya and South Africa. These diagnostic AI applications operate within the Applications and Services Layer (Layer 5) but rely on Layer 4 for the data infrastructure that trains, validates, and monitors their performance.

The critical analytics challenge for clinical AI in Africa is the availability of high-quality, representative training data. Most clinical AI models are trained on datasets from high-income countries that may not generalize well to African populations, disease presentations, or imaging equipment. Therefore, building African health data warehouses and curated clinical datasets is not only valuable for retrospective analytics but essential for developing and validating AI tools that perform reliably in African clinical settings (Wahl et al., 2018; Africa CDC, 2024).

10.9.3 Predictive Analytics for Public Health Surveillance

Machine learning models are being used to predict disease outbreaks, optimize resource allocation, and inform public health interventions across Africa. During the COVID-19 pandemic, predictive models helped several African countries anticipate case surges and plan the deployment of healthcare resources. The Africa CDC incorporated AI-driven analytics into its continental surveillance platforms, and several countries deployed WhatsApp-based rapid reporting systems and USSD-based data capture, which dramatically accelerated data flows from peripheral facilities (Labrique et al., 2021).

The EU's European Surveillance System (TESSy) and the European Health Data Space offer models for embedding predictive analytics into routine surveillance infrastructure. The Caribbean Public Health Agency operates event-based surveillance with 24-hour notification across 24 member states, increasingly supported by predictive models that analyze syndromic data to detect outbreaks early (CARPHA, 2023; European Commission, 2022).

10.9.4 Health System Performance Analytics

Beyond clinical and surveillance uses, Layer 4 analytics support health system performance monitoring. Dashboards that track facility-level performance against benchmarks, identify supply chain bottlenecks, monitor workforce deployment, and assess program coverage enable data-driven management at all levels of the health system. Brazil's SUS uses analytics dashboards integrated with its RNDS data network to track hospital performance, primary care coverage, and pharmaceutical supply chains across its federated system of over 5,400 municipalities (PAHO, 2021).

For African health systems, the most practical path to advanced analytics is to build incrementally on the DHIS2 platform already deployed across the continent. DHIS2's growing analytics capabilities—including the Climate App, Modeling App, and expanded tracker analytics—offer an accessible entry point to predictive analytics without the need for separate, expensive platforms. Countries should complement DHIS2 analytics with dedicated Business Intelligence tools for cross-system analysis and invest in the health informatics workforce needed to develop, interpret, and act on analytical outputs.

10.10 Data Governance Frameworks

Effective health data governance encompasses the policies, structures, and responsibilities that govern how health data is collected, managed, accessed, shared, and protected. Africa's health data governance landscape is changing rapidly: more than 40 African countries have enacted or are developing personal data protection laws, many modeled after the EU's GDPR—such as Kenya's Data Protection Act (2019), Nigeria's Data Protection Regulation (2019), and South Africa's POPIA (2021) (UNCTAD, 2023).

However, health-sector-specific governance frameworks, consent management systems, and enforcement capacity remain underdeveloped. The ethical dimensions are significant: concerns include the secondary use of health data by commercial actors without adequate consent, data colonialism through the extraction of African health data for external AI model training with limited local benefit, and the challenge of obtaining meaningful informed consent in contexts of low literacy and limited digital access (Tindana et al., 2021).

The principle of progressive data access—tiered regimes that provide open access to aggregated, de-identified data while protecting individual records through controlled-access frameworks—offers a practical balance between openness and privacy. The Africa CDC's Africa Health Data Observatory (AHDO) is a major continental effort to harmonize and publicly share national health data across AU Member States (WHO Africa, 2022).

10.11 Financing and Sustainability

Health data systems require substantial ongoing investment. A country with 30 million people needs about USD 4–8 million annually to maintain a functional HMIS—roughly 1–2% of total health spending (Broadband

Commission, 2019). Domestic financing remains critically low: fewer than 20% of African countries include a dedicated budget line for HMIS maintenance in their national health budgets (WHO, 2022).

Sustainable data financing requires integrating health information system costs into medium-term expenditure frameworks, building domestic technical capacity, and adopting open-source solutions to minimize licensing costs. Rwanda, Ghana, and Kenya have successfully transitioned from donor-funded pilots to government-financed systems, sharing common features: explicit government ownership, gradual absorption of recurrent costs, and strategic use of open-source platforms.

10.12 Strategic Priorities for Data Analytics

A phased roadmap to strengthen health data systems and analytics capacity should progress from data quality and digitization to advanced analytics and regional integration, aligned with broader digital transformation and AI strategies. In the short term (1–2 years), the focus should be on improving data quality and strengthening foundational systems. Priority actions include implementing validation rules in DHIS2 to reduce errors at the point of data entry, strengthening routine data quality audits, and investing in "data quality champions" at the facility and district levels to institutionalize accountability. Digitizing civil registration systems is another critical step, as it underpins accurate population data, vital statistics, and identity systems essential to effective health planning and service delivery.

In the medium term (3–5 years), the focus should shift from data collection to data integration, standardization, and governance. Countries are expected to adopt FHIR-based analytics architectures to enable interoperable, scalable data exchange across systems. The transition to ICD-11 further strengthens the standardization of health information for clinical and statistical use. At the institutional level, establishing national data governance bodies ensures oversight, coordination, and enforcement of data policies, while developing secondary data use frameworks enables the responsible use of health data for research, policy analysis, and innovation.

Table 10.3 Strategic Priorities for Data Management and Analytics in Africa

Timeframe	Priority Actions
Short-term (1–2 years)	Implement validation rules in DHIS2; strengthen data quality audits; invest in data quality champions at facility and district levels; digitize civil registration
Medium-term (3–5 years)	Adopt FHIR-based analytics architecture; begin ICD-11 transition; establish national data governance bodies; develop secondary use frameworks
Long-term (5–10 years)	Build integrated health data ecosystems with AI/ML capabilities; establish regional analytics platforms through AU/REC coordination; implement privacy-preserving data linkage

In the long term (5–10 years), the health data roadmap envisions the development of fully integrated, intelligence-driven health data ecosystems. This includes embedding AI and machine learning capabilities into health systems for predictive analytics, decision support, and system optimization. Regional coordination becomes increasingly important, with the establishment of shared analytics platforms at the AU and REC levels, enabling cross-country insights and benchmarking. At the same time, advanced techniques such as privacy-preserving data linkage can be introduced to balance data integration with strong safeguards for confidentiality and trust.

10.13 Conclusion

Layer 4 of the digital health technology stack transforms raw data flowing through Layer 3's interoperability infrastructure into actionable intelligence that informs clinical decisions, policy formulation, resource allocation, and improvements in health system performance. Africa's data landscape presents both remarkable strengths—global leadership in DHIS2 deployment, growing adoption of OpenHIE, and an increasingly robust legal framework for data governance—and persistent gaps in data quality, adoption of clinical standards, and analytical capacity.

The global evidence reviewed in this chapter shows that moving from data collection to data intelligence requires sustained investment across five interconnected domains: improving data quality within existing systems, harmonizing standards for interoperability, establishing governance frameworks that balance openness with privacy, strengthening analytical capacity, including AI/ML capabilities, and securing domestic financing for sustainability. Countries that address these domains in a coordinated, phased manner—building incrementally on existing infrastructure while aligning with continental frameworks such as the Smart Africa Digital Health Blueprint and the AU HIE Guidelines—will be best positioned to realize the full value of their investments across the entire digital health technology stack.

References

Australian Bureau of Statistics. (2024). Estimated Resident Population: Methodology. ABS.

Australian Digital Health Agency. (2024). My Health Record statistics and annual report. ADHA.

Australian Institute of Health and Welfare. (2024). Data linkage for population health intelligence. AIHW.

Balsari, S., Sesia, P., & Patnaik, S. (2024). India's evolving digital health strategy. npj Digital Medicine, 7, Article 285.

Bhattacharya, A. A., Umar, N., Audu, A., Felix, H., Allen, E., Schellenberg, J. R. M., & Marchant, T. (2019). Quality of routine facility data for monitoring priority maternal and newborn indicators in DHIS2. PLOS ONE, 14(1), e0211265.

Broadband Commission for Sustainable Development. (2019). The state of broadband 2019. ITU/UNESCO.

Canadian Institute for Health Information. (2024). Data quality framework and hospital reporting standards. CIHI.

Canadian Primary Care Sentinel Surveillance Network. (2024). Chronic disease surveillance from EMR data: Annual report. CPCSSN.

CARPHA. (2023). eHealth Caribbean Initiative: Regional surveillance and ICD-11 implementation. Caribbean Public Health Agency.

European Commission. (2022). Proposal for a Regulation on the European Health Data Space. COM(2022) 197 final.

HELINA. (2025). Africa on FHIR and SIL-Africa. Health Informatics in Africa.

Health Information Systems Programme. (2023). DHIS2 in numbers 2023. University of Oslo.

Kgasi, M., Ochieng, B., & Katurura, M. (2025). Adoption, barriers and opportunities of interoperability and eHealth standards in Africa. BMJ Health and Care Informatics, 32(1), e101210.

Ministry of Health New Zealand. (2024). National Health Index: Data quality and governance. Ministry of Health.

National Health Authority India. (2022). Ayushman Bharat Digital Mission: Annual report 2021–22. Government of India.

OECD. (2023). Health at a Glance: Asia/Pacific 2023. OECD Publishing.

PAHO. (2021). Digital health strategy of the Pan American Health Organization. PAHO.

PATH. (2021). Navigating the data ecosystem for health in sub-Saharan Africa. PATH.

Sharma, R. S., Rohatgi, A., Jain, S., & Singh, D. (2023). The ABDM: Making of India's digital health story. CSI Transactions on ICT, 11, 3–9.

Statistics New Zealand. (2024). Integrated Data Infrastructure: Health data linkage methodology. Stats NZ.

Tindana, P., Molyneux, C. S., Bull, S., & Parker, M. (2021). Constraints on community engagement in genomics research in Africa. PLOS ONE, 16(1), e0245351.

UNCTAD. (2023). Data protection and privacy legislation worldwide. United Nations.

Vital Wave. (2021). Interoperability in African health systems. Vital Wave.

Wagenaar, B. H., Gimbel, S., Hoek, R., Pfeiffer, J., Michel, C., Manuel, J. L., & Sherr, K. (2016). Stock-outs of essential health products in Mozambique. Tropical Medicine and International Health, 21(2), 246–258.

WHO. (2021). Global strategy on digital health 2020–2025. WHO.

WHO. (2022). World health statistics 2022: Monitoring health for the SDGs. WHO.

WHO Africa. (2022). State of digital health in the African region: 2022 report. WHO AFRO.

Africa CDC. (2024). Continental Artificial Intelligence Strategy: Health sector applications. Africa Centres for Disease Control and Prevention.

Boulle, A., Heekes, A., Tiffin, N., Smith, M., van de Merwe, L., & Fox, M. P. (2023). Record linkage for routinely collected health data in an African health information exchange. International Journal of Population Data Science, 8(1), 1771.

DHIS2. (2025). DHIS2 Climate Health Analytics Platform: Integrating predictive analytics into national health information systems. HISP Centre, University of Oslo.

HISP. (2024). DHIS2 Modeling App and Chap Platform: Machine learning for climate-sensitive disease forecasting. University of Oslo.

Jembi. (2024). OpenHIM Platform: Data warehousing and analytics for health information exchange. Jembi Health Systems.

Labrique, A., Wadhwani, C., Perakslis, E., & Bhatt, C. (2021). COVID-19 is a data crisis: Lessons from digital health responses to the pandemic. npj Digital Medicine, 4(1), 167.

Wahl, B., Cossy-Gantner, A., Germann, S., & Schwalbe, N. R. (2018). Artificial intelligence and global health: How can AI contribute to health in resource-poor settings? BMJ Global Health, 3(4), e000798.

PART 3

Enablers of Digital Health in Africa

Chapter 11 Digital Health Skills and Workforce Development

11.1 Introduction

The most sophisticated health information systems will fail without the human capacity to design, implement, manage, and improve them. Chapter 4 identified digital health skills and workforce development as a key enabler within the Digital Health Technology Stack (Figure 4.1), operating vertically across all five foundational layers—from physical infrastructure to applications and services. This chapter examines this enabler in depth, exploring the state of medical informatics as a discipline, the health IT workforce landscape in Africa, educational programs and their gaps, the compound challenge of brain drain, gender dimensions, and strategies for building sustainable human capacity at scale.

Drawing extensively on experiences from the Global South—including Latin America, the Caribbean, India, and Southeast Asia—as well as from Australia, Canada, and New Zealand, this chapter offers a comparative framework for workforce development that centers the African experience and distills transferable lessons from peer countries facing similar challenges of scale, resource constraints, and geographic disparity.

11.2 Medical and Health Informatics as a Discipline

Medical informatics—also called health informatics, clinical informatics, biomedical informatics, or digital health—is the interdisciplinary science focused on acquiring, storing, retrieving, communicating, and optimally using health-related data, information, and knowledge. Its goal is to support healthcare, biomedical research, and public health decision-making. As a formal academic discipline, it draws on computer science, information science, cognitive science, organizational behavior, and the full range of health and biomedical sciences (Shortliffe & Cimino, 2014). Within the Digital Health Technology Stack introduced in Chapter 4, this discipline provides the intellectual foundation for skills and workforce development across every layer of the stack—from network engineers who maintain connectivity infrastructure to data scientists who build analytical pipelines to clinical informaticians who design applications for frontline care.

The discipline has evolved substantially since the 1960s. Modern health informatics now encompasses a wide range of sub-disciplines, each with distinct methodological traditions and application domains. In Africa, the discipline has developed unevenly: public health informatics—especially as seen in DHIS2 implementation and management—and clinical informatics have received most investment and built the largest workforce. In contrast, other sub-disciplines, such as nursing informatics, pharmacy informatics, and health data science, remain in their early stages, with very limited formal training opportunities. This imbalance leaves health systems better equipped to collect and report aggregate data than to use patient-level clinical data to improve care or conduct advanced analytics.

The uneven pattern of disciplinary development is not unique to Africa. Latin America faces a similar challenge: digital health training and research programs are limited and poorly documented across the region, with health informatics capacity concentrated in a few institutions in Brazil, Mexico, Peru, and Chile, while most countries lack formal training infrastructure altogether (Curioso, 2019). In the Caribbean, the situation is exacerbated by the small size of individual island states, which cannot independently support the full range of health informatics sub-disciplines—a constraint that has led to a regional pooling approach. India, by contrast, has leveraged its established information technology sector to develop health informatics sub-disciplines more evenly, although a significant urban–rural knowledge gap persists (Balsari et al., 2024). The breadth of the field requires stratified competency frameworks with distinct training pathways for each sub-discipline.

The International Medical Informatics Association (IMIA) has articulated a global health informatics competency framework that distinguishes among the knowledge, skills, and attitudes required at different career levels and across sub-disciplines (Mantas et al., 2010). Several African universities have adapted this framework for local curricula design, though significant implementation gaps remain.

Table 11.1. Sub-disciplines of medical and health informatics and their primary applications in African health systems.

Sub-Discipline	Scope and Focus	Typical Applications in African Health Systems	Maturity in Africa
Clinical Informatics	Application of informatics to clinical care settings—hospitals, clinics, primary care	EMR workflow design and optimization; clinical decision support systems; digital prescription; hospital information systems	Moderate
Public Health Informatics	Use of information systems and data analytics to support population health, surveillance, and disease control	DHIS2 implementation and management; integrated disease surveillance; epidemic intelligence; health metrics dashboards	Most developed
Nursing Informatics	Integration of nursing science with information and communication technologies	Mobile nursing documentation; digital care planning; patient monitoring systems; nursing workflow optimization	Nascent
Pharmacy Informatics	Application of informatics to pharmaceutical and medication management	Electronic prescribing; e-LMIS; adverse drug reaction reporting; pharmacy supply chain management	Nascent
Consumer Health Informatics	Technologies that empower patients and communities to manage their own health	mHealth applications; patient portals; personal health records; digital health literacy platforms	Emerging
Biomedical Informatics	Interface between biological/clinical science and information science	Genomics data management; laboratory information systems; bioinformatics pipelines; precision medicine	Very limited
Health Data Science	Application of statistical and computational methods to health data	Machine learning for disease prediction; AI-driven diagnostics; big data analytics; NLP of clinical notes	Very limited

Source: Adapted from Shortliffe & Cimino (2014) and the author's elaboration.

The IMIA framework recognizes three competency tiers—IT user, health informatics specialist, and IT manager/chief information officer—that map onto the multi-level capacity building approach advocated throughout this chapter. In the Global South, adaptation of these competency tiers has been uneven: India's ABDM has formally codified new professional roles aligned with national digital health architecture, whereas most Latin American countries still lack nationally recognized health informatics professional categories (Curioso, 2019; National Health Authority India, 2022).

Australia's Health Informatics Competency Framework is organized into six domains of expertise, comprising 50+ competency statements that reflect the multidisciplinary nature of health informatics. These domains include health and biomedical knowledge; information and communication technologies; data and information management; governance and ethics; system design and lifecycle management; and leadership and change management. The framework also incorporates multiple levels of proficiency, enabling its application across a wide range of roles—from clinicians and administrators to specialist informaticians—while emphasizing critical capabilities such as interoperability, data quality, privacy, and safe system use (Digital Health Australia, 2022).

11.3 Current State of the Health IT Workforce in Africa

Africa faces a severe and widening health informatics workforce deficit. A 2020 assessment estimated that sub-Saharan Africa has about one health informatics professional per 100,000 people, compared with 10–15 per 100,000 in high-income countries—a gap of an order of magnitude (Nutley et al., 2020). This aggregate figure obscures profound regional and country-level variation. South Africa, with its relatively developed higher education system and substantial private health sector, has the continent's most developed health informatics workforce, at about 2.1 professionals per 100,000. Central African countries have fewer than 0.5 professionals per 100,000 and very limited training infrastructure. The gap between current and required workforce levels underscores the scale of the capacity challenge, with Central Africa facing the most acute deficit.

Figure 11.1. Estimated Health Informatics Workforce per 100,000 Population, Comparing African Regions with Global Benchmarks

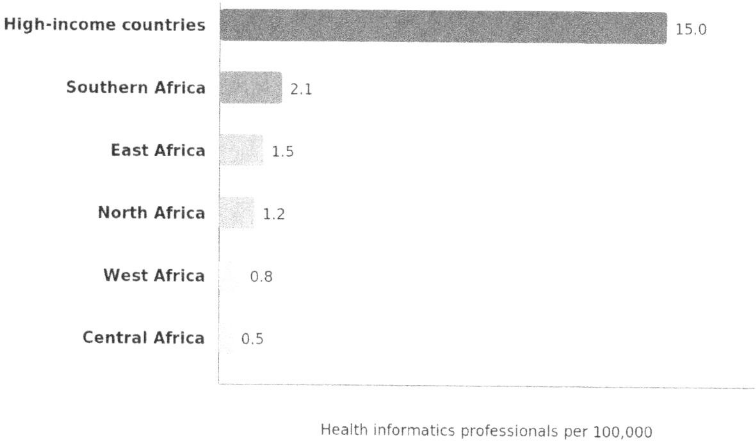

Source: Adapted from Nutley et al. (2020); WHO (2022); Expert Estimates

11.3.1 Workforce Distribution and Urban Concentration

The health informatics workforce in Africa is heavily concentrated in capital cities and major urban centers, mirroring the broader pattern of skilled health worker distribution. In Ethiopia, over 60% of health informaticians work in Addis Ababa or major regional capitals, while tens of thousands of rural health posts lack data management support. In Nigeria, Lagos and Abuja account for a disproportionate share of health IT professionals, while northern states, which carry some of the highest disease burdens, have near-zero local capacity. This geographic concentration has systemic consequences: data quality is generally better at central and urban facilities, peripheral facilities receive less supervision and technical support, and national aggregate data systematically overestimates system performance (WHO Africa, 2022).

The urban–rural digital health workforce gap is a feature shared across the Global South. In Brazil, health informatics professionals are concentrated in São Paulo, Rio de Janeiro, and Brasília, while the vast northern and northeastern regions—home to some of the country's greatest health needs—have minimal capacity. India faces an analogous pattern: despite the ABDM's national ambitions, adoption of electronic health records, AI diagnostics, and remote monitoring remains uneven outside metropolitan areas, and hospitals in smaller cities and rural areas continue to rely on legacy paper-based workflows (Digital Health News, 2025). Australia and Canada, despite their vastly greater resources, also struggle with the distribution of the rural digital health workforce: Canada's 2024 State of the Health Workforce report found that 5.7 million adults lacked a regular healthcare provider, with the deficit most acute in rural and remote communities (CIHI, 2024). The pattern is universal, but the consequences are most severe where the overall workforce supply is lowest—precisely the situation in sub-Saharan Africa. The urban–rural gap is consistent across all cadres, with community health workers and laboratory technicians in rural settings showing the most critical deficits.

Figure 11.2. Digital Literacy Rates by Health Worker Cadre and Facility Setting Across Sub-Saharan Africa (Composite Estimates, 2022)

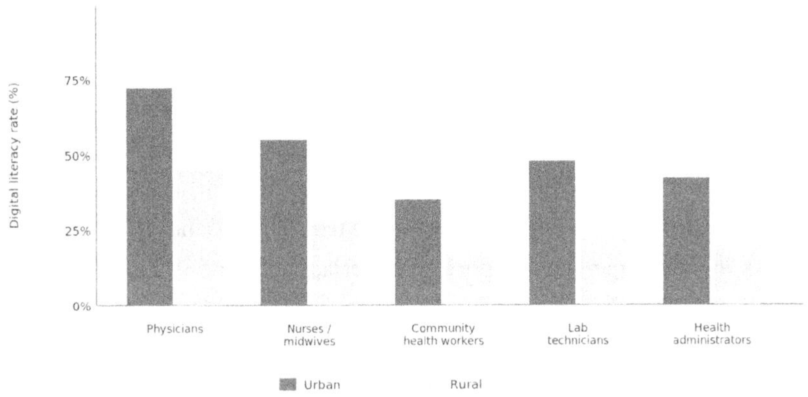

Source: Adapted from WHO (2022); ITU (2022); National Health Workforce Assessments

Digital literacy—a prerequisite for effective use of any digital health tool—varies substantially across cadres and settings. Studies across sub-Saharan Africa consistently show that physicians have higher digital literacy than nurses and midwives, who in turn outperform community health workers, laboratory technicians in remote settings, and health administrators in district offices. Urban–rural differentials are particularly pronounced, with rural health workers often unfamiliar with basic devices or Internet use (ITU, 2022).

11.3.2 Private Sector Absorption and Workforce Dynamics

A growing challenge is the absorption of trained health IT professionals by the private sector—both domestic private health organizations and international technology companies. As digital health investment accelerates, demand for health informatics skills has expanded well beyond the public health sector. Graduates are increasingly recruited by mHealth startups, international NGOs, consulting firms, and technology companies offering salaries that the public sector cannot match. While financially sensible for individuals, this domestic brain drain—from the public to the private sector—reduces the pool available to strengthen public health systems, which require the largest numbers and need them most.

Rwanda has systematically addressed this challenge: the Rwanda Biomedical Center has established a clear career ladder for health informatics professionals in the public health system, featuring competitive salary scales benchmarked to the private sector, structured professional development programs, and defined pathways from junior data manager to senior informatics specialist. This strategy has helped Rwanda retain a relatively high level of public-sector health informatics capacity (Ministry of Health, Rwanda, 2021).

India's experience offers valuable lessons: the National Health Authority's ABDM established new government-recognized professional roles—Health Data Manager and Digital Health Analyst—with defined career structures, generating demand signals that influenced training institutions' responses (National Health Authority India, 2022). In 2024, UNICEF India, the International Institute of Health Management Research, Delhi, and IIT Bombay jointly launched a comprehensive Digital Health Enterprise Planning Course, a ten-week program covering digital health governance, procurement, health informatics, and data management—demonstrating how institutional partnerships can quickly expand workforce capacity when aligned with national infrastructure goals (UNICEF India, 2024).

11.4 Educational Programs and Training Institutions

The formal education infrastructure for health informatics in Africa has expanded substantially over the past two decades. From fewer than five dedicated programs continent-wide in the early 2000s, Africa now hosts more than 78 university-level programs offering degrees or diplomas in health informatics, health information management, or closely related fields—with the pace of program creation accelerating sharply after 2015 (WHO, 2022; AfHIMA, 2022). This acceleration reflects the influence of national digital health strategies and increased donor support. Online and blended programs are the fastest-growing modality, driven by adaptations to COVID-19.

Figure 11.3 Growth of Health Informatics Academic Programs in Africa (2005-2023)

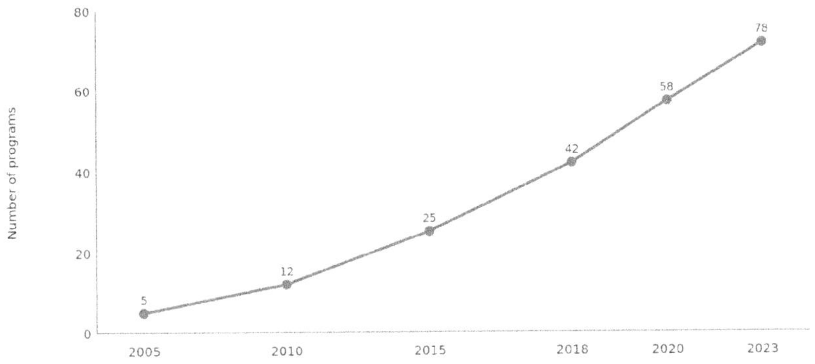

Source: WHO (2022); AfHIMA (2022); University Registries

11.4.1 University Degree Programs in Africa

Bachelor's degree programs in health informatics or health information management are now available in most African countries, though program density and curriculum quality vary widely. Ethiopia stands out as a continental leader: following a strategic decision by the Federal Ministry of Health to integrate health informatics into the national scale-up of health professional training, over 30 Ethiopian universities now offer Bachelor of

Science degrees in Health Informatics, producing over 2,000 graduates annually who are deployed to health facilities, district health offices, and national programs (Federal Ministry of Health Ethiopia, 2020). At the postgraduate level, options are more limited. A small number of institutions offer MSc programs, including Muhimbili University of Health and Allied Sciences (MUHAS) in Tanzania; the University of Cape Town and the University of the Witwatersrand in South Africa; Jomo Kenyata University of Agriculture and Technology (JKUAT) and the University of Nairobi in Kenya; and Kwame Nkrumah University of Science and Technology (KNUST) in Ghana. Doctoral programs—essential for producing faculty and researchers—are even rarer, with South Africa and Tanzania having the most established PhD tracks. Ethiopia and South Africa offer the most developed ecosystems; Central and Francophone West Africa show the most acute gaps.

Table 11.2 Selected African Country Profiles for Health Informatics Education.

Country	Key Institutions	Programmes Offered	Professional Body	Notes
South Africa	UCT, Wits, UNISA, UP	BSc, MSc, PhD Health	ITHS; IMIA member	Strongest ecosystem; high private sector absorption
Ethiopia	AAU, Jimma, Haramaya + 27 more	BSc Health Informatics (national	Ethiopian HIM Assoc.	30+ universities; 2,000+ graduates/ year; continental leader in pre-service
Kenya	U. of Nairobi, Strathmore, KCA	BSc Health Informatics, MSc eHealth	KHIMA	Growing ecosystem; shortage of PhD-level faculty constrains postgraduate
Ghana	KNUST, UG, Ashesi	BSc Health Info Mgt,	GHIMA	Good undergraduate base; limited postgraduate and research capacity
Rwanda	U. of Rwanda, CMU-Africa	BSc, MSc programmes	RBC digital health unit	High quality, small scale; CMU partnership model widely cited
Nigeria	UNILAG, ABU, OAU	BSc Health Info Mgt	AHIMA Nigeria	Large number of programmes; significant quality variation across
Tanzania	MUHAS	BSc, MSc Health	MUHAS Centre for HI	East African research pioneer; strong international partnerships

Source: WHO (2022); AfHIMA (2022); Author's Compilation

11.4.2 Comparative Perspectives: Training Infrastructure in the Global South

Africa's educational infrastructure challenges become more pronounced when compared with those in other Global South regions. Latin America's health informatics training landscape shares many structural features with Africa's: programs are scarce, poorly documented, and concentrated in a small number of institutions. Brazil's Fundação Oswaldo Cruz (Fiocruz) offers nationally recognized short courses in health informatics that count toward professional certification within the Unified Health System (SUS), directly aligning training with the national interoperability framework (PAHO, 2021). Peru has pioneered digital health workforce capacity building through partnerships between universities and PAHO, developing culturally relevant training programs that address the sociocultural and organizational challenges of digital health implementation in resource-constrained environments (Curioso et al., 2024). However, only a handful of Peruvian universities offer accredited programs in health informatics, underscoring the gap between aspiration and institutional capacity that characterizes much of the region.

India offers a contrasting model of scale. The IIT Bombay Health Informatics track and the Indian Institute of Management's healthcare analytics programs have produced a substantial cohort of health data scientists who are transforming India's healthcare AI landscape. In 2024, a new Digital Health Enterprise Planning Course, jointly developed by UNICEF India, IIHMR Delhi, and IIT Bombay, began equipping healthcare professionals—including doctors, nurses, administrators, and IT professionals—with skills in digital health governance, data management, and patient engagement across nine modules over ten weeks (UNICEF India, 2024). India's healthcare hiring rose by 62% in March 2025 compared with the previous year, driven by emerging requirements for AI and machine learning engineers, data scientists, and health informatics specialists (Digital Health News, 2025). Africa needs analogous investments, embedding health data science tracks within leading universities.

The Caribbean Public Health Agency has developed a regional approach that pools training resources across 24 small island developing states, offering shared curricula, faculty, and certification frameworks that no single country could afford—achieving substantial scale with limited per-country investment (PAHO, 2021). This regional pooling model is particularly relevant to Africa's Regional Economic Communities, which could host shared health informatics training hubs serving clusters of countries with similar linguistic and health system characteristics.

Indonesia illustrates yet another emerging model in Southeast Asia: rather than relying solely on post-employment training, the country has piloted integrated digital health curricula for public health, nursing, and medical students, recognizing that health workers entering the workforce have limited prior exposure to digital health tools and concepts. This pre-service curriculum integration approach parallels Ethiopia's strategy and offers a complementary model for African countries seeking to embed digital competencies before health workers enter practice.

11.4.3 Short Courses, Certification Programs, and Online Learning

Given the long timelines of pre-service degree programs and the urgent need to equip existing health workers with digital skills, short courses and certification programs play a vital complementary role. The DHIS2 Academy, coordinated by HISP at the University of Oslo, has trained more than 50,000 participants from over 100 countries, with most enrollees from Africa. Country-level DHIS2 academies have been established in Kenya, Ghana, Uganda, Ethiopia, and Mozambique. The IntraHealth International Capacity Plus initiative has reached tens of thousands of health information managers across sub-Saharan Africa through iHRIS training. iHRIS Train enables training institutions to track progress in curriculum implementation and student performance, and to collect information on faculty and tutors, as well as the training experience of individual health workers. The Africa CDC's e-Learning platform offers short courses in public health informatics, integrated disease surveillance, and health data management in English, French, and Portuguese (HISP, 2023; Africa CDC, 2021).

The expansion of MOOCs and online platforms has dramatically broadened access to health informatics education for learners across the Global South. However, online learning faces distinct challenges in African, Caribbean, and parts of Latin American and Asian contexts: unreliable Internet access, power supply disruptions, low completion rates without institutional support, and the dominance of English-language content that disadvantages Francophone, Lusophone, Arabophone, and Spanish-speaking learners. Promising innovations include the African Union's Harmonization of African Higher Education Quality Assurance and Accreditation (HAQAA) initiative, the development of regional quality standards for online health education, Ethiopia's e-Learning center, the development of offline-capable digital learning platforms, and Peru's collaboration with PAHO to develop culturally relevant digital health courses in Spanish (WHO, 2022; Curioso et al., 2024). Figure 11.4. Comparative assessment of health informatics training modalities across three dimensions: knowledge retention, geographic reach, and cost-effectiveness.

Figure 11.4. Assessment of Health Informatics Training Modalities

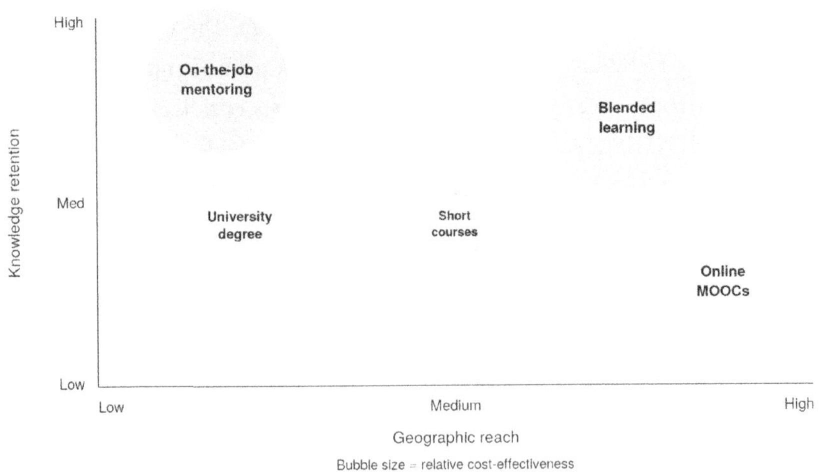

Source: Expert assessment based on Manders et al. (2021); WHO (2022).

No single training modality is sufficient, and effective capacity-building strategies—particularly in digital health and AI—require a portfolio approach that combines high-retention methods (mentoring, blended learning) with scalable platforms (online learning) to balance depth, reach, and cost.

On-the-job mentoring achieves the highest knowledge retention but has limited geographic reach, reflecting its intensive, localized nature. Blended learning emerges as a strong, balanced approach, combining high retention with medium-to-high reach and strong cost-effectiveness, making it particularly suitable for scaling skills development. Traditional university degrees and short courses occupy the middle ground, offering moderate retention and reach, while online MOOCs provide the widest geographic reach but relatively lower retention, despite being highly cost-effective.

11.5 Skills Gaps and Training Needs Assessment

A comprehensive, evidence-based training needs assessment is the foundation of any effective capacity-building strategy. Yet across Africa, health informatics training needs are more often assumed than rigorously assessed: programs are frequently designed around available faculty expertise and donor funding priorities rather than documented workforce gaps and health system demand. A systematic review by Manders et al. (2021) found that the most consistently identified skill gaps across sub-Saharan Africa were data quality management, DHIS2 administration and customization, data analysis and interpretation for decision-making, interoperability and health information exchange, and health information system governance and policy.

Emerging skills—such as health data science, AI and machine learning, cybersecurity for health systems, and digital health product management—are largely unmet by African training infrastructure. These competencies are increasingly in demand from the digital health startup ecosystem, international programs, and national digital health agencies, yet the supply remains very limited.

WHO/Europe's 2025 policy brief on digital skills for the health workforce confirms that training remains insufficient even in European countries, especially in advanced areas like AI, robotics, and genomics—highlighting that the skills gap is not only an African issue but a global one, though far more severe where baseline workforce capacity is lowest (WHO/Europe, 2025).

Figure 11.5. Health Informatics Skills Gap Analysis Comparing System Demand with the Current Workforce Supply Across Ten Critical Competency Areas

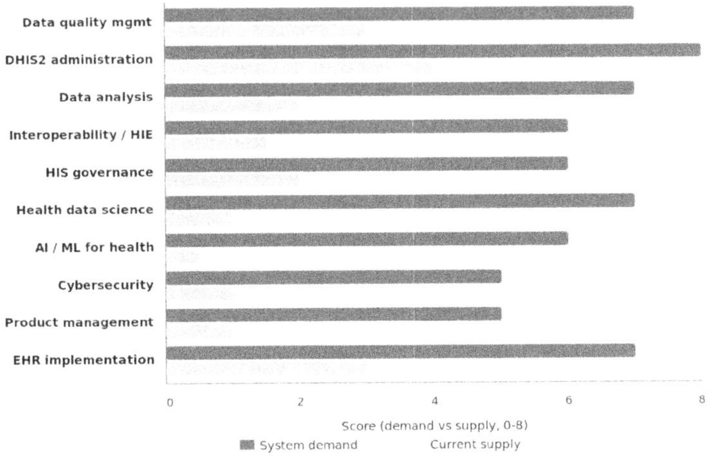

Source: Adapted from Manders et al. (2021); WHO (2022); AfHIMA (2022).

India's experience demonstrates the potential of integrating health data science into leading academic institutions: ABDM-aligned training requirements for facility registration created large-scale demand signals, and demand for health-tech talent increased by 62% in early 2025 as roles in AI, data science, and clinical informatics expanded (Digital Health News, 2025). However, even in India, workforce upskilling remains a major challenge, with hospitals citing capability building and IT upskilling as critical barriers to digital transformation. The lesson for Africa is clear: expanding supply-side training without demand-side policy signals risks producing graduates the system cannot absorb.

Table 11.3 presents a proposed multi-level health informatics competency framework for African health systems. Each level requires distinct training pathways, professional recognition mechanisms, and enabling institutional environments. At the base is foundational digital literacy, applicable to all health workers and focusing on essential skills such as device use, basic Internet navigation, digital record handling, and awareness of data privacy.

Table 11.3 A proposed Multi-level Health Informatics Competency Framework for African Health Systems.

Competency Level	Target Audience	Core Competencies	Primary Application
Foundational Digital Literacy	All health workers	Device operation; email and Internet; digital record navigation; data privacy awareness	Frontline service delivery—nurses, CHWs, laboratory staff, pharmacists
Health Information Management	HI officers, records managers	HIM principles; ICD-10/11 coding; data quality; facility reporting; register management	Facility data management; HMIS reporting; patient record stewardship
Health Informatics Specialist	Informaticians, system analysts	EHR design; standards implementation; system integration; DHIS2 admin; workflow analysis	HMIS management; digital health project implementation; troubleshooting
Health IT Professional	Developers, engineers, network admins	Health software development; API design; data exchange protocols; security; cloud infrastructure	HIS development, deployment, maintenance; infrastructure management
Health Data Scientist	Data scientists, epidemiologists	Statistical analysis; ML for health; data visualization; NLP; GIS health analytics	Population health analytics; AI diagnostics; surveillance intelligence
Health Informatics Leader	CIOs, digital health directors	Strategic planning; stakeholder management; governance; policy; change management	National digital health strategy; ministerial units; hospital CIO roles

Source: Adapted from IMIA (Mantas et al., 2010); ABDM India; Author's Elaboration.

This level is critical for frontline service delivery, enabling nurses, community health workers, laboratory staff, and pharmacists to operate effectively in increasingly digitized care environments. Building on this, the health information management (HIM) level targets records officers and data managers, emphasizing competencies in coding systems such as ICD-10/11, data quality assurance, reporting, and patient record stewardship. Together, these two levels form the operational backbone of digital health systems, ensuring that data is accurately captured, managed, and utilized at the point of care and within facility-level reporting systems.

The more advanced tiers focus on specialized and strategic roles that drive system design, innovation, and governance. The health informatics specialist and health IT professional levels focus on technical and systems-oriented capabilities, including EHR design, interoperability standards, software development, API integration, cybersecurity, and cloud infrastructure. These roles are central to the development, deployment, and maintenance of health information systems and digital platforms. Further up the hierarchy, the health data scientist level introduces advanced analytics, including machine learning, natural language processing, and geospatial analysis, supporting applications such as disease surveillance, population health insights, and AI-driven diagnostics. At the top, the health informatics leader level emphasizes strategic competencies—policy development, governance, stakeholder coordination, and change management—required to lead national digital health programs and institutional transformation.

11.5.1 Gender Dimensions of the Health Informatics Workforce

The health informatics workforce in Africa shows a distinct gender pattern. Women are concentrated at the community health worker and health information management levels—making up over 65% of CHWs and about 55% of health information officers. However, at the health IT professional and health data science levels, the gender distribution shifts sharply: women account for fewer than 30% of health software developers and data scientists, mirroring the broader gender gap in technology professions (WHO, 2022; ITU, 2022). As a result, rising salaries and career advantages associated with data science, software development, and health IT leadership tend to favor men, while lower-paid roles such as data entry and health information management remain female-dominated.

The gender gap in health informatics is a widespread issue across the Global South. At the ninth Summit of the Americas, the Regional Agenda for Digital

Transformation recognized that the COVID-19 pandemic deepened digital divides that disproportionately affect women, children, and persons with disabilities. It called for inclusive workforce development strategies that focus on traditionally marginalized groups (Atlantic Council, 2024).

Figure 11.6 Gender Distribution Across Health Informatics Roles in Africa

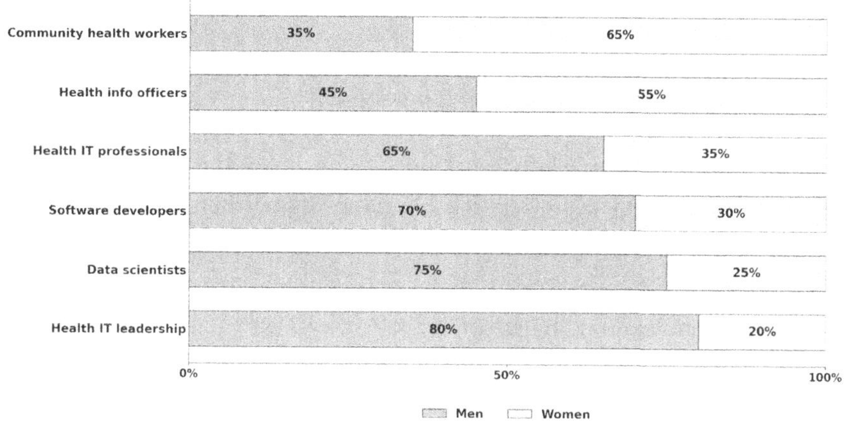

Source: WHO (2022); ITU (2022); AfHIMA (2022)

Closing the gender gap requires deliberate effort: targeted scholarships for women in health data science, structured mentoring programs, and the cultivation of visible role models. The EU's Digital Education Action Plan includes specific targets for women in digital health professions and is backed by funding for women-focused digital skills programs across member states, offering a governance model that African continental institutions could adapt (European Commission, 2022).

11.6 Building Capacity at Different Levels

An effective approach to health informatics human capacity development must target all levels of the health system simultaneously—ranging from the frontline health worker using a mobile data form to the national technical team designing the country's digital health ecosystem. Within the Digital Health Technology Stack (Figure 4.1), each foundational layer requires distinct competencies: the infrastructure layer requires network engineers and cloud administrators; the identity and registries layer requires database architects and identity management specialists; the interoperability layer requires standards experts and integration engineers; the analytics layer requires data scientists and visualization specialists; and the application layer requires software developers, user experience (UX) designers, and clinical informaticians. These levels are interconnected: gaps at any level can cascade both upward and downward, undermining the integrity and usefulness of the entire system.

11.6.1 Healthcare Provider Digital Literacy

For most of Africa's health workforce, digital health capacity building primarily focuses on achieving reliable basic digital literacy: the ability to operate a device, navigate digital systems, enter and retrieve data, and maintain data privacy and security. Several countries have made significant progress in embedding digital literacy in pre-service curricula. Ethiopia's revised health professional training curriculum incorporates digital health competencies across all cadres, including a dedicated health informatics module for nurses and health extension workers. Kenya's Medical Training Colleges have integrated basic digital literacy into nursing and clinical officer programs. Tanzania's Ministry of Health launched a nationwide health worker digital literacy program from 2019 to 2021, reaching more than 15,000 health workers through a cascade training model (Federal Ministry of Health, Ethiopia, 2020; WHO Africa, 2022).

11.6.2 Global Approaches to Promoting Health Workers' Digital Literacy

Cross-regional evidence shows that the most effective health systems view digital literacy not as a single ICT course but as an ongoing workforce skill linked to patient safety, data protection, service redesign, and quality improvement. Countries typically promote health workers' digital literacy through six linked mechanisms: embedding digital competencies in pre-service education; integrating digital health training into licensing or continuing professional development; providing role-specific training for tools such as EHRs, e-prescribing, and telehealth; establishing 'super-user' or clinical champion models within facilities; providing national online learning platforms and accredited short courses; and supporting these efforts with implementation assistance, including workflow redesign, help desks, interoperability standards, and dedicated training time.

In Europe, the trend is shifting toward competency-based, system-level approaches. WHO/Europe's 2025 policy brief emphasizes that training remains inadequate in many European countries, particularly in advanced fields such as AI, robotics, and genomics. It also highlights enablers such as national digital health strategies, legislation that incorporates skills into education requirements, sustainable funding, and coordination between the health and education sectors. European countries are increasingly integrating undergraduate curriculum reform, in-service training, and knowledge-sharing networks into broader digital health reforms, including the European Health Data Space (WHO/Europe, 2025).

In Canada, the approach is more focused on profession- and competency-driven practices. Canada Health Infoway, the Registered Nurses' Association of Ontario, and academic institutions have collaborated to define the competencies health professionals need for digital practice, including patient-centered technology use, privacy, workflow integration, and reducing technology-related burdens. Canada relies primarily on professional guidance, curriculum updates, and ongoing education rather than a single national mandatory program for all workers (Digital Health Canada, 2023).

In Latin America, the most prominent pattern is regional scaling through PAHO, paired with workforce training focused on telehealth. In April 2025, PAHO launched a Digital Literacy Program for Health Sector Personnel to improve the digital skills of health workers across the Americas. PAHO's approach is practical and comprehensive: it covers digital tools, data management, and emerging technologies, and offers telehealth training resources to enhance health teams' ability to implement and use telehealth services. In Latin America, workforce digital literacy is often promoted through regional virtual training, tele-education, and continuing professional development, especially in countries where expanding access in remote or underserved areas is needed (PAHO, 2025). India has linked capacity building under the ABDM to formal courses and new programs to strengthen AI and broader digital competencies among medical professionals, emphasizing that doctors, nurses, frontline workers, paramedics, and students all need extensive training and awareness for digital health to work at scale.

Five common implementation practices emerge across these diverse regional approaches. First, countries define a competency framework to ensure that 'digital literacy' is not vague. Second, they tailor training by cadre and use case, recognizing that nurses, community workers, hospital managers, and specialist physicians do not need identical skills. Third, they combine pre-service education with continuous in-service learning. Fourth, they link training to real systems being deployed—EHRs, telehealth, e-prescribing, decision support, and patient portals—rather than teaching digital skills in isolation. Fifth, they support adoption through change management, local champions, and workflow redesign. When countries do this well, digital literacy becomes part of health system transformation rather than a stand-alone IT project. For Africa, these five practices provide an actionable template: competency frameworks adapted to the IMIA model; cadre-specific training aligned with DHIS2 and emerging EMR platforms; blended pre- and in-service modalities; training anchored to real national digital health infrastructure; and sustained change management support.

11.6.3 IT Professionals in Healthcare Settings

Health IT professionals—software developers, system administrators, network engineers, database managers, and cybersecurity specialists—are the technical backbone of digital health systems. Across Africa, this group is severely underrepresented in the public health sector. Health IT requires specialized expertise at the intersection of general IT and health-specific knowledge—familiarity with clinical workflows, health data standards (HL7 FHIR, ICD, SNOMED CT), regulatory requirements, and the challenges of deploying systems in low-bandwidth, high-reliability healthcare environments. South Africa's Western Cape eHealth initiative has developed an innovative approach: a structured graduate recruitment program that provides computer science graduates with an intensive 12-month health informatics orientation—including clinical placement, health data standards training, and mentored system development—before assigning them to the provincial health IT infrastructure team (Western Cape Government, 2022).

11.6.4 Health Information Managers

Health information managers—professionals responsible for the collection, organization, coding, retrieval, and reporting of health data—are among the most critical yet least recognized roles in Africa's digital health ecosystem. In most African countries, they hold diplomas or bachelor's degrees in health records and information management and are certified by national bodies affiliated with the American Health Information Management Association (AHIMA). However, this group faces significant structural challenges: low salaries relative to clinical cadres, poorly defined career progression pathways, and frequent task shifting to general administrative duties. Professionalizing the group through improved salary scales, clear career ladders, and mandatory continuing professional development is a priority identified across multiple African national digital health strategies (AHIMA, 2023).

11.6.5 Data Scientists and Analysts

The rise of large-scale health data is creating demand for a vital new skill: the ability to analyze complex health information, produce actionable insights, and communicate findings effectively to decision-makers. Formal training programs in health data science are scarce in Africa. Notable exceptions include the African Institute for Mathematical Sciences (AIMS), the African Center for Excellence in Bioinformatics at the University of Cape Town, the Epidemic Intelligence and Data Science Program at Makerere University, and the Data Science for Health (DS4H) initiative, supported by the Wellcome Trust and IDRC across five African universities. India's experience—where IIT Bombay's Health Informatics track and IIM's healthcare analytics programs have helped create a large group of professionals shaping India's healthcare AI field—demonstrates the potential of integrating health data science into top academic institutions (AIMS, 2022; National Health Authority India, 2022).

11.7 Brain Drain and Retention Strategies

The international migration of skilled health workers—brain drain—is among the most serious challenges facing African health systems. For health informatics professionals, the situation is particularly acute: their skills are highly marketable worldwide; remote work opportunities have grown significantly since COVID-19; and salary gaps between African public-sector roles and positions in Europe, North America, and the Gulf states are considerable. A 2022 survey of health informatics graduates from three East African universities found that 35% had emigrated within five years of graduation, and another 28% reported active plans to emigrate (Haile et al., 2022). It is estimated that 10–15% of graduates currently work remotely for international employers while physically remaining in Africa—a form of 'virtual brain drain' that preserves their physical presence but removes their economic and intellectual contributions from the local community.

Brain drain in digital health is not limited to Africa. The OECD reports that several high-income countries—including Australia, Canada, Ireland, New Zealand, the United Kingdom, and the United States—have historically recruited health professionals from abroad, and the share of foreign-trained doctors and nurses has risen in most OECD countries since 2010 (OECD, 2024). This recruitment pattern directly affects African training investments: health workers trained at significant public expense in African institutions migrate to systems that did not bear those costs. PAHO's 2023 Workforce Policy for the Americas projects a shortage of 600,000 health professionals in Latin America and the Caribbean by 2030, with part of this gap addressed through cross-border recruitment that further destabilizes smaller Caribbean and Central American health systems. In Africa, where the overall workforce supply is the lowest, this brain drain is disproportionately damaging. Rwanda scores most favorably across the retention dimensions of brain drain; Nigeria's high emigration rate coexists with significant potential for diaspora engagement.

11.7.1 Retention Strategies

Effective retention strategies must address root causes—primarily economic (salary and career advancement), professional (opportunities for growth, recognition, and contribution), and quality-of-life factors (infrastructure, stability, and security). No single intervention is sufficient; retention requires a systemic approach. Competitive compensation, including supplementary allowances, performance bonuses, housing assistance, and non-monetary benefits, can help close the salary gap. Clear career pathways from junior data manager to digital health director, with transparent criteria and professional development support, signal long-term prospects. Recognition through formal credentialing, association membership, conference participation, and publication opportunities strengthens professional identity. Notably, enabling public-sector workers to work remotely on international projects part-time may reduce the need to emigrate while building skills that benefit the home system. Rwanda's structured incentive scheme—including performance-linked bonuses and preferred mortgage rates—has helped achieve above-average retention (Ministry of Health, Rwanda, 2021).

Figure 11.7 Brain Drain and Retention Factors for Health Informatics Professionals Across Selected African Countries

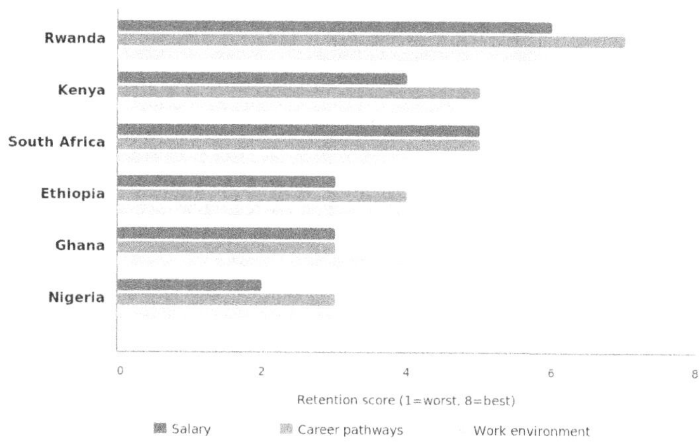

Source: Haile et al. (2022); WHO (2022); Expert Assessment

11.7.2 Diaspora Engagement

Africa's health informatics diaspora is a vast, underutilized resource. Structured diaspora engagement can partially offset brain drain through knowledge transfer, mentoring, research collaboration, and investment. The Ethiopian diaspora health informatics initiative—coordinated by the Ethiopian North American Health Professionals Association (ENAHPA) and the Federal Ministry of Health—has facilitated virtual mentoring, contributed to curriculum development, and supported grant applications for digital health research. Rwanda's Diaspora Global Convention features a technology track that brings together diaspora health IT professionals and national authorities. The AMIA Africa working group, founded in 2018, promotes research collaboration and peer mentoring.

The Caribbean model is especially instructive for Africa. CARPHA's regional approach explicitly integrates diaspora professionals into training and technical assistance, treating them as an extension of the regional health informatics workforce rather than a lost resource (PAHO, 2021). This shift—from 'brain drain' to 'brain circulation'—recognizes that, when deliberately structured, diaspora engagement can foster two-way flows of knowledge, mentorship, and investment that partially offset the effects of emigration. African organizations should establish similar frameworks by creating health informatics diaspora registries, virtual mentoring platforms, and structured sabbatical programs that encourage periodic returns.

11.8 Professional Associations and Communities of Practice

Professional associations play essential roles in the health informatics ecosystem: setting standards for practice and education, providing ongoing professional development, advocating for the profession within health systems, and connecting African professionals with global networks. At the national level, health information management associations exist in most African countries—Kenya's KHIMA, Ghana's GHIMA, Nigeria's AHIMA chapter, and South Africa's HIASA are among the most active. At the continental level, the Africa Health Information Management Association

(AfHIMA), founded in 2013, aims to coordinate national associations and unify professional standards, though it remains underfunded (AfHIMA, 2022).

The HISP network—a global community of practice for DHIS2 implementation—has a particularly strong African presence, with nodes in more than 20 countries that provide technical support, training, research, and advocacy. HISP's model of collaborative problem-solving and open-source solution development is among the most successful pan-African health informatics communities of practice (HISP, 2023).

The Health and Biomedical Informatics Association of Sub-Saharan Africa (HELINA), the International Medical Informatics Association's regional member for Africa, plays a key role in connecting African health informatics professionals with global networks. It organizes biennial scientific conferences and, through its Digital Health Applied Leadership Program in Burkina Faso, Rwanda, and Zambia, provides one of the few dedicated continental capacity-building initiatives for health informatics leadership (HELINA, 2025).

Table 11.4 presents a global comparison of health informatics workforce development, including professional bodies, certification systems, estimated workforce size, and key contextual notes. High-income regions such as the United States and the European Union lead in scale and institutional maturity, with large, well-established certification systems (e.g., AMIA, EFMI) and workforces of 40,000–65,000 professionals. Their growth has been strongly driven by national or regional policy mandates—such as electronic health record (EHR) adoption and emerging frameworks like the European Health Data Space—which have created sustained demand for informatics, data governance, and digital health expertise. Similarly, countries such as India, Brazil, Australia, Canada, and New Zealand demonstrate strong national-level institutionalization, with tailored certification pathways and workforce expansion linked to flagship digital health programs, including ABDM in India and My Health Record in Australia. In contrast, regions such as Latin America and the Caribbean and Sub-Saharan Africa exhibit smaller workforce sizes and more fragmented institutional arrangements, though notable progress is emerging through regional cooperation mechanisms. Sub-Saharan

Africa's estimated 8,000 professionals fall far short of those in comparator regions of similar population size.

Table 11.4 Global Comparison of Health Informatics Workforce Development

Region/ Country	Professional Body	Certification System	Est. Workforce	Key Notes
United States	AMIA	ONC HIT Certification; RHIA/RHIT	65,000+	Federal EHR mandate drove rapid growth; AMIA 10x10 expanded online training
European Union	EFMI	National certifications; EFMI-EDiHE	40,000+	EHDS driving new demand for data engineers and governance specialists; WHO/Europe 2025 policy brief on digital skills
India	HISI	ABDM national certification	25,000+	ABDM created Health Data Manager and Digital Health Analyst roles at scale; 62% hiring surge in 2025
Brazil	SBIS	CFM/CFN guidelines; SBIS certification	18,000+	SUS digitalization and RNDS created large civil servant demand; Fiocruz training pipeline
Australia	ACHI / AIDH	ACHI Fellowship; CHIA; HIMAA; Digital Health Hub	12,000+	My Health Record drove workforce; Digital Health Hub as capability platform; HIKM conferences since 2007
Canada	Digital Health Canada	DHC competency framework; co-op programmes	15,000+	Health Workforce Canada (est. 2023); Quintuple Aim competency framework; RNAO digital nursing guideline
New Zealand	HINZ	Cross-institutional model; primer workshops	3,000+	Grassroots workforce awareness programme; strong primary care informatics; 2024 Health Workforce Plan
Latin America / Caribbean	PAHO eHealth; CARPHA	CARPHA regional curriculum; PAHO Digital Literacy Program (2025)	~10,000	PAHO trained 70,000+ in 2025; regional cooperation compensates for small national pools; diaspora integration
Sub-Saharan Africa	AfHIMA; HELINA; nascent national bodies	AHIMA international adaptation ongoing	~8,000	Severe shortage; largely donor-funded; no pan-African certification framework yet

Source: Author's Compilation from Multiple Sources

11.9 Continuing Professional Development

Continuing professional development (CPD)—the ongoing learning that keeps professionals current with evolving technologies, standards, and practices—is crucial in a rapidly changing field such as health informatics. In Africa, CPD infrastructure remains underdeveloped, fragmented, and heavily reliant on donors. Where frameworks exist, they typically require 15–20 continuing education units annually through approved activities. Kenya's KHIMA mandates 20 Continuing Education Units (CEUs) annually for professional registration; Nigeria's AHIMA chapter has similar requirements. Yet enforcement remains weak, and the availability of affordable, high-quality CPD content relevant to African settings is limited (AfHIMA, 2022).

The COVID-19 pandemic disrupted in-person CPD but accelerated the development of online CPD infrastructure. Virtual conferences—including the HISP Global Conference, the Africa Health Informatics Conference, and the WHO Digital Health Webinar Series—significantly improved accessibility. Australia's Health Informatics Knowledge Management (HIKM) conference, held annually since 2007 and drawing submissions from across the Asia-Pacific region, offers a model for sustained academic CPD that Africa's HELINA conferences could emulate more regularly with greater institutional support (HIKM, 2025). Canada's 2024 effort to update public health core competencies, including digital skills, demonstrates how CPD frameworks can be systematically refreshed to keep pace with evolving technology (BMC Public Health, 2025).

Looking ahead, a continental CPD framework developed by the African Health Information Management Association, featuring harmonized minimum standards and mutual recognition across African countries, could provide the consistency and quality assurance that individual national frameworks lack. The EU's approach to CPD in regulated professions—with harmonized minimum standards across member states and mutual recognition of certifications—offers a relevant governance model. This model is complemented by WHO/Europe's emphasis on coordination between the health and education sectors as a key enabler of sustainable digital skills development (WHO/Europe, 2025). Table 11.5 summarizes the comparative strengths and limitations of various capacity-building approaches.

Table 11.5. Comparative Analysis of Health Informatics Capacity Building Approaches

Approach	Strengths	Limitations	Examples (Africa and Global South)
Pre-service Degrees	Foundational; broad competencies; workforce pipeline	Long lead time (3–5 yrs); high cost; faculty shortages	Ethiopia BSc scale-up; MUHAS MSc; CMU-Africa Rwanda; IIT Bombay/IIHMR India; Indonesia curriculum pilots
In-service Short Courses	Rapid skill update; targeted; minimal service disruption	Knowledge decay without follow-up; difficult to sustain quality at scale	DHIS2 Academy; WHO AFRO workshops; Fiocruz Brazil; PAHO/Peru digital health courses; PAHO 2025 Digital Literacy Program
Online / eLearning	Scalable; geographically equitable; low marginal cost	Requires reliable Internet; high dropout; limited hands-on practice	Africa CDC e-Learning; Coursera Global Health MOOCs; India ABDM course; Australia Digital Health Hub
On-the-Job Mentoring	Contextualized; immediate application; high retention	Requires skilled mentors; difficult to scale; quality varies	PEPFAR SIMS mentoring; Rwanda iHMS facility coaches; Western Cape eHealth graduate programme; clinical champion models
Regional Cooperation	Achieves scale; shares costs; harmonizes standards	Requires political coordination; linguistic barriers	CARPHA Caribbean; PAHO regional training; WHO/Europe multi-country partnerships; ECOWAS/EAC potential hubs
Diaspora Engagement	High expertise; cultural connection; network effects	Engagement fragility; tensions with local institutions	Ethiopian diaspora initiative; Ghana Health IT diaspora; CARPHA diaspora integration

Source: Author's Compilation from Multiple Sources

11.10 Lessons from the Global South: Implications for Africa

The experiences of Latin America, the Caribbean, India, Southeast Asia, and the broader Asia-Pacific region in health informatics workforce development offer valuable lessons—not because these regions have solved the challenge, but because they face similar constraints to Africa related to scale, resources, and institutional capacity. This section summarizes key lessons that apply across different contexts. Six common themes emerge from these comparative experiences, which have direct implications for African strategies.

First, policy mandates are the most powerful accelerators of workforce development. The United States' ONC HITECH Act mandated EHR adoption and funded 50,000 health IT training positions. India's ABDM established mandatory digital registration requirements, creating demand for tens of thousands of trained professionals. Brazil's RNDS requires data managers at all levels of the health system. In each case, a regulatory requirement generated immediate, large-scale demand that the training sector was able to meet. Africa's national digital health strategies should include explicit workforce mandates aligned with the requirements for digital health deployment.

Second, regional cooperation is essential for achieving scale in fragmented systems. CARPHA's model shows that small states can access high-quality training by pooling resources. PAHO's 2025 Digital Literacy Program reached a continental audience within weeks. Africa's Regional Economic Communities—ECOWAS, EAC, SADC, and ECCAS—could host shared health informatics training hubs, with curricula tailored to linguistic and health-system clusters. A Francophone West African hub led by UCAD in Senegal, an East African hub at MUHAS in Tanzania, and a Southern African hub at the University of Cape Town could serve as primary training centers across the continent.

Third, aligning training with the national digital health infrastructure creates the strongest incentives. Brazil's Fiocruz courses count toward SUS certification because they align with the RNDS interoperability framework. India's ABDM-aligned training is mandatory for facility registration. Australia's Digital Health Hub connects learning directly to My Health Record and other national platforms. When certification requirements are tied to the systems professionals will actually use, completion rates rise and knowledge application improves.

Fourth, the private sector can be both a threat and an opportunity. In India, health-tech hiring increased by 62% in early 2025, attracting trained professionals at rates the public sector cannot keep up with. The same trend exists in Africa's expanding healthTech sector. Instead of viewing private-sector talent acquisition as merely brain drain, African governments should create structured public–private workforce exchange programs—such as secondments, joint appointments, and co-funded training—that enable the public sector to benefit from private-sector innovation while preserving essential public-sector workforce capacity.

Fifth, facility-level adoption models are as important as national training programs. The 'super-user' and clinical champion models used across Europe, Australia, and parts of Asia create internal advocates within health facilities who support colleagues through the transition to digital workflows. These models complement formal training with informal, peer-to-peer support that influences whether digital tools are consistently used in practice. Africa's facility-level capacity building—particularly in EMR and DHIS2 adoption—should systematically incorporate champion networks.

Sixth, professional identity and communities of practice support long-term growth. Australia's CHIA certification and Canada's competency framework help build a professional identity that retains people in the field. Africa's health informatics professional associations—AfHIMA, HELINA, and their national affiliates—require ongoing investment to fulfill this role. A pan-African health informatics certification framework with mutual recognition across countries would establish professional standards that enhance mobility within Africa and reduce incentives to emigrate.

11.11 Priority Interventions for Digital Health Skills and Workforce

Translating the foregoing analysis into action requires a strategic, phased approach that builds on existing strengths, addresses the most critical gaps, and establishes institutional foundations for long-term, self-sustaining workforce development.

In the short term (1–2 years), the top priorities are to assess training needs, align curricula, and adopt facility-level champion models. Countries should conduct systematic evaluations of health informatics workforce gaps—considering level, cadre, geographic distribution, and sub-discipline—to replace assumption-based training with evidence-based program planning. Existing pre-service curricula should be reviewed and updated to include digital health skills at all health worker levels, following the Indonesian and Ethiopian models that integrate digital literacy before health workers begin practicing. National professional associations should be strengthened through secretariat support, governance development, and the fostering of international partnerships to provide the institutional foundation for professional recognition and CPD. Facility-level super-user and clinical champion networks should be established at sites that use EMRs and DHIS2 to accelerate adoption.

In the medium term (3–5 years), investments should prioritize scaling effective models and strengthening regional collaboration. Countries that have succeeded in pre-service health informatics training—such as Ethiopia, Kenya, and Tanzania—should share curricula, faculty development methods, and deployment strategies with those at earlier stages. Regional training centers supported by MUHAS in East Africa, KNUST in West Africa, and the University of Cape Town in Southern Africa could serve multiple nations through regional student admissions, faculty exchanges, and shared online platforms. A pan-African health informatics certification system should be established through AfHIMA, with mutual recognition agreements. The CARPHA Caribbean, PAHO's Digital Literacy Program, and India's ABDM initiatives should be examined and adapted for African regional cooperation. A continental digital health workforce capability platform, modeled on Australia's Digital Health Hub, should be created to provide self-assessment tools, educational content, and career-pathway guidance.

Over the long term (5–10 years), the goal is to develop a self-sustaining, institutionally embedded health informatics workforce capable of leading Africa's digital health transformation from within. This includes establishing PhD programs at leading African universities to build a local faculty and research base for sustainable training; offering competitive salaries and career paths to retain talent within African public health systems; and fostering a vibrant continental community of practice connected through AfHIMA, HELINA, HISP, and emerging platforms that continuously improve the quality and relevance of health informatics across the continent. By this stage, digital literacy should be integrated not as a separate IT topic but as a core component of patient safety, data protection, service redesign, and quality improvement—the approach adopted by the strongest health systems worldwide.

11.12 Conclusion

This chapter has explored digital health skills and workforce development—the key enabler of the Digital Health Technology Stack introduced in Chapter 4—drawing on experiences from Africa, Latin America, the Caribbean, India, Indonesia, Australia, Canada, New Zealand, and the European Union to develop a comprehensive framework for building human capacity. The evidence is clear: Africa faces a health informatics workforce gap that is much larger than in high-income countries, making it the biggest obstacle to sustainable digital health progress on the continent.

The comparative analysis shows that no country in the Global South has fully solved the health informatics workforce challenge. India's ABDM has created significant demand and built institutional infrastructure, but adoption remains inconsistent and upskilling challenges persist. Brazil's Fiocruz–RNDS alignment highlights a strong link between training and infrastructure, yet the workforce remains heavily concentrated. The Caribbean's regional pooling model achieves scale from small beginnings but depends on ongoing political coordination. Peru's culturally relevant training methods address key contextual barriers, yet institutional capacity remains limited. PAHO's 2025 Digital Literacy Program demonstrates that, with institutional support, regional training can reach a large number of professionals quickly—over 70,000 in just weeks. Indonesia's integration of digital skills into pre-service curricula shows that embedding these skills before health workers begin practice helps build a stronger foundation.

These experiences reveal a key insight: deploying technology without parallel investment in the workforce leads to systems that are difficult to maintain, data that cannot be used, and innovations that are hard to sustain. Across all regions, the most successful implementation practices emphasize five principles: establishing competency frameworks, tailoring training to different roles and use cases, combining pre-service and ongoing in-service learning, linking training to systems in use, and supporting adoption through change management and local champions. The most successful national strategies—such as Ethiopia's pre-service scale-up, India's demand-driven policy mandates, CARPHA's regional collaboration, Brazil's alignment of training and infrastructure, and Australia's capability platform approach—combine supply-side training expansion with demand-side institutional signals, professional recognition with career incentives, and national investment with regional cooperation.

As Africa's digital health ecosystem evolves—with rising healthTech investments, expanding DHIS2 and EMR deployments, growing AI applications, and increasing data volumes—the need for workforce investment will become even more urgent. The foundational layers of the technology stack, described in Chapters 7 through 10, outline the technical architecture; this chapter has focused on the human architecture that determines whether those investments succeed or fail. The remaining cross-cutting enablers—research and development (Chapter 12), the healthtech ecosystem (Chapter 13), and financing and sustainability (Chapter 14)—are closely linked to workforce capacity, and their analysis will build on the frameworks established here.

References

Africa CDC. (2021). Africa CDC digital health strategy 2021–2025. African Union / Africa CDC.

Africa Health Information Management Association (AfHIMA). (2022). Africa Health Informatics Workforce Report. AfHIMA.

African Institute for Mathematical Sciences (AIMS). (2022). Data science for health initiative: Annual report. AIMS.

American Health Information Management Association (AHIMA). (2023). AHIMA International Health Informatics Competency Framework. AHIMA Press.

Atlantic Council. (2024). The future of digital transformation and workforce development in Latin America and the Caribbean. Adrienne Arsht Latin America Center.

Australian Digital Health Agency. (2024). Digital Health Hub and professional development resources. ADHA.

Balsari, S., Sesia, P., & Patnaik, S. (2024). India's evolving digital health strategy. npj Digital Medicine, 7, Article 285.

BMC Public Health. (2025). Considerations for adapting digital competencies and training approaches to the public health workforce: Practitioners' perspectives in Canada. BMC Public Health.

Canadian Institute for Health Information (CIHI). (2024). The state of the health workforce in Canada, 2024. CIHI.

Curioso, W. H. (2019). Building capacity and training for digital health: Challenges and opportunities in Latin America. Journal of Medical Internet Research, 21(12), e16513.

Curioso, W. H., Coronel-Chucos, L. G., & Oscuvilca-Tapia, E. (2024). Empowering the digital health workforce in Latin America: The Peruvian case. Informatics for Health and Social Care, 49(1), 73–82.

Digital Health Canada. (2023). Health Informatics Core Competencies Framework. Digital Health Canada.

Digital Health News. (2025). India's healthtech surge 2025: Capital, talent and new models. Digital Health News.

Digital Health Australia (2022). Australian Health Informatics Competency Framework. Digital Health Australia

European Commission. (2022). Proposal for a Regulation on the European Health Data Space (COM/2022/197 final). European Commission.

Federal Ministry of Health, Ethiopia. (2020). Health Sector Transformation Plan II 2020/21–2024/25. Federal Democratic Republic of Ethiopia.

Haile, T., Kebede, M., & Abebe, Y. (2021). Health informatics education and workforce development in Ethiopia. Ethiopian Journal of Health Development, 35(1), 12–21.

Haile, T., Mekonen, T., Tesfaye, W., & Kebede, M. (2022). Brain drain of health informatics professionals in East Africa. Global Health: Science and Practice, 10(3), e2100623.

Health Information Systems Programme (HISP). (2023). DHIS2 global report 2023. University of Oslo.

HELINA. (2025). Digital Health Applied Leadership Programme. Health Informatics in Africa.

HIKM. (2025). Health Informatics Knowledge Management Conference proceedings. HIKM.

International Telecommunication Union (ITU). (2022). Measuring digital development: ICT price trends 2021. ITU.

Manders, E., Yamey, G., & Shroff, Z. (2021). Health informatics training needs in sub-Saharan Africa: A systematic review. BMJ Global Health, 6(1), e003695.

Mantas, J., Ammenwerth, E., Demiris, G., et al. (2010). Recommendations of the IMIA on education in biomedical and health informatics. Methods of Information in Medicine, 49(2), 105–120.

Ministry of Health, Rwanda. (2021). National digital health strategic plan 2019–2024: Progress report 2021. Republic of Rwanda.

National Health Authority India. (2022). Ayushman Bharat Digital Mission: Annual report 2021–22. Government of India.

Nutley, T., et al. (2020). A practical guide to health systems strengthening through health information use. Global Health: Science and Practice, 8(3), 350–369.

OECD. (2024). Health workforce. Organization for Economic Co-operation and Development.

Office of the National Coordinator for Health IT (ONC). (2014). Health IT workforce development programs: Final evaluation report. US DHHS.

Pan American Health Organization (PAHO). (2021). Digital health strategy 2016–2025: Evaluation and update. PAHO.

PAHO. (2023). Policy on the Health Workforce 2030: Strengthening Human Resources for Health. PAHO.

PAHO. (2025). Digital Literacy Program for Health Sector Personnel: Launch and progress report. PAHO.

Shortliffe, E. H., & Cimino, J. J. (Eds.). (2014). Biomedical informatics (4th ed.). Springer.

UNICEF India. (2024). Digital Health Enterprise Planning Course: Launch announcement. UNICEF India.

Western Cape Government. (2022). eHealth implementation report 2021/22. Department of Health, Western Cape Government.

WHO. (2022). World health statistics 2022: Monitoring health for the SDGs. WHO.

WHO Africa. (2022). State of digital health in the African region: 2022 report. WHO AFRO.

WHO/Europe. (2025). Digital skills for the health and care workforce: Policy brief. WHO Regional Office for Europe.

Chapter 12 Research, Innovation, and Frontier Technologies

12.1 Overview

This chapter explores research and development—the second key enabler in the Digital Health Technology Stack—by examining the research landscape, innovation trends, and frontier-technology studies that are shaping digital health's future in Africa. It highlights research priorities, profiles leading academic and research institutions, and discusses how implementation science can translate evidence into practice. The chapter offers an in-depth analysis of studies on artificial intelligence and machine learning applications in healthcare, genomics and bioinformatics research, digital health technology assessment methods, and the ethical issues that should guide research and innovation.

Drawing systematically on practices from Latin America, the Caribbean, India, Southeast Asia, Australia, Canada, New Zealand, and Europe, this chapter outlines a course for developing a strong, ethical, and impact-oriented digital health research ecosystem that links Africa to global knowledge flows and ensures that African evidence drives African digital health policy and practice.

12.2 Research Priorities for Digital Health in Africa

Establishing clear, contextually relevant research priorities is essential to guide limited resources toward the most important questions for Africa's digital health transformation. The global digital health research landscape is extensive and expanding rapidly—PubMed indexed more than 15,000 digital health publications in 2023 alone—yet African contributions remain disproportionately small. A bibliometric analysis by Agarwal et al. (2022) found that sub-Saharan Africa accounted for less than 5 percent of global digital health publications from 2015 to 2022, despite bearing a disproportionate share of the global disease burden and being one of the fastest-growing markets for digital health technologies.

The gap between global research priorities and African needs is clear. Global research focuses on drug discovery, artificial intelligence for clinical decision support, and precision medicine—domains that require large-scale infrastructure, data, and expertise, largely concentrated in high-income countries. Africa's most pressing digital health research questions center on implementation challenges, adapting applications to local settings, community health worker platforms, mobile health for maternal and child health, optimizing existing systems such as DHIS2, and analyzing the effectiveness of telemedicine services (Wahl et al., 2018; Mehl et al., 2018). Latin America faces a similar challenge: a bibliometric analysis of AI research in the region found that between 2019 and 2023, the number of AI papers published each year increased 19-fold, yet the average citations per article dropped by 70 percent—showing a pattern of high volume but low impact, especially in health-related applications (De Gruyter, 2025). Brazil and Mexico are at the forefront of regional AI research, but incorporating AI into health policy remains in its early stages.

Figure 12.1. Comparative Research Activity Levels Across Digital Health Domains in Africa

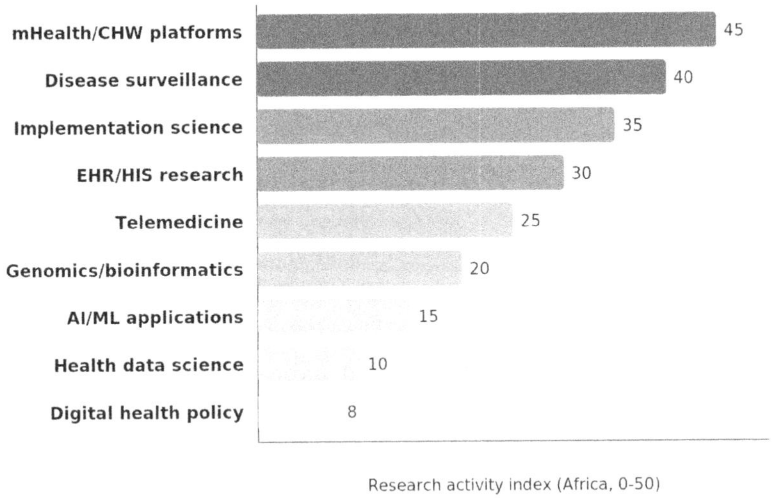

Source: Agarwal et al. (2022); Author's Assessment

Priority research areas for Africa's digital health agenda can be grouped into five interconnected domains:

- Implementation science research to understand how digital health interventions work across diverse African settings,
- Health systems research examining how digital technologies reshape governance, financing, human resources, and service delivery.
- Data science and AI research that address algorithmic bias, data quality, and local validation,
- Genomics and bioinformatics research to build Africa's capacity in precision medicine, and
- Research into ethical, legal, and social implications (ELSI), anticipating challenges in contexts with low digital literacy and diverse cultural norms regarding health information.

The implications of digital health research are widely recognized worldwide. The WHO's Global Strategy on Digital Health 2020–2025 highlights research as one of four main objectives (WHO, 2021). The European Commission's Horizon Europe program has dedicated more than EUR 1 billion to health research and innovation, including targeted calls on digital health in low- and middle-income countries (European Commission, 2023). The International Digital Health and AI Research Collaborative (I-DAIR), based in Geneva with global hubs in Singapore, Cambodia, India, Kenya, Chile, and Tunisia, represents a new model for building research capacity across Africa, Asia, and Latin America through collaborative 'pathfinder projects' (I-DAIR, 2024). Australia's National Health and Medical Research Council (NHMRC) and Canada's International Development Research Center (IDRC) have both increased funding for digital health research partnerships with institutions in the Global South.

12.3 Academic and Research Institutions Leading Innovation

Africa's digital health research landscape is anchored by a growing network of academic institutions that combine technical expertise with contextual understanding. The University of Cape Town's H3D has pioneered computational drug discovery for neglected tropical diseases. Makerere University's AI Lab has produced globally recognized research on machine learning for TB detection. The University of Nairobi/Strathmore's @iLabAfrica drives innovation in mHealth and health information systems. The University of Ghana/WACCBIP leads genomics research within the H3Africa network. The African Institute of Mathematical Science (AIMS) provides advanced data science training across six African countries. DHIS2 implementation research is anchored by the Health Information System Program nodes across the continent, and the Institut Pasteur Africa network drives pathogen genomics and digital surveillance (AIMS, 2023; Makerere AI Lab, 2023; H3D, 2023).

Table 12.1. Selected Leading Digital Health Research Institutions in Africa.

Institution	Country	Key Research Areas	Notable Contributions
UCT / H3D	South Africa	Drug discovery, biomedical engineering,	AI for neglected tropical diseases; computational drug design
Makerere University	Uganda	AI/ML diagnostics, health informatics,	Deep learning for TB and malaria detection; globally recognized AI Lab
U. Nairobi / Strathmore	Kenya	HIS, mHealth, AI diagnostics, telemedicine	@iLabAfrica; DHIS2 research; community health platforms
U. Ghana / WACCBIP	Ghana	Genomics, bioinformatics, pathogen	H3Africa leadership; malaria genomics; digital pathogen
AIMS Network	Pan-African	Data science, ML, mathematical modelling	Training pipeline; epidemic modelling; climate-health analytics
HISP (Africa nodes)	Multi-country	HIS, DHIS2, data quality	DHIS2 development; implementation research in 40+ countries
Institut Pasteur (Africa)	Multi-country	Pathogen genomics, digital surveillance	COVID-19/Ebola sequencing; Africa PGI

Source: Author's Compilation.

Compared with other regions, Latin America's biomedical research capacity is constrained by low R&D investment and limited integration into global networks, although Brazil, Mexico, and Argentina lead in output (Huete-Perez et al., 2025). India's research ecosystem features institutions such as IIT Bombay, the Indian Institute of Science, and CSIR-IGIB that contribute to the ABDM framework. Australia's Digital Health CRC and CSIRO, Canada's Vector Institute and Mila, and New Zealand's health informatics centers have developed research programs with explicit components for Global South collaboration.

12.4 Implementation Science for Digital Health

Implementation science—the study of methods to promote the systematic uptake of evidence-based practices into routine practice—is arguably the most critical research discipline for Africa's digital health transformation. The continent's challenge is not primarily a technology deficit but rather a knowledge deficit in effectively implementing, adapting, scaling, and sustaining these technologies within complex, resource-constrained health systems (Peters et al., 2013; Theobald et al., 2018).

The implementation science framework for digital health in Africa emphasizes that digital health interventions should be grounded in rigorous evidence, data, and learning, ensuring that technologies are not only introduced but also effective, safe, and contextually relevant. The framework positions implementation as a continuous, learning-driven process rather than a one-time deployment, emphasizing feedback loops and adaptation over time. The key components of evidence-informed implementation are:

- Context assessment examines political, economic, social, and technological conditions to ensure interventions align with country realities.
- Stakeholder engagement that emphasizes the inclusion of users, providers, policymakers, and communities to promote ownership and usability.

- Adaptation and localization to ensure that solutions are tailored to cultural, linguistic, and infrastructural contexts.
- Outcome evaluation, which focuses on measuring effectiveness, cost, equity, and sustainability, while
- Scale-up pathways that address how successful interventions can expand horizontally, vertically, or functionally.
- Knowledge translation that ensures that evidence is synthesized into actionable policies, guidelines, and practices.

Figure 12.2. Implementation Science Framework for Digital Health in Africa

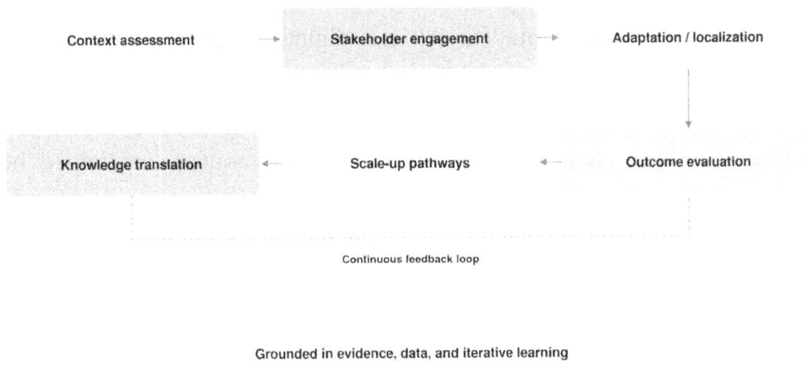

Source: Adapted from Damschroder et al. (2009); Peters et al. (2013); Author's Elaboration.

Several implementation science frameworks have been used in African digital health contexts. The Consolidated Framework for Implementation Research (CFIR) has been used to evaluate the deployment of electronic health records in South African primary care, highlighting leadership engagement, usability, and workflow compatibility as key factors (Katurura & Cilliers, 2018). The Reach, Effectiveness, Adoption, Implementation, Maintenance (RE-AIM) framework has been adapted for digital health assessments across the Global South: in Tanzania for mHealth antenatal care (Lund et al., 2014) and in Brazil to expand teleconsultation services within its primary care system (Harzheim et al., 2016).

India's ABDM implementation offers further insights: a phased rollout beginning with six pilot states, 'sandbox' environments to test interoperability standards, and a dedicated implementation support unit (National Health Authority India, 2022). Australia's shift of My Health Record to share-by-default in 2025, after years of low opt-in uptake, demonstrates that implementation strategies must evolve in response to real-world evidence.

12.5 Artificial Intelligence and Machine Learning Research

12.5.1 Disease Diagnosis and Prediction

AI-powered diagnostic tools can help address Africa's severe shortage of specialists by extending diagnostic capabilities to primary care. The Makerere AI Lab's work on automated TB detection has achieved accuracy comparable to radiologists' on African datasets (Nakasi et al., 2021). Qure.ai, an Indian AI company, has deployed chest X-ray AI tools in Kenya, Ghana, and South Africa, demonstrating South–South technology transfer (Qure.ai, 2023). In Latin America, AI diagnostics are used for TB screening in Peru, cervical cancer screening via Colombia's CITOBOT device, and diabetic retinopathy detection in Mexico—each tailored to resource-limited settings with disease burdens similar to those in Africa (Rios-Garcia et al., 2025).

Figure 12.3 highlights six key application areas of AI and machine learning in African healthcare: medical imaging and diagnostics (including TB and cancer detection), predictive analytics (for outbreak prediction and patient risk assessment), natural language processing (clinical text analysis and multilingual chatbots), drug discovery and repurposing, genomics and precision medicine, and supply chain optimization (including forecasting and logistics). These domains span clinical care, research, and health system management, underscoring AI's wide-ranging transformative potential. Critical cross-cutting factors—data quality, algorithmic bias, regulatory frameworks, local validation, and ethics—are essential to ensuring AI solutions are safe, equitable, and effective in African settings.

Figure 12.3. Six Major Domains of AI/ML Applications in African Healthcare with Cross-cutting Challenges

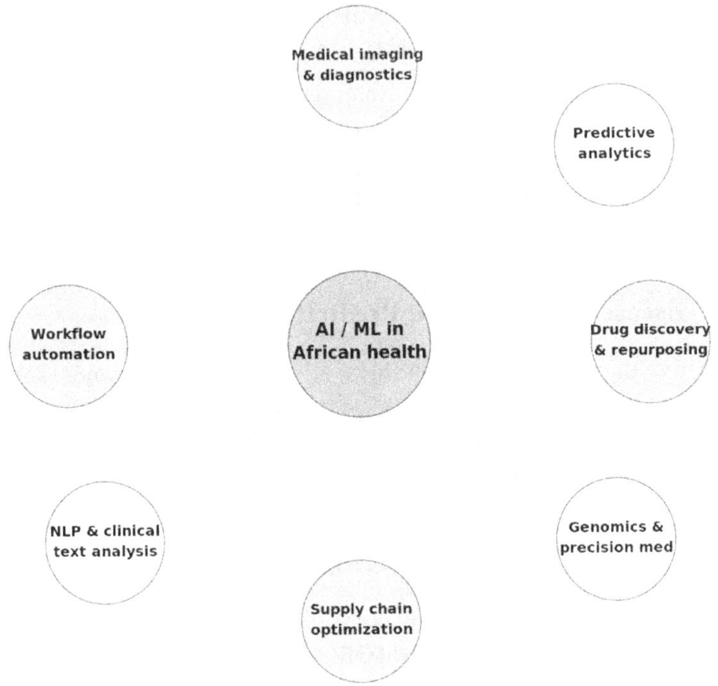

Source: Author's Elaboration

Algorithmic bias is the most significant challenge to AI adoption in Africa and is a growing area of research. Most AI models are trained on data from high-income countries, raising concerns about their effectiveness for African, Latin American, or South Asian populations. Obermeyer et al. (2019) demonstrated significant racial bias in widely used US clinical prediction algorithms. Latin American initiatives such as LatinCells are creating inclusive, AI-ready genomic data to address this bias, and researchers are moving from simply providing samples to leading in equitable genomics-based medicine (Nature Reviews, 2025). The Africa CDC has also invested in AI-driven epidemic intelligence platforms that aggregate data from multiple sources for early outbreak detection (Africa CDC, 2023).

12.5.2 Drug Discovery and Personalized Medicine

The University of Cape Town's H3D has pioneered computational drug discovery for neglected diseases. Partnerships with Open Source Malaria and DNDi advance the use of machine learning for drug-target interactions (DNDi, 2023). Genomic datasets from the H3Africa Consortium provide a foundation for pharmacogenomics—research into how genetic variation affects drug responses. Research at UCT and Stellenbosch focuses on developing pharmacogenomic models for Southern African populations (Dandara et al., 2019). India's Genome India project and the UK's Genomics England also demonstrate how population-specific genomics can be translated into clinical applications.

12.6 Genomics and Bioinformatics Research

Africa's genomics capacity has grown significantly through H3Africa, which has supported more than 50 projects across 30 countries. African populations harbor more genetic variation than all others combined yet accounted for less than 3 percent of participants in Genome-Wide Association Studies (GWAS) until recently (Gurdasani et al., 2019). Latin America faces a similar gap: a 2024 Wellcome report highlighted reluctance to share genetic data, limited infrastructure, and low political priority as barriers. Initiatives such as Project JAGUAR are generating population-specific data that parallel H3Africa's mission (Sanger Institute, 2025).

Pathogen genomics, accelerated by COVID-19, has been transformative. The Africa Pathogen Genomics Initiative built continent-wide sequencing capacity, which contributed to the identification of the Omicron variant (Viana et al., 2022). The UK's Genomics England and Australia's Genomics Health Alliance serve as models for translating genomics into clinical practice, supported by ongoing government investment and integration with digital health infrastructure.

Figure 12.4. Leading African Countries in Genomics and Bioinformatics Research Output, 2018–2024

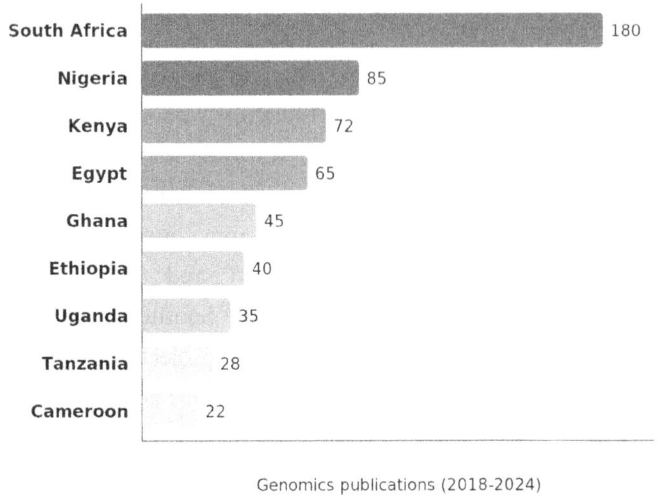

Source: H3Africa Consortium (2023); Author's Compilation

12.7 Digital Health Technology Assessment

Digital Health Technology Assessment (DHTA) involves several steps for evaluating and implementing digital health solutions. It begins with technology identification through horizon scanning and stakeholder input, followed by evidence evaluation focused on clinical effectiveness, safety, and data quality. The process then includes economic assessment to determine cost-effectiveness, budget impact, and return on investment, and proceeds to ethical, legal, and social analysis covering issues such as equity, privacy, consent, and cultural acceptability.

The final stages assess implementation feasibility—considering infrastructure, workforce, and scalability—and conclude with recommendations and monitoring, including policy guidance and post-market evaluation. A key feature of the framework is its emphasis on continuous feedback, in which real-world evidence informs updated assessments and adaptive decision-making, making DHTA an iterative process that supports sustainable, context-specific digital health adoption.

Figure 12.5. The Six-stage Process for Digital Health Technology Assessment

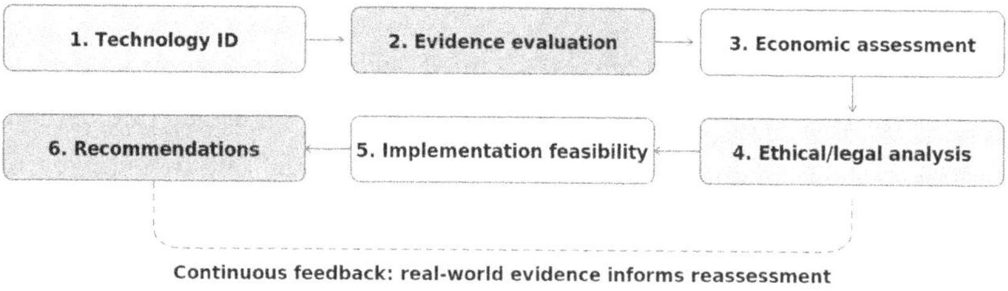

Source: Adapted from Kidholm et al. (2012); Author's Elaboration

The EU's Model for Assessment of Telemedicine (MAST) framework, which parallels the DHTA, evaluates telemedicine across seven domains (Kidholm et al., 2012). It begins with health problems and application characteristics, which define the clinical condition being addressed and the technology's operation. This is followed by safety, which minimizes clinical and technical risks, and clinical effectiveness, which examines the impact on patient outcomes and life expectancy. The framework also considers patient perspectives, capturing user experience, satisfaction, and the service's acceptability. In addition, economic aspects assess costs, cost-effectiveness, and broader financial implications, while organizational aspects evaluate how the intervention affects workflows, staff roles, training needs, and institutional coordination. Finally, socio-cultural, ethical, and legal aspects address critical issues such as privacy, equity of access, cultural acceptability, and regulatory compliance, ensuring that digital health solutions are not only effective but also equitable and contextually appropriate.

Thailand's Health Intervention and Technology Assessment Program (HITAP), established in 2007, has become a globally recognized LMIC-led HTA center, providing technical support to Ghana, Kenya, and Tanzania (HITAP, 2023). Chile's GES program links evidence reviews to national coverage decisions (Vargas & Poblete, 2017). The African Health Economics and Policy Association (AfHEA) and the international Decision Support Initiative (iDSI) have also created platforms for HTA capacity building, but dedicated digital health assessment units remain rare on the continent.

12.8 Ethical Considerations in Digital Health Research

Digital health research ethics in Africa must account for communal decision-making, low digital literacy, power asymmetries, and the legacy of exploitative research. Dynamic consent—allowing participants to update their preferences over time—has been proposed but is difficult to implement in low-resource settings (Kaye et al., 2015). In Latin America, similar colonial legacies create barriers to sharing genetic data (Sanger Institute, 2025).

The ethical framework for digital health research in Africa, grounded in human dignity and justice, underpins all research and innovation activities. Digital health projects must respect individual rights, promote equity, and prevent harm, especially in settings marked by inequality and vulnerability. Six key ethical pillars guide responsible research and deployment. These pillars include informed consent, tailored to varying levels of digital literacy; privacy and confidentiality, ensuring robust data protection, especially for vulnerable groups; and data sovereignty, which emphasizes community and national ownership of data.

The framework also emphasizes community involvement, encouraging participatory research design and governance; algorithmic fairness, including testing AI systems for bias among African populations; and benefit sharing, advocating for an equitable distribution of research results. Collectively, these elements constitute a comprehensive, context-aware ethical approach that aligns digital health research with African values, governance goals, and social justice priorities.

Data sovereignty has become increasingly important—an area of research expected to advance as digital health adoption grows across the continent. The Human Heredity and Health in Africa (H3Africa) framework mandates storage on African servers and African-led governance. New Zealand's Te Mana Raraunga—Māori Data Sovereignty Network—asserts indigenous rights over community-derived data, shaping global discussions directly relevant to African communities. The Montreal Declaration (2018) and WHO's AI Ethics guidance (2021) serve as references; however, Africa-specific research and guidelines are still needed.

12.9 Research Collaboration and Networks

The ecosystem of digital health research collaboration networks in Africa can be structured around three complementary models: South–South collaboration, North–South partnerships, and multi-stakeholder platforms. South–South collaboration focuses on intra-African and Global South cooperation, strengthening local capacity, promoting knowledge exchange, and supporting context-driven innovation. North–South partnerships connect African institutions with global funders and research organizations, providing resources, technical expertise, and access to advanced infrastructure. Multi-stakeholder platforms bring together governments, international organizations, private-sector actors, and NGOs to coordinate efforts, mobilize funding, and scale solutions. Together, these interconnected models demonstrate how diverse partnerships enhance research capacity, foster innovation, and enable more impactful and sustainable digital health development across Africa.

Figure 12.6. Three Principal Modes of Digital Health Research Collaboration in Africa

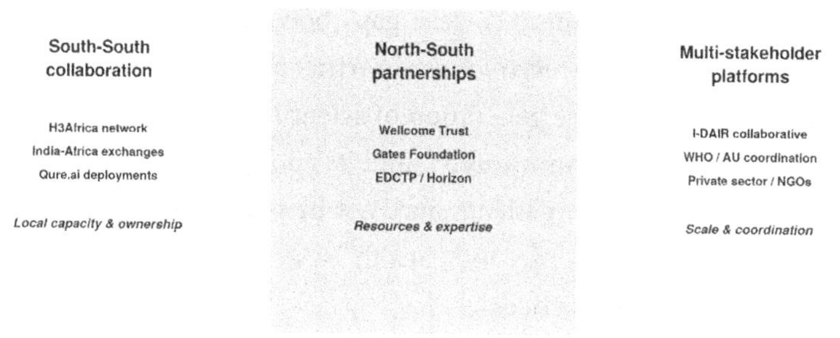

Source: Author's Elaboration

South–South collaboration has expanded significantly in recent years. The Human Heredity and Health in Africa (H3Africa) initiative links researchers from more than 30 countries. India–Africa health exchanges are growing through the India–Africa Health Sciences Cooperation. Qure.ai's deployments in Africa demonstrate South–South technology transfer. Brazil's Fiocruz collaborates with Lusophone Africa through CPLP (Fiocruz, 2023). Latin American genomics initiatives such as LatinCells and Project JAGUAR develop approaches similar to those of H3Africa and could benefit from structured exchanges between Africa and Latin America.

North–South partnerships remain dominant, with major funders such as the Wellcome Trust, Gates Foundation, NIH/Fogarty, Horizon Europe, UK NIHR, and Canada's IDRC providing the platform. The European and Developing Countries Clinical Trials Partnership (EDCTP) has invested more than EUR 2.3 billion, and EDCTP3 explicitly includes digital health innovation (EDCTP, 2023). However, growing criticism of power imbalances has sparked calls to decolonize global health research (Abimbola, 2019). Deliberations by the International Digital Health & AI Research Collaborative and a 2024 Lancet Digital Health article warning against colonialism in pathogen genomics point to studies that encourage a shift toward more equitable research structures (Saha et al., 2024).

12.10 Translating Research into Practice

On average, it takes about 17 years for research evidence to be translated into routine clinical practice. This "17-year gap" between evidence and practice (Morris et al., 2011) is likely even longer in African health systems. It implies a significant delay between the generation of scientific knowledge—such as new treatments, guidelines, or innovations—and its adoption and use in real-world health systems. As a result, patients may not benefit from the most effective and up-to-date interventions, and health systems may continue to use outdated or less efficient practices.

The concept highlights systemic barriers, including weak knowledge translation mechanisms, limited health system capacity, inadequate training, regulatory delays, and resistance to change among practitioners and institutions. It underscores the importance of implementation science, which seeks to narrow this gap by promoting faster, more effective uptake of evidence through strategies such as stakeholder engagement, context-sensitive adaptation, continuous learning, and policy alignment—particularly relevant in resource-constrained settings, including many African health systems.

Knowledge translation platforms, including the African Institute for Development Policy (AFIDEP), Evidence-Informed Policy Network (EVIPNet) Africa, and the Cochrane Africa Network, work to bridge the "17-year gap" by ensuring that health policies and clinical practices are grounded in high-quality research rather than intuition or outdated traditions. AFIDEP serves as a "knowledge translator," working directly with governments to bridge gaps among research, policy, and practice across sectors such as health, environment, and education. EVIPNet establishes national partnerships among policymakers, researchers, and civil society. Its primary tool is the "Evidence Brief for Policy," which packages complex data into actionable summaries for health system managers. The Cochrane Africa Network serves as a regional hub of the global Cochrane collaboration, focusing on identifying research gaps specific to Africa (e.g., malaria, TB, and HIV/AIDS) and on building the capacity of local researchers to lead these studies. These platforms can improve the dissemination of digital health research, thereby increasing uptake and influencing policy decisions.

Thailand's Health Intervention and Technology Assessment Program (HITAP) offers a model for translating Health Technology Assessment (HTA) into coverage decisions. In Africa, evidence-based procurement guidelines offer a practical way to integrate research evidence into digital health investment decisions.

12.11 Conclusion

This chapter has examined research and development—a key cross-cutting enabler of the Digital Health Technology Stack—drawing on Africa's growing research ecosystem and experiences from Latin America, India, Southeast Asia, Australia, Canada, New Zealand, and Europe. Africa's research output is growing but remains disproportionately small. The most critical gaps are in implementation science, AI validation using representative datasets, and the translation of genomic discoveries into clinical applications.

No region has fully resolved the tension between global collaboration and local ownership. Latin America's genomics initiatives face the same bias challenges as H3Africa. India's ABDM offers implementation lessons. Thailand's HITAP demonstrates LMIC-led HTA. In Africa, the path forward requires simultaneous investment in research capacity, governance, and the translation of evidence into digital health investment practice.

References

Abimbola, S. (2019). The foreign gaze. BMJ Global Health, 4(5), e002068.

Africa CDC. (2023). Epidemic intelligence: Digital tools. Africa CDC.

Agarwal, S., et al. (2022). Evidence on mHealth strategies. TMIH, 20(8), 1003-1014.

AIMS. (2023). Annual report 2023. AIMS.

Canada Health Infoway. (2024). Pan-Canadian interoperability strategy. CHI.

Dandara, C., et al. (2019). Pharmacogenomics in Africa. Pharmacogenomics, 20(7), 515-527.

Damschroder, L. J., et al. (2009). CFIR. Implementation Science, 4, 50.

De Gruyter. (2025). AI research trends in Latin America. Open Political Science.

DNDi. (2023). Annual report 2023. DNDi.

EDCTP. (2023). Portfolio and impact report. EDCTP.

European Commission. (2023). Horizon Europe Health cluster. EC.

EVIPNet. (2023). Annual review. WHO.

Fiocruz. (2023). CPLP partnerships. Fundação Oswaldo Cruz.

Genomics England. (2023). Annual report 2022-2023. Genomics England.

Glasgow, R. E., et al. (1999). RE-AIM. AJPH, 89(9), 1322-1327.

Government of India. (2022). Genome India project. DoB.

Gurdasani, D., et al. (2019). Uganda Genome Resource. Cell, 179(4), 984-1002.

H3Africa Consortium. (2023). Consortium report 2023. H3Africa.

H3D. (2023). Annual report. UCT.

Harzheim, E., et al. (2016). Telehealth in Brazil. Telemed e-Health, 22(11), 938-944.

Hedt-Gauthier, B. L., et al. (2019). Research capacity strengthening. Ann Glob Health, 85(1), 146.

HITAP. (2023). Institutional profile. HITAP Thailand.

Huete-Perez, J. A., et al. (2025). Biomedical research in Latin America. Front Res Metr Anal, 10.

I-DAIR. (2024). Institutional profile. I-DAIR / Fondation Botnar.

Katurura, M. C., & Cilliers, L. (2018). EHR in South Africa. Afr J Prim Health Care, 10(1), e1–e8.

Kaye, J., et al. (2015). Dynamic consent. EJHG, 23(2), 141–146.

Kidholm, K., et al. (2012). MAST. IJTAHC, 28(1), 44–51.

Lund, S., et al. (2014). Mobile phones in Zanzibar. BMC Pregnancy Childbirth, 14, 29.

Makerere AI Lab. (2023). Annual report. Makerere University.

Mehl, G., et al. (2018). Harnessing mHealth. Springer.

Montreal Declaration. (2018). Responsible AI. U. de Montréal.

Morris, Z. S., et al. (2011). The 17-year gap. JRSM, 104(12), 510–520.

Mulder, N. J., et al. (2018). Bioinformatics infrastructure. Global Heart, 12(2), 91–98.

Nakasi, R., et al. (2021). Malaria diagnosis. SN Applied Sciences, 3, 340.

NHA India. (2022). ABDM implementation report. NHA India.

Nature Reviews. (2025). Single-cell research in LAC. Nat Rev Mol Cell Biol.

NICD. (2022). COVID-19 forecasting. NICD.

Obermeyer, Z., et al. (2019). Racial bias in algorithms. Science, 366, 447–453.

PANCAP. (2022). Benefit-sharing framework. PANCAP.

Peters, D. H., et al. (2013). Implementation research. BMJ, 347, f6753.

Qure.ai. (2023). Africa deployment report. Qure.ai.

Rios-Garcia, W., et al. (2025). AI for chronic disease in LAC. J Med Syst, 49, 82.

Saha, S., et al. (2024). Colonialism in pathogen genomics. Lancet Digit Health, 6, e520–e525.

Sanger Institute. (2025). Genomics research in Latin America. Wellcome Sanger Blog.

Theobald, S., et al. (2018). Implementation research. Lancet, 392, 2214–2228.

Vargas, V., & Poblete, S. (2017). Chile health prioritization. Global Network for Health Equity.

Viana, R., et al. (2022). Omicron variant. Nature, 603, 679–686.

Wahl, B., et al. (2018). AI and global health. BMJ Glob Health, 3(4), e000798.

WHO. (2021). Global strategy on digital health. WHO.

WHO. (2021). Ethics and governance of AI for health. WHO.

Chapter 13 The HealthTech Ecosystem in Africa

13.1. Overview

This chapter examines the healthTech ecosystem—the third cross-cutting enabler in the Digital Health Technology Stack (Figure 4.1). HealthTech comprises private-sector companies, startups, social enterprises, and innovation hubs that develop, deploy, and sustain digital health products and services. The chapter charts the rapidly evolving digital health market across Africa and discusses the innovation ecosystems that nurture startups and technology ventures. It analyzes the diverse business models that promote sustainability and scale, and examines intellectual property, technology transfer, and the creation of enabling environments that foster digital health innovation.

Drawing systematically on experiences from India, Southeast Asia, Brazil, Latin America, the Caribbean, Australia, Canada, New Zealand, and Europe, the chapter provides a comprehensive guide for entrepreneurs, investors, policymakers, and development partners seeking to build a healthTech ecosystem that is locally rooted, commercially viable, and aligned with public health priorities.

13.2 Digital Health Market Landscape in Africa

Africa's digital health market has grown rapidly, driven by rising mobile adoption, expanding Internet access, and the catalytic effects of the COVID-19 pandemic. The market was expected to exceed USD 11 billion by 2025. Africa's healthTech industry was the only sector to post year-over-year funding growth during the 2023–2024 global downturn, recording a 7 percent rise while other tech sectors declined (Founders Factory Africa, 2024; Healthcare Digital, 2025). In 2025, African healthTech funding reached about USD 215 million, a substantial 232 percent increase from the previous year, signaling that the sector had moved past its lowest point and was entering a phase of recovery and growth (Partech Partners, 2025).

Figure 13.1. Africa's Digital Health Market Growth

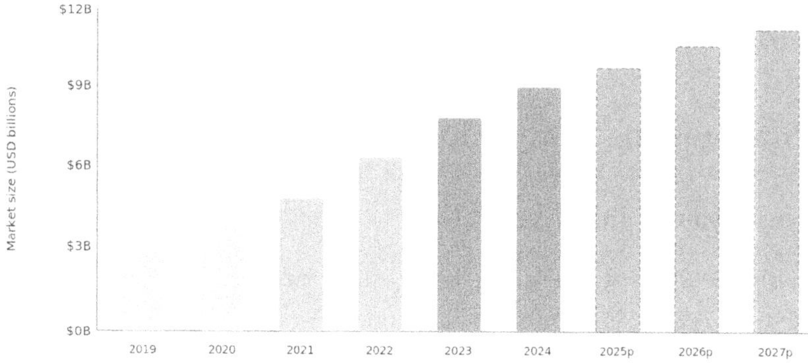

Source: Research & Markets (2023); Frost & Sullivan (2023); Author's Update.

The market is highly diverse. Nigeria, South Africa, Kenya, and Egypt together account for about 83 percent of startup funding, reflecting their larger economies, more developed tech ecosystems, and higher concentrations of venture capital and talent (Partech Partners, 2025). However, smaller markets such as Rwanda, Ghana, Senegal, and Tanzania are emerging as key innovation hubs, often fueled by progressive government policies and targeted support from development partners. By segment, telemedicine and virtual care account for the largest share, at roughly 28 percent of market value, followed by health financing and insurtech at 22 percent, and electronic health records and health information systems at around 16 percent (Disrupt Africa, 2023).

Compared with India's digital health market—estimated at around USD 12 billion in 2023 and driven by the ABDM and substantial government investment in digital public infrastructure—and Brazil's market, valued at roughly USD 8 billion and supported by the unified health system (SUS) and a vibrant startup ecosystem concentrated in São Paulo and Belo Horizonte, Africa's market potential remains largely underexploited (NASSCOM, 2023; ABStartups, 2023). Latin America's digital health market was valued at USD 12.82 billion in 2024 and is expected to reach USD 66.40 billion by 2033, reflecting a CAGR of over 20 percent (Market Data Forecast, 2024). Southeast

Asia attracted around USD 1.8 billion in healthTech investment from 2020 to 2023 (Tracxn, 2023). These examples suggest that deliberate policy interventions and ecosystem investments could significantly accelerate Africa's growth trajectory.

13.3 Startups and Innovation Ecosystems

13.3.1 Incubators and Accelerators

Africa's digital health startup ecosystem is supported by a rapidly expanding network of technology incubators, accelerators, and innovation hubs. As of 2024, the continent had more than 1,000 active technology hubs, with an estimated 120 focused specifically on health technology or health-sector apps (AfriLabs, 2023; GSMA, 2023). The HealthTech Hub Africa (HTHA) in Rwanda, supported by the Novartis Foundation and the Global Fund, awarded USD 400,000 to seven startups in Nigeria, Kenya, Rwanda, Tanzania, and Ghana through its 2024 Innovation Challenge. These companies collectively reached more than 905,000 patients, engaged 2,865 healthcare providers, and integrated their solutions into 1,811 public health facilities (HTHA, 2025). HTHA's 2025 cohort grew to 21 enterprises, building on the 2024 cohort's success in raising USD 7.85 million in additional funding and reaching more than 1.6 million people.

The Investing in Innovation (i3) Africa program—a partnership of donors, pharmaceutical companies, and African government agencies—has supported over 60 early- and growth-stage innovators from 21 African countries over 36 months. It provides risk-tolerant grants of USD 50,000 for early-stage innovators and up to USD 225,000 for growth-stage innovators, along with commercialization support and facilitation of market access(i3 Africa, 2025). The UNDP's Timbuktoo Innovation Fund, working with eight African countries including Rwanda, Nigeria, Kenya, and Egypt, aims to invest USD 1 billion to support 1,000 African tech startups over the next decade, with a dedicated healthTech hub based in Kigali.

In Latin America, comparable programs include the Inter-American Development Bank's (IDB) WeXchange accelerator and Brazil's Eretz.bio health-tech incubator at Albert Einstein Hospital in São Paulo, which provides startups with direct access to clinical settings for testing and validation—a hospital-embedded innovation model that Africa can learn from (IDB, 2022). In Asia, Singapore's Health Sciences Authority sandbox for AI-based medical devices and India's Atal Innovation Mission, which has established more than 10,000 Atal Tinkering Labs nationwide, demonstrate how government-supported innovation infrastructure can foster health-tech entrepreneurship at the national level.

13.3.2 Venture Capital and Funding Landscape

Venture capital and impact investment in African digital health have grown significantly, though from a low base and subject to the global funding cycle. Cumulative investment in African health technology startups from 2019 to 2024 exceeded USD 4 billion, with funding peaking in 2022 before moderating during the 2023–2024 global contraction (Salient Advisory, 2024; Partech Partners, 2025). In Q1 2025, AVCA data indicated the decline was stabilizing, with seed deals up 48 percent year-over-year—a crucial signal for early-stage healthTech startups (Healthcare Digital, 2025). Helium Health raised USD 30 million in Series B funding in 2023, the second-largest ever for African healthTech, and extended its footprint to eight countries (Springer Nature, 2025).

Key investors include pan-African and global funds with clear health mandates. Impact-oriented investors such as the Skoll Foundation, Omidyar Network, and the Bill & Melinda Gates Foundation have been especially active in supporting early-stage, high-impact ventures. Compared with Asia, where digital health funding in India alone surpassed USD 2.5 billion in 2021, and where the global digital health market continues to concentrate capital in North America, Africa's share remains disproportionately small relative to its disease burden.

Addressing this gap requires strengthening the pipeline of investable enterprises, expanding access to patient capital for early-stage ventures, and building investor confidence through successful exits—such as RapidDeploy's acquisition by Motorola Solutions, which is among the most significant African healthTech exits to date (HealthCap Africa, 2024).

Figure 13.2. Venture Capital and Impact Investment in African Digital Health, 2018–2024

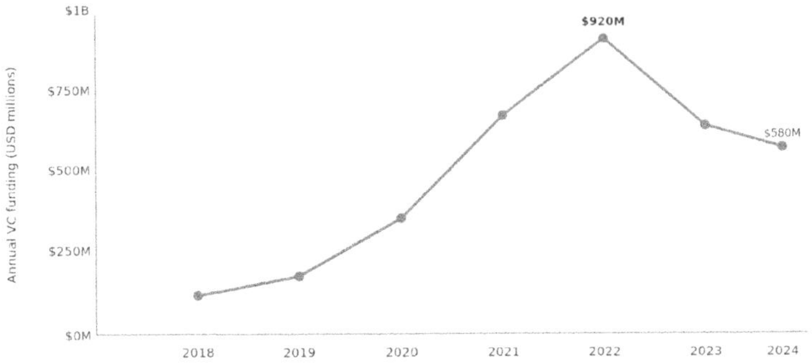

Source: Partech Partners (2023); Briter Bridges (2023); Author's Update

13.3.3 Success Stories and Emerging Leaders

Africa's digital health landscape is characterized by both the regional distribution of startups and the allocation of funding across solution areas, indicating highly concentrated innovation activity. The 2023 Disrupt Africa and Partech Partners survey shows that West Africa leads with 210 startups, followed by East Africa with 185, making them the dominant hubs of digital health entrepreneurship on the continent. Southern Africa (95) and North Africa (65) show moderate levels of activity, while Central Africa (20) lags significantly, reflecting persistent structural constraints, including weaker infrastructure, limited access to finance, and less-developed innovation ecosystems. Overall, the data highlight a clear geographic imbalance, with a few regions driving most of the continent's digital health innovation.

The 2023 survey also shows that investment funding is skewed toward scalable, technology-driven solutions. Telemedicine and virtual care attract the largest share ($320M), followed by health financing ($280M), indicating strong investor interest in remote service delivery and fintech-enabled healthcare access. Mid-level investments are seen in EHR and data systems ($195M) and diagnostics & AI ($175M), reflecting a growing emphasis on data-driven healthcare. Meanwhile, pharmacy and supply chain solutions ($140M) receive moderate support, and maternal and child health ($85M) receives the least funding despite its critical importance. This pattern reveals a sectoral imbalance in which commercial scalability tends to outweigh public health priorities, suggesting the need for more targeted policy and financing interventions.

Figure 13.3. Distribution of Digital Health Startups Across African Regions

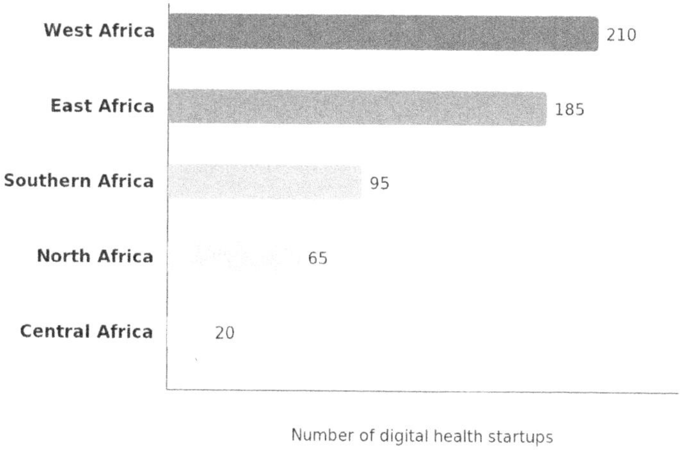

Source: Disrupt Africa (2023); Partech Partners (2023)

Several African digital health enterprises have achieved significant scale. mPharma (Ghana) has built a pharmacy and drug supply chain platform across nine African countries, serving more than 800 pharmacies and backed by more than USD 65 million in financing. Vezeeta (Egypt) offers integrated telemedicine and appointment platforms that serve more than 5 million patients. Helium Health (Nigeria) provides cloud-based hospital management solutions across West Africa.

LifeBank (Nigeria) uses technology to address challenges in blood and medical commodity supply chains. Access Afya (Kenya) operates digitally enabled micro-clinics in Nairobi's informal settlements. Vula Mobile (South

Africa) connects 7,000+ healthcare providers for specialist referrals. mPedigree (Ghana) combats counterfeit medicines using mobile authentication.

Table13.1. Selected Leading African Digital Health Enterprises

Enterprise	Country	Focus Area	Scale & Impact	Funding
mPharma	Ghana	Pharmacy & supply chain	800+ pharmacies across 9 countries	USD 65M+ (equity & debt)
Vezeeta	Egypt	Telemedicine &	5M+ patients, 30,000+ providers	USD 40M+
Helium Health	Nigeria	EHR & hospital	10,000+ providers; 8 countries	USD 30M+ (Series B 2023)
LifeBank	Nigeria	Blood & medical	Major cities across Nigeria & Kenya	USD 10M+
Access Afya	Kenya	Primary care micro-clinics	Underserved urban communities	USD 7M+
Vula	South Africa	Specialist	7,000+ providers	Grant & social enterprise
Zipline	Rwanda/ multi	Drone medical	10M+ health products delivered	USD 400M+

Source: Company reports; Disrupt Africa (2023); Author's Compilation

13.4 Local vs. International Technology Vendors

The African digital health market features a dynamic interplay between locally developed solutions and international technology platforms. Local vendors have critical advantages in understanding the context, including local disease profiles, health system workflows, cultural norms, language diversity, and infrastructure constraints such as intermittent connectivity and power supply issues. Solutions like Helium Health (Nigeria), Savics (Rwanda), and OpenFn (South Africa) include offline capabilities, low-bandwidth optimization, USSD-based interfaces, and mobile money integration. International vendors —Microsoft, Google Health, AWS, Oracle Health—bring technical maturity, established support ecosystems, and the ability to invest at scale.

However, reliance on international platforms raises concerns about data sovereignty, long-term cost sustainability, and vendor lock-in. India's ABDM, which mandates open standards and interoperability to prevent vendor lock-in, provides a relevant policy model. Brazil's SUS digital platform emphasizes open-source and locally developed solutions where feasible, while integrating international components through standardized APIs (National Health Authority India, 2021; Ministry of Health Brazil, 2020). An increasing number of African countries are adopting hybrid approaches: Rwanda's health information exchange uses the OpenHIE framework as the integration layer, while individual applications may be developed locally or sourced internationally. Australia's National Healthcare Interoperability Plan and Canada's Connected Care for Canadians Act also mandate the use of open standards to ensure vendor neutrality across their health information ecosystems.

13.5 Social Enterprises and Impact-Driven Organizations

Social enterprises occupy a distinctive position in Africa's digital health landscape, defined by a dual-purpose mission: achieving measurable health impact while maintaining financial sustainability through earned revenue. Access Afya's micro-clinic model generates revenue through affordable fee-for-service primary care and uses digital tools to optimize operations. mPedigree combines commercial drug authentication with a public health mission to combat counterfeit medicines. Jacaranda Health delivers digitally supported maternity care at prices accessible to low-income women in Kenya

In Latin America, Fundación Carlos Slim's CASALUD program in Mexico provides a parallel example, using mobile technology to manage chronic diseases in underserved communities through a blended funding model that combines philanthropic capital with government reimbursement (Fundación Carlos Slim, 2021). The Caribbean Fintech Association has promoted digital health insurance and mobile money platforms that enable micro-insurance for informal-sector workers (Caribbean Fintech Association, 2022). In Southeast Asia, Halodoc (Indonesia) and Ping An Good Doctor (China) have demonstrated that digitally enabled health models can achieve large-scale impact when supported by integrated payment systems and insurance partnerships.

13.6 Business Models for Digital Health Sustainability

The key business models that sustain digital health ecosystems in Africa can be grouped into six distinct yet complementary categories.

- The primary market-facing grouping models include: **B2G (Business-to-Government)**, which relies on public procurement, PPPs, and donor-supported systems (e.g., DHIS2, mTrac); **B2B (Business-to-Business)**, in which companies provide software and services (such as SaaS) to hospitals, clinics, pharmacies, and insurers; and B**2C (Business-to-Consumer)**, which focuses on direct-to-patient services via apps, subscriptions, and freemium models (e.g., telehealth and e-pharmacy platforms). These models reflect distinct revenue streams and customer bases, ranging from governments to enterprises and individual users.

- Three enabling or hybrid models enhance sustainability and scalability. I**mpact-driven or hybrid** models combine grants with earned revenue, often targeting underserved populations whilè maintaining financial viability. **Platform or marketplace models** act as intermediaries, connecting providers and patients through two-sided digital ecosystems to improve access and efficiency. **Data monetization models** leverage anonymized health data to create value across pharmaceuticals, insurance, and public health, though they require robust data governance frameworks.

Across all models, cross-cutting enablers—including regulatory compliance, interoperability, user trust, and adaptation to local contexts—highlight that long-term sustainability depends not only on business strategy but also on the broader institutional and policy environment.

Freemium models provide basic features for free while charging for premium options—Vezeeta uses this approach, though conversion rates in African markets generally range from 2–10 percent, compared with 5–15 percent in more mature markets (Disrupt Africa, 2023). B2B models sell solutions directly to healthcare facilities and institutional buyers—Helium Health's SaaS model exemplifies this approach and has been validated at scale in Europe by companies like Doctolib (France). B2C models offer services directly to consumers, supported by Africa's mobile money revolution—similar to Halodoc (Indonesia) and Ping An Good Doctor (China) in Asia.

Figure 13.4. Business Models for Digital Health Sustainability in Africa

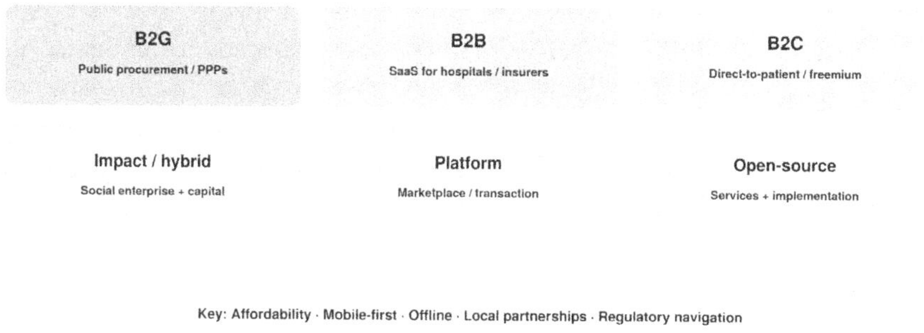

Source: Author's Elaboration

Government procurement and public-private partnerships are key revenue sources, especially for infrastructure solutions. DHIS2's open-source model has created a sustainable network of African service providers offering implementation, customization, and support. Data monetization models generate income from anonymized health data insights. The EU's European Health Data Space is developing a regulatory framework for the secondary use of health data that could inform African approaches (European Commission, 2022). Each model has strengths and limitations; enterprises must align their business model with local market conditions, regulatory contexts, and users' purchasing power.

13.7 Intellectual Property and Technology Transfer

Three principal intellectual property (IP) and technology transfer pathways shape the development, adoption, and scaling of digital health solutions in Africa.

- The first pathway, **Open Source & Commons,** focuses on technologies that are freely available for use and adaptation, driven by community collaboration and shared innovation. This model supports localization and cost-effective deployment, as demonstrated by OpenMRS, DHIS2, and OpenHIE. It is particularly well suited to public health systems seeking flexibility, interoperability, and reduced dependence on proprietary vendors.

- The second pathway, **Licensed Technology,** relies on proprietary solutions accessed via fees or royalties, typically with vendor support and structured service agreements. This includes commercial electronic health record systems and SaaS platforms, which provide reliability and technical support but often carry higher costs and offer less flexibility.

- The third pathway, **Joint Ventures & Partnerships**, represents a collaborative model involving co-development and shared intellectual property rights, often between universities, governments, and private industry. This approach fosters local capacity building and innovation ecosystems while enabling technology transfer through partnerships.

Together, these pathways highlight the trade-offs between openness, control, cost, and sustainability in Africa's digital health transformation.

Open-source approaches have been particularly influential. DHIS2, deployed in over 80 countries, has supported local adaptation and community-led development. OpenMRS has been deployed in over 40 countries. The OpenHIE framework provides an open architecture for health information exchange. Licensed commercial transfer operates through vendor agreements and franchise models. Joint ventures blend external expertise with local ownership—UCT's d.school and Makerere University's partnerships illustrate how academic-private collaborations generate locally owned IP.

Figure 13.5. Three Principal Pathways for Intellectual Property and Technology Transfer in African Digital Health

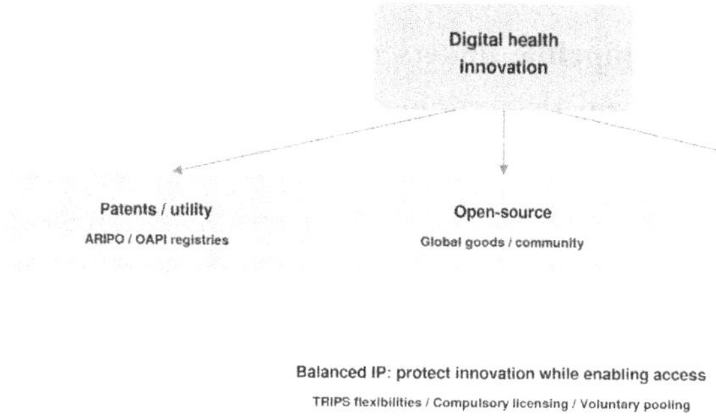

Source: Author's Elaboration

The African Continental Free Trade Area (AfCFTA), with provisions on intellectual property and digital trade, has the potential to create a more coherent continental framework. India's experience with compulsory licensing for essential medicines offers lessons on balancing innovation incentives with access. Estonia's X-Road data exchange platform—now adopted by more than 20 countries, including pilot programs in Chile, Australia, and South Africa—demonstrates how open, interoperable data infrastructure can drive private-sector innovation while remaining under public governance. The Digital Public Goods Alliance (DPGA), co-hosted by UNICEF and Norad, maintains a registry of recognized DPGs, including DHIS2, OpenMRS, and OpenCRVS, which provide shared foundations for ecosystem development.

13.8 Creating Enabling Environments for Innovation

Six interconnected pillars underpin robust digital health innovation environments.

- **Policy and regulatory sandboxes** emphasize the importance of flexible regulation, innovation-friendly licensing, and sandbox mechanisms for securely testing new solutions.

- **Infrastructure and connectivity,** including broadband, cloud services, open APIs, and health data exchanges, form the technical backbone of digital health systems.

- **Talent and capacity pipeline** underscores the importance of STEM education, health informatics training, and diaspora engagement to ensure a skilled workforce capable of developing and managing digital health innovations.

- **Financing and investment**, including seed funding, venture capital, blended finance, and public procurement, are essential to sustaining innovation throughout its lifecycle.

- **Market access and demand** are equally important, with governments serving as anchor buyers and insurance integration and user adoption promoting scale.

- D**ata and standards ecosystem** supports the entire framework by emphasizing open data, interoperability standards, and data protection, thereby building trust and enabling system integration.

Together, these pillars illustrate that successful digital health innovation depends on a coordinated ecosystem approach in which policy, infrastructure, skills, finance, market dynamics, and data governance are aligned.

13.8.1 Regulatory Sandboxes and Adaptive Regulation

Rwanda's drone-delivery sandbox for medical supplies (Zipline) and Mauritius's broader regulatory sandbox framework demonstrate how controlled environments can accelerate innovation while managing risk. In Asia, Singapore's Health Sciences Authority has implemented an AI-based medical device sandbox. The UK's Medicines and Healthcare products Regulatory Agency (MHRA) sandbox has enabled companies such as Babylon Health to test AI-driven triage tools before obtaining full regulatory approval. Africa can adopt these models by leveraging the African Medicines Regulatory

Harmonization (AMRH) Initiative to facilitate cross-border sandbox arrangements.

13.8.2 Government as Anchor Buyer

Government procurement policies can catalyze private-sector development. Kenya's Access to Government Procurement Opportunities program reserves procurement for youth, women, and persons with disabilities, thereby supporting local health technology companies. Brazil's SUS procurement framework favors locally developed solutions and requires international vendors to engage local partners and transfer technology—a model that could inform African procurement reform. A key insight from the 2024 HealthTech Hub Africa Innovation Challenge is that although African governments are eager to engage with healthTech startups, formal agreements and funding are slow to materialize—policy design is not the problem; implementation is (HTHA, 2025). Australia's approach to procurement through the Australian Digital Health Agency, which mandates conformance testing against national standards, provides a quality-assurance model that African countries could adapt.

13.8.3 Talent Pipeline and Open Data

Building the talent pipeline for digital health entrepreneurship requires investment in STEM education, health informatics training, and entrepreneurship programs—as outlined in Chapter 11. Diaspora engagement is an underused resource: the CARICOM Caribbean diaspora model and Africa's diaspora engagement programs can catalyze local innovation by providing technical expertise, professional networks, and access to capital.

The Digital Health Innovation Ecosystem is supported and shaped by a range of interconnected actors. These include incubators and accelerators, which nurture startups and early-stage innovation; venture capital and impact investors, which provide critical financing; and universities and research labs, which contribute to knowledge creation, research, and talent development. Together, these actors form the supply side of innovation, enabling the development and scaling of digital health solutions. The demand side includes government policy and regulation, which provide the enabling framework through laws, standards, and strategic direction, while health system demand drives the adoption and practical use of digital solutions.

Development partners and donors play a catalytic role by providing funding, technical assistance, and capacity building, particularly in underserved contexts. Finally, the private sector and corporations contribute through technology development, partnerships, and service delivery. Effective digital health transformation in Africa depends on coordinated collaboration among these diverse stakeholders, ensuring that innovation is both responsive to health needs and supported by sustainable financing, policy, and institutional ecosystems.

Figure 13.6. Actors and Resources for Africa's Digital Health Innovation Ecosystem

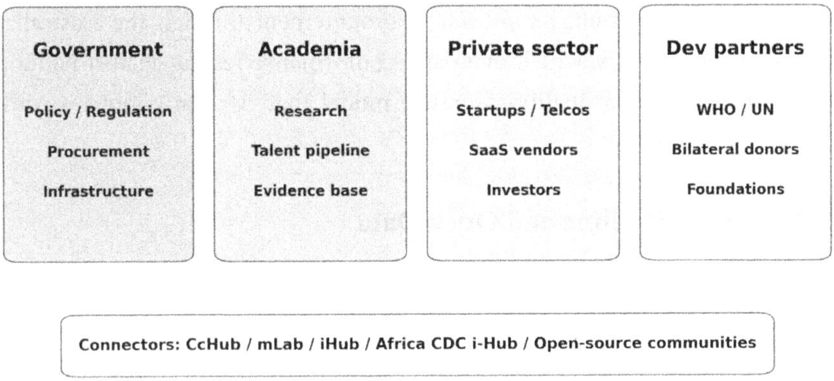

Source: Author's Elaboration

Open data and digital public goods lay the foundation for innovation by lowering barriers to entry. Kenya's Open Data Initiative, South Africa's Data Portal, and Estonia's X-Road platform illustrate how government-led open data programs can be leveraged by digital health innovators. Canada's open health data initiatives through the Canadian Institute for Health Information (CIHI) and New Zealand's health data catalogs similarly demonstrate how systematized access to open data can stimulate research and commercial innovation in digital health.

13.9 Conclusion

This chapter has examined the healthTech ecosystem—the enterprise-focused, cross-cutting enabler within the Digital Health Technology Stack—drawing on Africa's rapidly maturing innovation landscape and comparative experiences from India, Brazil, Latin America, Southeast Asia, Australia, Canada, and Europe. Africa's healthTech ecosystem has demonstrated remarkable resilience, with the sector the only technology vertical to see year-over-year funding growth during the 2023–2024 global contraction. HealthTech equity funding surged by 232 percent in 2025. The companies in the 2024 HealthTech Hub Africa Innovation Challenge collectively reached more than 905,000 patients and integrated their solutions into 1,811 public health facilities, demonstrating that African healthTech startups can achieve measurable impact at scale.

Yet significant challenges remain. Funding remains concentrated in Egypt, Kenya, Nigeria, and South Africa. The gap between policy design and implementation frustrates startups seeking government partnerships. Regulatory fragmentation across 54 jurisdictions increases compliance costs. Data governance frameworks are incomplete. The global funding contraction exposed the fragility of investor-dependent business models. The comparative analysis shows that the most successful healthTech ecosystems worldwide—such as those in India, Brazil, Singapore, and Estonia—have been developed through deliberate government actions: mandating digital health infrastructure to create market demand, establishing regulatory sandboxes to reduce innovation risks, procuring from local innovators to strengthen the supply chain, and investing in open data and digital public goods to lower entry barriers. Africa's path forward requires the same deliberate combination of market creation, enabling regulation, talent investment, and ecosystem coordination.

References

ABStartups. (2023). Brazilian Startup Ecosystem Report 2023. ABStartups.

Access Afya. (2023). Impact report 2023. Access Afya.

AfriLabs. (2023). Building a connected African innovation ecosystem. AfriLabs.

Caribbean Fintech Association. (2022). Digital health and financial inclusion in the Caribbean. CFA.

Disrupt Africa. (2023). African tech startups funding report 2023. Disrupt Africa.

European Commission. (2022). Proposal for a Regulation on the European Health Data Space. EC.

Founders Factory Africa. (2024). How Africa's health tech industry is stacking up in 2024. FFA.

Frost & Sullivan. (2023). Digital health in Africa: Market analysis 2023–2027. Frost & Sullivan.

Fundación Carlos Slim. (2021). CASALUD: Digital health for chronic disease management. FCS.

GSMA. (2023). The mobile economy: Sub-Saharan Africa 2023. GSMA.

HealthCap Africa. (2024). HealthTech unicorns insight paper 2024. HealthCap Africa.

Healthcare Digital. (2025). HealthTech Africa emerges in 2025. Healthcare Digital.

HTHA. (2025). Catalysing health innovation in Africa: Lessons from the 2024 Challenge. HTHA.

i3 Africa. (2025). Investing in Innovation: Programme overview. i3 Africa.

IDB. (2022). Health innovation in Latin America and the Caribbean. IDB.

Market Data Forecast. (2024). Latin America digital health market size and forecasts. MDF.

Ministry of Health, Brazil. (2020). Digital health strategy for Brazil 2020–2028. MoH Brazil.

mPharma. (2023). Annual report 2023. mPharma.

NASSCOM. (2023). India Digital Health Market Report 2023. NASSCOM.

National Health Authority India. (2021). ABDM strategy document. NHA India.

Partech Partners. (2025). 2025 Africa tech venture capital report. Partech Partners.

Research & Markets. (2023). Africa digital health market forecast 2023–2028. R&M.

Salient Advisory. (2024). African healthTech: Innovators kick-off 2024. Salient Advisory.

Springer Nature. (2025). Beyond seed funding: Nigerian digital health startups. Health Economics Review.

Tracxn. (2023). Southeast Asia healthTech landscape 2023. Tracxn.

WEF. (2024). Investing in African health tech can transform health systems. World Economic Forum.

Chapter 14 National Digital Health Strategies

14.1 Overview

National digital health strategies provide essential roadmaps for countries to systematically transform their health systems by purposefully adopting and integrating technology. Chapter 4 identified digital health strategy as the primary cross-cutting enabler in the Digital Health Technology Stack (Figure 4.1), providing the vision, roadmap, and coordination mechanism that align digital health investments with health system priorities. This chapter examines the state of national digital health strategy development across the African continent, analyzes successful country approaches, identifies common implementation challenges, and distills lessons for effective strategy formulation and execution.

Drawing systematically on comparative insights from the European Union, India, Brazil, Latin America and the Caribbean, Asia, Australia, Canada, and New Zealand, the chapter situates Africa's experience within the global strategy landscape and highlights both transferable lessons and distinctive features of the African context. Country deep dives are presented in summary form, recognizing that situations evolve rapidly and that structural lessons matter more than point-in-time status descriptions.

14.2 Overview of National Digital Health Strategies Across Africa

National eHealth strategies have become critical tools for guiding the digital transformation of health systems across Africa. The WHO eHealth Resolution (WHA58.28), adopted in 2005, catalyzed global attention to strategic planning for health information systems, and the WHO/ITU National eHealth Strategy Toolkit provided structured guidance widely adopted across the continent (WHO, 2012). In May 2025, the Seventy-eighth World Health Assembly endorsed extending the WHO's Global Strategy on Digital Health (2020–2025) to 2027 and requested the development of a successor strategy for 2028–2033, informed by Member State priorities and inclusive stakeholder engagement—a process in which African voices are actively participating through regional consultations convened by WHO AFRO (WHO, 2025).

The landscape of national digital health strategies across Africa is diverse and rapidly evolving. As of 2024, the Global Digital Health Monitor reported that 48 AU Member States had some form of digital health strategic plan, though maturity levels varied widely. A comprehensive assessment using the WHO-ITU eHealth Strategy Rating Tool found that only 9 countries had 'complete' implementation plans, while 24 had 'incomplete' plans; only 14 had complete monitoring and evaluation frameworks (Oladele et al., 2024).

A separate 2025 analysis of 11 recent African digital health strategic plans identified recurring gaps in workforce development, legal frameworks, financing, and interoperability, and found that more than half of the strategies did not adequately describe the health system challenges they aimed to address (Nikiema et al., 2025). These findings confirm a persistent pattern across almost all types of digital strategies on the continent: the number of strategies far outpaces their implementation effectiveness.

Figure 14.1. Status of National Digital Health Strategy Development Across African Countries as of 2024

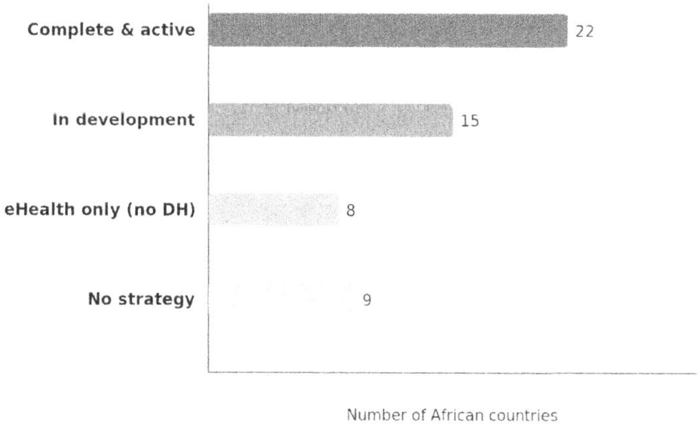

Source: Adapted from WHO AFRO (2024); Global Digital Health Index (2023)

Regional variations are notable. East Africa stands out as the most advanced region, with the highest number of countries that have comprehensive strategies and are actively implementing them. East African countries—Kenya, Rwanda, Tanzania, and Uganda—typically show the highest strategy maturity, reflecting both strong national institutions and support from development partners. Southern Africa follows, with fewer countries having comprehensive strategies, but more actively implementing or having developed strategies with limited implementation, indicating a transition from policy design to execution. Southern African nations have well-articulated strategies, though interoperability and provincial coordination challenges persist.

West Africa shows strong policy formulation, with most countries classified as "developed but limited implementation," alongside moderate levels of comprehensiveness and active implementation, indicating that operationalization remains a key challenge. Across the region, progress is mixed: Ghana, Senegal, and Nigeria have made significant advances, while others struggle with resource and governance constraints. Central African countries generally lag due to broader health system fragmentation. North African countries have developed strategies, but implementation often occurs through sector-specific initiatives rather than within integrated frameworks.

Figure 14.2. Digital Health Strategy Maturity in the African Regions (2024)

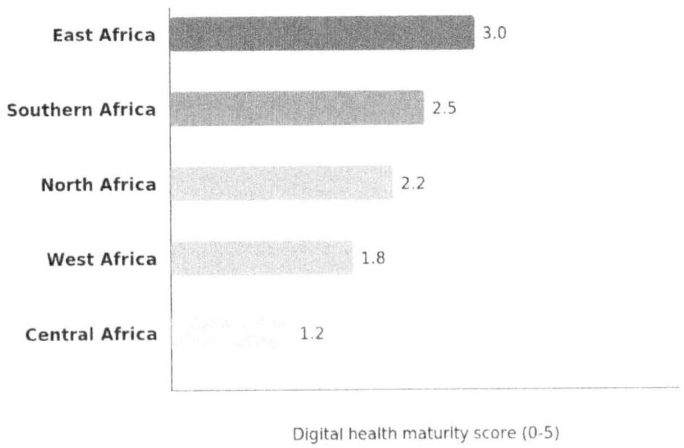

Source: WHO AFRO (2024); Country Reports

Globally, national digital health strategies have accelerated across all regions. In the European Union, the European Health Data Space (EHDS) regulation provides a continental framework for cross-border interoperability of health data. India's Ayushman Bharat Digital Mission, launched in 2020, generated unique health identifiers for more than 770 million citizens by April 2025 and registered more than 679,000 healthcare professionals—making it one of the most ambitious national digital health architectures worldwide.

Thailand's Health 4.0 strategy integrates digital health into broader economic transformation efforts. Brazil's Estratégia de Saúde Digital (2020–2028) provides a comprehensive framework supported by the SUS. Indonesia's SATUSEHAT health data exchange platform, launched in 2022, mandates integration for government-funded health facilities. Australia's National Digital Health Strategy (2023–2028) and Canada's Connected Care for Canadians Act exemplify mature frameworks in high-income federated systems. These global experiences confirm that strategic frameworks are necessary—but not sufficient—for transformation; successful implementation, ongoing funding, and political support are critical for strategies to make an impact.

Figure 14.3. Core Components of Comprehensive National Digital Health Strategies

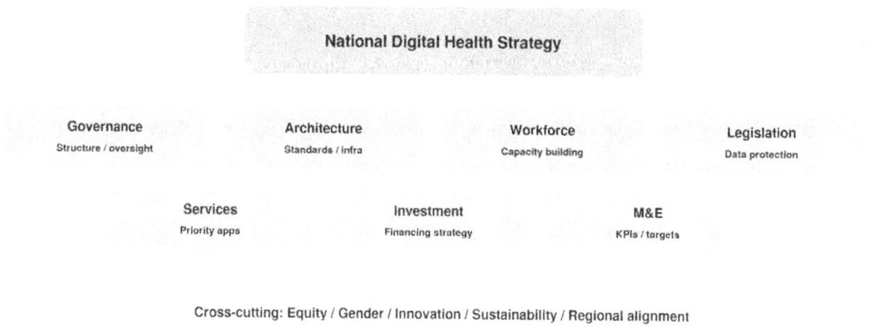

Source: Adapted from WHO (2012); Scott & Mars (2013)

Effective national digital health strategies typically encompass six core components: leadership and governance structures; infrastructure and standards frameworks; legal and regulatory components; human capacity development; financing and sustainability plans; and monitoring and evaluation frameworks. Each component must be addressed coherently for a strategy to succeed (Scott & Mars, 2013).

- Leadership and governance emphasize accountability, stakeholder coordination, and strategic alignment, ensuring that digital health initiatives are guided by clear institutional mandates.

- Infrastructure and standards focus on connectivity, hardware, and interoperability, forming the technical backbone of effective digital health systems.

- The legal and regulatory pillar covers data protection, privacy, licensing, and quality assurance, all essential to building trust, ensuring compliance, and safeguarding patient information.

- Human capacity development underscores the importance of digital literacy, workforce training, and long-term workforce planning to support the system's adoption and use.

- Financing and sustainability focus on funding sources, cost-recovery mechanisms, and broader resource mobilization strategies essential for long-term viability.

- Monitoring and evaluation provide mechanisms for tracking progress, assessing performance, and enabling adaptive management, ensuring strategies remain responsive and effective over time.

Together, these six pillars form an integrated ecosystem, indicating that a successful national digital health strategy depends not only on technical solutions but also on governance, capacity, financing, and continuous learning.

14.2 Country Experiences: Strategic Approaches Across Africa

Six African countries illustrate the diversity of approaches to developing and implementing digital health strategies. These summaries highlight structural lessons and governance models rather than exhaustive status updates, recognizing that implementation contexts evolve rapidly.

Countries such as Kenya, Rwanda, Ghana, and Ethiopia adopt largely centralized governance approaches, often complemented by multi-stakeholder coordination mechanisms, whereas South Africa and Nigeria operate more federal or hybrid systems with decentralized implementation. In terms of achievements, several countries have made significant progress in building digital health infrastructure and platforms.

Kenya's digital health strategy exemplifies comprehensive, well-governed implementation, featuring a national Health Information Exchange connecting more than 850 facilities, KenyaEMR in more than 5,000 facilities, and a Master Patient Index covering 28 million citizens—paralleling India's ABDM approach to unique health identifiers at the national level.

Rwanda demonstrates how a small, resource-constrained country can achieve significant impact through disciplined governance and integrated architecture—with over 90 percent insurance coverage and 95 percent facility connectivity facilitated by centralized coordination by the Rwanda Biomedical Center, mirroring Estonia's X-Road success in small-country digital integration.

South Africa's experience highlights the complexity of digital health in federal systems, where provincial autonomy creates coordination challenges similar to those in Brazil's SUS (which manages 5,570 municipalities) and in Germany's Telematikinfrastruktur (which negotiates with Länder and self-governing medical associations).

Ghana exemplifies a phased approach—consolidating DHIS2 coverage before expanding to facility-level EHRs—while innovating with mPedigree drug authentication, a system replicated in Nigeria and India. Nigeria's strategy faces the challenge of coordinating at scale across 36 states, addressed through

SORMAS disease surveillance and a vibrant technology ecosystem—with lessons drawn from India's ABDM (open standards for federal adoption) and Indonesia's SATUSEHAT (incentive-driven facility integration).

Table 14.1. Comparative analysis of national digital health strategies across six African countries.

Country	Strategy	Governance	Key	Main	Global Parallel
Kenya	2017/2021	Centralized + multi-stakeholder TWG	National HIE (850+ facilities); KenyaEMR (5,000+ sites);	Sustainability funding; rural connectivity	India (ABDM unique IDs)
Rwanda	2016	Centralized through RBC	Integrated HIE (OpenHIE); 90% insurance; 95% connectivity; Zipline drones	Limited local technical capacity; sustainability	Estonia (X-Road small-country)
South Africa	2012/2019	Federal with provincial autonomy	Comprehensive NHLS (260+ labs); POPIA data protection; NHI	Provincial fragmentation; legacy systems	Germany (TI), Brazil (SUS federalism)
Ghana	2021	Centralized coordination	90%+ DHIS2; digital NHIS; mPedigree; E-	EHR scaling; interoperabilit y gaps	Jamaica (pharma tracking)
Nigeria	2020	Federal coordination, state implementation	Nationwide DHIS2 (30,000+ facilities); SORMAS; vibrant	Scale complexity; 36-state coordination	India/Indonesia (federal digital health)
Ethiopia	2021	Centralized strategy	National DHIS2; HEW digital tools; SmartCare	Infrastructure; connectivity; electricity	Bangladesh (CHW digitalization)

Source: Country strategy documents; WHO AFRO (2024)

Ethiopia's Digital Health Strategy 2021–2025 prioritizes digitally empowering over 38,000 Health Extension Workers through the FamilyConnect platform —sharing features with Bangladesh's community health workforce digitalization and India's ASHA worker mobile tools.

14.3 Common Elements in Successful Strategies

Analysis of successful digital health strategy implementation across Africa and comparator countries reveals recurring enabling factors that distinguish sustained progress from aspirational documentation.

Figure 14.4. Achievement of Critical Success Factors for Digital Health Strategy Implementation Across African Countries (2024)

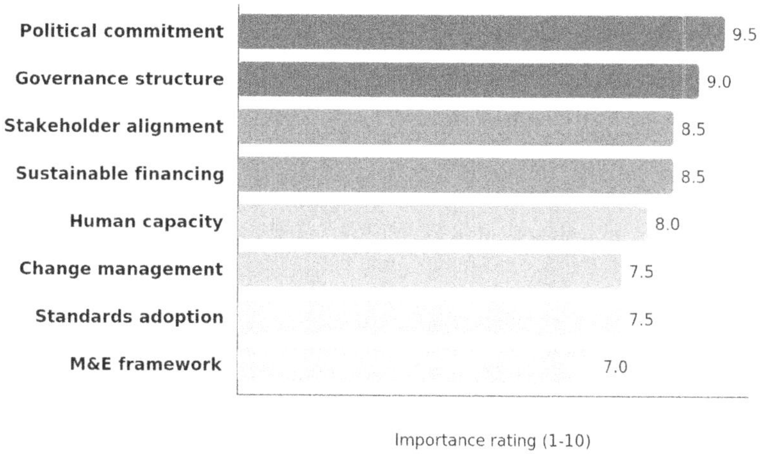

Source: WHO AFRO (2024) Assessment Data

Strong political leadership and governance are essential to turning strategy into action. Countries that implement effectively have ministerial champions, adequate budget allocations, and clear governance structures with defined roles. Rwanda and Kenya demonstrate strong governance through empowered digital health units. India's ABDM benefited from the Prime Minister's direct endorsement. Thailand's Health 4.0 strategy is embedded in the national economic transformation agenda. Australia's strategy is guided by the Australian Digital Health Agency, a dedicated national agency with a clear legislative mandate.

Phased implementation using incremental approaches, rather than attempting a full-scale transformation all at once, remains a critical success factor. Countries typically start with basic elements—governance, policies, and

DHIS2—and then expand to EHRs, HIE, and advanced analytics. Ghana and Senegal exemplify this method. Brazil's digital health development followed a similar path: the CADSUS patient registry came first, then the e-SUS primary care platform, and later the RNDS health data network. New Zealand's phased approach to its National Health Information Platform also prioritizes establishing core data standards before moving on to more advanced interoperability.

Standards and interoperability prevent fragmentation, which can later lead to costly remediation. Kenya's Health Data Standards and South Africa exemplify early adoption of frameworks such as HL7, FHIR, ICD, and SNOMED CT. The EU's decade-long effort toward cross-border interoperability through the EHDS highlights both the importance and the challenges of harmonizing standards at scale. Canada's Connected Care for Canadians Act mandates interoperability standards across provincial health systems.

Capacity development as a strategic priority is a hallmark of successful implementations, as detailed in Chapter 11. Countries such as Rwanda integrate health informatics into medical curricula. Kenya's Digital Health Academy offers structured certification. South Korea's 20+ university health informatics programs strongly correlate with the maturity of its digital health systems.

Sustainable financing models require a gradual shift away from donor reliance toward domestically funded programs. Ghana's allocation of National Health Insurance Scheme resources to information systems and Kenya's Digital Health Investment Case demonstrate commitment. Even within the EU, the European Court of Auditors has noted significant variation in digital health investment levels among member states.

14.4 Policy Implementation Challenges

Despite remarkable progress in strategy development, implementation faces persistent challenges across African contexts that are similarly shared, to varying extents, across the Global South. Limited and unpredictable funding is the most frequently cited barrier. Digital health investments often compete with immediate clinical needs and are given lower priority in budget allocation. Many strategies exist only as policy documents without corresponding resource commitments.

Figure 14.5. Most Frequently Reported Challenges in Implementing Digital Health Strategies Across African Countries (2024)

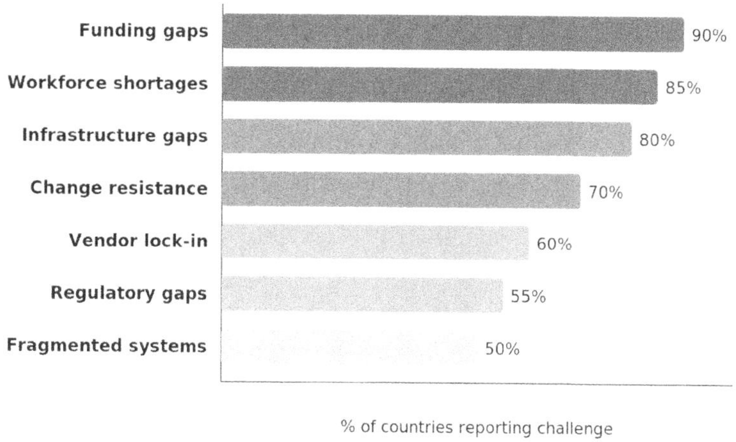

Source: WHO AFRO (2024); Country Assessment Reports

Technical capacity gaps constrain implementation across the continent. The African health informatics workforce gap is estimated at more than 50,000 professionals—a deficit that cannot be closed quickly through conventional pipelines, as discussed in Chapter 11. Fragmented governance and coordination lead to duplicative efforts and incompatible systems, particularly when disease programs implement separate digital systems without shared standards.

Infrastructure limitations, including unreliable electricity and limited connectivity, constrain the deployment of digital health, especially in rural areas. Resistance to change among health workers who perceive digital systems as increasing their workload or threatening routines can derail even well-funded initiatives—the UK's abandoned National Program for IT, which cost £10 billion, is a cautionary example. A 2025 analysis of 11 recent African strategic plans found that more than half did not adequately describe the challenges facing health systems, suggesting that strategies are sometimes developed without sufficient contextual analysis (Nikiema et al., 2025).

These challenges are not unique to Africa. In Latin America, PAHO assessments identified similar implementation gaps across Caribbean and Central American countries, despite well-articulated strategies (PAHO, 2021). In Indonesia, the SATUSEHAT platform faces adoption challenges in smaller cities and rural areas, even with national mandates. In Canada, 5.7 million adults lacked a regular healthcare provider in 2024, despite a sophisticated digital health infrastructure. The lesson is universal: strategy is necessary but not sufficient; sustained political commitment, adequate resources, and effective governance are required to translate strategic plans into health system improvements.

14.5 Africa in Global Perspective

Africa's achievement in strategy formulation—with the vast majority of countries possessing some form of digital health strategy—is comparable to, or even exceeds, that of other developing regions. However, the gap between the existence of strategies and their implementation effectiveness remains more pronounced in Africa than in Europe or high-income Asia, driven primarily by financing constraints, capacity deficits, and infrastructure limitations. Asia's performance is highly variable—ranging from digitally advanced systems in South Korea and Singapore to nascent efforts in low-income countries—making regional averages potentially misleading. Latin America demonstrates moderate, uneven progress, with standout performers (Brazil, Uruguay) coexisting alongside significant gaps in Central America and the Caribbean islands.

Africa's unique strengths include the widespread use of open-source platforms (DHIS2, OpenMRS, OpenHIE) that help avoid vendor lock-in; vibrant health technology startup ecosystems; a proven ability to adapt quickly during crises; and strong South–South collaboration networks. However, emerging challenges are intensifying. The 2025 reorganization of global health funding —especially the restructuring of PEPFAR and modifications to USAID support—has raised serious concerns about data sovereignty. New bilateral agreements reportedly require African countries to share pathogen specimens and genetic data under terms that may conflict with the WHO's multilateral pathogen-sharing framework and the Africa CDC's Health Security and Sovereignty Agenda (ICTworks, 2026). These developments underscore the need for African countries to embed data governance, digital sovereignty, and financing sustainability into their national digital health strategies—rather than treating them as peripheral concerns.

14.6 Recommendations for Strengthening National Digital Health Strategies

Addressing the implementation gap requires coordinated action across multiple areas. Countries should prioritize securing sustained political commitment by demonstrating measurable value through rigorous impact evaluations and investment cases. Strategy documents must be accompanied by costed implementation plans that identify funding sources and include multi-year budget commitments. Investing in local capacity development—from community health workers to system architects—should be treated as a core strategic pillar rather than an afterthought.

Governance mechanisms must be strengthened through clear accountability, regular coordination meetings, and effective enforcement of standards. Countries should adopt proven open-source solutions and prioritize adaptation over building from scratch. Regional collaboration—enabled by the African Union's Digital Transformation Strategy (2020–2030) and regional economic communities—offers opportunities to share experiences, pool resources, and harmonize standards. The WHO Global Strategy on Digital Health 2028–2033, informed by African regional consultations, offers a critical opportunity for the continent to shape global digital health governance in ways that prioritize African interests.

Data sovereignty and digital governance must be core strategic priorities rather than peripheral concerns. National strategies should clearly define ownership of health data, international data-sharing policies, pathogen-specimen governance, and the regulatory framework governing the commercial use of health data. New Zealand's Māori data sovereignty framework (Te Mana Raraunga) and the H3Africa Consortium's data governance model serve as reference points, but African countries need to develop frameworks tailored to their unique political, cultural, and institutional contexts.

Above all, strategies must balance ambitious vision with practical execution and remain flexible to adapt to implementation experience, technological changes, and evolving health system priorities. The most successful digital health strategies—in Rwanda, Kenya, India, Brazil, Estonia, and Australia—are living documents that are regularly reviewed, honestly evaluated, and continually refined, rather than static plans that become outdated as circumstances shift.

14.7 Conclusion

This chapter has examined national digital health strategies—the primary cross-cutting enabler in the Digital Health Technology Stack—highlighting Africa's impressive progress in developing these strategies, alongside experiences from India, Brazil, Indonesia, the EU, Australia, Canada, and New Zealand. The evidence shows a continent with nearly universal strategy coverage, yet still facing a significant and impactful implementation gap. Only a small number of countries have turned strategy documents into detailed, funded, governed, and monitored programs that deliver real improvements in their health systems.

The experiences of six countries—Kenya's multi-stakeholder governance and interoperability efforts, Rwanda's centralized integration, South Africa's federal coordination challenges, Ghana's phased approach, Nigeria's scale management, and Ethiopia's digitalization of community health workers—each offer transferable lessons for the continent. Global comparisons show that implementation challenges are common, but they are often more severe in Africa due to resource constraints. The five critical success factors—political leadership, phased implementation, standards adoption, capacity development, and sustainable financing—provide an evidence-based framework for countries developing or updating their strategic plans.

As Africa shapes its input for WHO's upcoming Global Strategy on Digital Health (2028–2033) and navigates a changing global health funding landscape, the clear strategic need is for national digital health strategies to move from policy papers to real institutional practices—integrated into health system governance, linked to the other five enablers discussed in this book (governance, skills, research, ecosystem, and financing), and rooted in the foundational layers of the technology stack.

References

African Union. (2020). Digital transformation strategy for Africa (2020–2030). AU Commission.

Binagwaho, A., et al. (2014). Rwanda 20 years on: Investing in life. The Lancet, 384(9940), 371–375.

Braa, J., Heywood, A., & Sahay, S. (2012). Improving the quality and use of data. Bull WHO, 90(5), 379–384.

Federal Ministry of Health, Ethiopia. (2021). Digital health strategy 2021–2025. Government of Ethiopia.

Federal Ministry of Health, Nigeria. (2021). National health ICT strategic framework. Government of Nigeria.

ICTworks. (2026). African digital health data is a condition of global health funding. ICTworks.

Katurura, M. C., & Cilliers, L. (2018). EHR in South Africa. Afr J Prim Health Care, 10(1), e1–e8.

Ministry of Health, Kenya. (2021). National digital health strategic framework 2021–2025. Government of Kenya.

Ministry of Health, Ghana. (2022). National eHealth strategy 2021–2025. Government of Ghana.

Ngabo, F., et al. (2012). SMS-based alert system in Rwanda. Pan Afr Med J, 13, 31.

Nikiema, J. N., et al. (2025). African digital health strategic plans analysis. npj Digital Medicine, 8, 748.

Oladele, R., et al. (2024). National eHealth strategy frameworks in Africa. Oxford Open Digital Health.

PAHO. (2021). Digital health strategy evaluation and update. PAHO.

Scott, R. E., & Mars, M. (2013). Principles for eHealth strategy. JMIR, 15(7), e155.

WHO. (2012). National eHealth strategy toolkit. WHO Press.

WHO. (2025). Shaping the next global strategy on digital health (2028–2033): African Region stakeholder consultation. WHO AFRO.

WHO AFRO. (2024). Assessment of national digital health strategies: Status report 2024. WHO AFRO.

Chapter 15 Governance, Policy, and Standards

15.1. Overview

Without institutions, policies, and standards, strategies that outline enablers and aim to build foundations will not succeed. Chapter 4 identified governance, policy, and standards as the critical cross-cutting enabler in the Digital Health Technology Stack (Figure 4.1). This encompasses data protection legislation, health data standards and policies, cybersecurity frameworks, ethical guidelines for artificial intelligence, institutional oversight arrangements, and the regulatory environment for digital health products and services. This chapter examines these governance dimensions in depth, providing the institutional architecture that connects strategy (Chapter 14) to the other enablers—workforce (Chapter 11), research (Chapter 12), and the healthTech ecosystem (Chapter 13)—and underpins the foundation layers described in Chapters 7 through 10.

Drawing systematically on experiences from Asia, Europe, India, Brazil, Latin America, the Caribbean, Australia, Canada, and New Zealand, the chapter provides a comprehensive analysis of how to build robust, accountable, and sustainable digital health governance.

15.2 Governance Structures for Digital Health

The quality of governance structures—dedicated digital health units, multi-stakeholder steering committees, and cross-sectoral coordination mechanisms —is the most important determinant of whether digital health strategies translate into implementation and yield results.

15.2.1 Ministries of Health Digital Health Units

The creation of a dedicated digital health unit within the Ministry of Health is increasingly viewed as a precondition for effective governance. Kenya's Division of Digital Health, established in 2019, is among Africa's most advanced models, with dedicated staff, a clear mandate, and direct reporting to the Director General of Health (Ministry of Health, Kenya, 2020).

Organizational positioning matters: units higher in the hierarchy tend to exert more influence over policy and budget decisions. Thailand's Digital Health Development Division, located within the Office of the Permanent Secretary, illustrates how strategic placement enhances authority and coordination (Ministry of Public Health Thailand, 2019). Australia's approach goes even further, establishing a dedicated statutory agency—the Australian Digital Health Agency—with its own legislation, board, and budget, providing a level of institutional permanence that ministerial units within African governments typically lack.

15.2.2 Multi-Stakeholder Steering and Coordination

National steering committees provide multi-stakeholder oversight for coordinated governance. Rwanda's eHealth Steering Committee, co-chaired by the Ministry of Health and the Rwanda Biomedical Center, meets quarterly and has the authority to reallocate resources based on evidence (Ministry of Health, Rwanda, 2018). In the Caribbean, PAHO has supported multi-country steering mechanisms through its eHealth Strategy for the Caribbean, promoting cross-border governance for shared platforms (PAHO, 2021). South Korea's Presidential Committee on the Fourth Industrial Revolution emphasizes health within a cross-sectoral framework. In Africa, Nigeria's NITDA collaborates with the Federal Ministry of Health on data governance and cybersecurity, while Senegal's Ministry of Digital Economy partners with the Ministry of Health on infrastructure planning.

The digital health governance maturity model is a five-level progression that illustrates how countries or health systems evolve from fragmented governance toward fully optimized, innovation-driven systems. The model can be visualized as a horizontal sequence of stages, each representing higher levels of institutional capacity, coordination, and system sophistication. At Level 1 (Ad Hoc), governance is absent or minimal, and digital health initiatives are fragmented and uncoordinated. Level 2 (Emerging) introduces basic coordination mechanisms and some strategic direction, though both remain limited in scope and implementation. By Level 3 (Defined), a formal governance body is established, and a national digital health strategy is approved, signaling a transition to structured, policy-driven coordination.

Figure 15.1. A Five-level Maturity Model for Assessing the Evolution of Digital Health Governance Structures

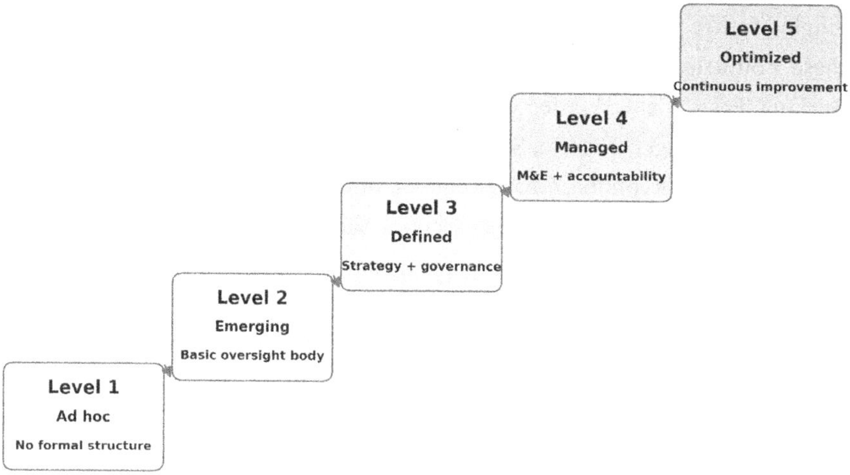

Source: Author's Elaboration

The model then advances to higher levels of maturity. Level 4 (Managed) signifies active oversight, with monitoring and evaluation (M&E) systems in place to track implementation, performance, and outcomes. Governance at this stage becomes institutionalized and operational. Finally, Level 5 (Optimized) reflects a mature system characterized by continuous improvement, adaptive governance, and innovation-driven approaches. At this level, digital health governance is not only stable but also responsive, using data, feedback loops, and emerging technologies to refine policies and maximize impact. Most digital health governance in African countries remains at the emerging and defined levels, with only a few countries reaching the managed level—a reflection of the need to strengthen governance capacity as a core element of digital health transformation.

15.3 Data Protection and Privacy

Protecting personal health data is a foundational requirement for trusted digital health systems. By 2026, more than 4African countries had enacted some form of data protection and privacy legislation, reflecting significant progress toward implementing the principles of the African Union Data Policy Framework and enabling cross-border data governance under the Digital Single Market agenda. According to the UNCTAD Global Cyberlaw Tracker, these countries include: Algeria, Egypt, Libya, Morocco, Tunisia; Benin, Burkina Faso, Cabo Verde, Côte d'Ivoire, Ghana, Guinea, Guinea-Bissau, Liberia, Mali, Niger, Nigeria, Senegal, Sierra Leone, Togo; Angola, Cameroon, Central African Republic, Chad, Republic of the Congo, Democratic Republic of the Congo, Equatorial Guinea, Gabon, São Tomé and Príncipe; Djibouti, Ethiopia, Kenya, Rwanda, Somalia, Tanzania, Uganda; Botswana, Lesotho, Madagascar, Malawi, Mauritius, Mozambique, Namibia, Seychelles, South Africa, Zambia, and Zimbabwe. This represents roughly three-quarters of African Union member states and signals that the continent has reached a critical threshold in establishing the legal foundations for data protection, although variations remain in scope, alignment with global standards, and enforcement readiness.

Of these countries, about 38 have established Data Protection Authorities (DPAs) responsible for oversight, enforcement, and compliance, marking an important shift from legal adoption to institutionalization. Countries with operational or formally designated DPAs include: Algeria, Egypt, Morocco, and Tunisia; Benin, Burkina Faso, Cabo Verde, Côte d'Ivoire, Ghana, Guinea, Mali, Niger, Nigeria, Senegal, Sierra Leone, and Togo; Angola, Cameroon, the Republic of the Congo, the Democratic Republic of the Congo, Gabon, and São Tomé and Príncipe; Djibouti, Ethiopia, Kenya, Rwanda, Somalia, Tanzania, and Uganda; Botswana, Lesotho, Madagascar, Malawi, Mauritius, Mozambique, Namibia, Seychelles, South Africa, Zambia, and Zimbabwe. A smaller group—such as Libya, Liberia, Guinea-Bissau, the Central African Republic, Chad, and Equatorial Guinea—has adopted legislation but still faces gaps in establishing fully operational or independent authorities. Overall, while Africa has largely completed the legislative phase of data protection reform, the next challenge is to strengthen enforcement capacity, regulatory independence, and regional harmonization to support trusted data ecosystems and digital health, trade, and AI applications.

Analysis of Africa's digital health policy and regulatory landscape shows that health-specific regulatory areas lag behind. Telemedicine regulations show moderate progress, with mixed adoption and ongoing development, indicating growing recognition but uneven implementation across countries. Health data-sharing policies, especially digital health product certification frameworks, remain underdeveloped, and many countries have yet to establish formal mechanisms. This suggests that while Africa has made significant strides in horizontal enablers such as data protection and cybersecurity, a substantial gap remains in sector-specific governance frameworks needed to operationalize digital health systems. A few countries are developing guidelines and rules based on their data protection laws. Kenya's Office of the Data Protection Commissioner introduced industry-specific directives for the healthcare, education, and digital lending sectors in 2024. South Africa's Information Regulator has issued enforcement notices and fines, heightening compliance awareness.

Regionally, the African Union's Malabo Convention on Cyber Security and Personal Data Protection, adopted in 2014, and the AU Data Policy Framework provide a continental framework. Globally, the EU's GDPR has served as a reference model, particularly for its emphasis on lawful processing, data subject rights, and data protection officers. The European Health Data Space, which builds on the GDPR, establishes a unified legal, technical, and governance framework for the secure sharing and use of health data across member states, supporting both primary use (healthcare delivery) and secondary use (research, innovation, and policymaking). It enables citizens to access and control their electronic health records across borders, allows healthcare providers to exchange patient data seamlessly, and facilitates the reuse of anonymized data through trusted institutions such as Health Data Access Bodies. EHDS combines strong data protection with interoperability standards, cross-border infrastructure, and governance mechanisms to create a single European health data ecosystem. By moving beyond data protection toward data utilization, it supports AI development, evidence-based policymaking, and more efficient healthcare systems, offering an important model for Africa seeking to operationalize data governance under the AU Data Policy Framework and the Digital Single Market.

Australia's My Health Records Act 2012 and its 2025 amendment, which transition to a share-by-default model, illustrate the governance complexity of balancing data access with privacy protection. Canada's Personal Information Protection and Electronic Documents Act (PIPEDA) and provincial health information privacy legislation (such as Ontario's PHIPA) demonstrate how federated systems manage health data governance across jurisdictions. In Latin America, Brazil's Lei Geral de Proteção de Dados (LGPD), modeled on the GDPR, has influenced health data governance across the region.

15.4 Cybersecurity for Health Systems

The digitalization of health systems expands the attack surface for cyber threats. The Ghana Health Service's COVID-19 test results breach, the SingHealth breach in Singapore, and the WannaCry ransomware attack that disrupted parts of the UK's National Health Service underscore the urgent need for robust cybersecurity governance in health (Conduah et al., 2025). Africa's health systems are especially vulnerable: limited cybersecurity expertise, outdated IT infrastructure, insufficient investment in security, and the rapid deployment of digital health tools during COVID-19 without adequate security evaluations have created significant risks.

The latest International Telecommunication Union Global Cybersecurity Index (GCI) 2024 provides the most comprehensive assessment of countries' cybersecurity readiness, measuring performance across five pillars: legal, technical, organizational, capacity development, and cooperation. Globally, the average score reached 65.7/100, while Africa's regional average rose significantly to around 57, reflecting rapid progress over recent years and a narrowing gap with global performance. The index categorizes countries into five tiers—from Tier 1 (Role Modeling) to Tier 5 (Building)—highlighting maturity levels. In Africa, a small group of countries has reached Tier 1 leadership status, including Mauritius (100), Ghana (~99.3), Tanzania (~99.3), Kenya (~98.6), Rwanda (~98.1), Morocco (~97.5), and Egypt, demonstrating near-comprehensive cybersecurity frameworks.

A second group of "advancing" countries (Tier 2) includes South Africa (~86), Zambia (~92.6), Togo (~88.8), and Benin (~91.5). A larger cluster of countries falls into Tier 3 (establishing)—such as Nigeria (~82.4), Uganda (~82.9), Tunisia (~82), Botswana (~78.6), Côte d'Ivoire (~78.8), and Malawi (~80.4)—indicating solid but still developing cybersecurity systems. However, many countries, particularly in Central Africa and fragile contexts, remain in Tier 4 and Tier 5, with scores often below 50, reflecting limited institutional capacity, weak incident response systems, and enforcement gaps.

The implications of these findings for Africa's health sector are profound. As countries digitize health systems—through electronic health records, telemedicine, and health information exchanges—cybersecurity is critical to trust, safety, and system resilience. Countries in Tier 1 and Tier 2 are better positioned to secure sensitive health data, implement robust identity and access controls, and support cross-border data-sharing frameworks (e.g., digital health platforms and regional disease surveillance). In contrast, countries in Tier 3–5 face heightened risks of data breaches, ransomware attacks, and system disruptions, which can directly affect patient safety, continuity of care, and national health security.

The GCI also shows that Africa's strengths are concentrated in legal frameworks and basic technical measures, but gaps persist in capacity building, workforce skills, and operational readiness, all essential for protecting increasingly complex digital health ecosystems. For digital health transformation, the priority is therefore shifting from adopting laws to building sector-specific cybersecurity capabilities, including health-sector CERTs, secure interoperability standards, and integrated governance between ministries of health and national cybersecurity agencies.

Effective cybersecurity governance for health requires national cybersecurity strategies with health-sector-specific provisions; mandatory security standards for health information systems; incident reporting and response protocols; regular security audits and vulnerability assessments; cybersecurity training for health workers; and data encryption and access control standards. Nigeria's National Information Technology Development Agency (NITDA) has collaborated with the Federal Ministry of Health to develop cybersecurity frameworks.

The EU's Network and Information Security (NIS2) Directive explicitly covers health-sector entities and mandates incident reporting. Australia's Essential Eight cybersecurity framework, although not health-specific, provides a practical, incremental approach to mitigating cyber risk. In 2024, Health New Zealand (Te Whatu Ora) centralized its cybersecurity governance, recognizing that the cybersecurity of a fragmented health system poses unacceptable risks. These experiences underscore the importance of a health-specific cybersecurity framework that integrates strategy, standards, incident-reporting mechanisms, and capabilities aligned with the national cybersecurity strategy and frameworks.

15.5 Artificial Intelligence Ethics and Governance

The rapid expansion of AI applications in African healthcare—from diagnostic imaging to epidemic forecasting to drug discovery, as examined in Chapter 12—demands governance frameworks that ensure safety, fairness, transparency, and accountability. In July 2024, the African Union Executive Council formally endorsed the Continental AI Strategy, which focuses on five areas: maximizing AI's benefits, building capabilities, mitigating risks, encouraging investment, and fostering cooperation. The strategy includes a five-year implementation roadmap (2025–2030) covering intellectual property, data protection, cybersecurity, consumer rights, and competition law (Future of Privacy Forum, 2024). It proposes a multi-tiered governance approach that includes amending existing laws, sector-specific guidelines, regulatory sandboxes, and dedicated AI governance institutions.

At the national level, several African countries have developed AI strategies. By 2025, fourteen countries — Benin, Cote d'Ivoire, Democratic Republic of Congo, Egypt, Ethiopia, Ghana, Lesotho, Kenya, Mauritius, Rwanda, Senegal, South Africa, Zambia, and Zimbabwe — had developed dedicated AI strategies or policies, while others were integrating AI with other emerging technologies, such as blockchain and IoT. Kenya launched its AI Strategy 2025–2030, explicitly citing data privacy, cybersecurity, and ethics as core enablers and naming healthcare a strategic AI priority sector. South Africa published its National AI Policy Framework in August 2024, built on nine pillars that emphasize ethical design, transparency, and human oversight. It ranked highest in Africa on the 2024 Global Index on Responsible AI. Egypt unveiled its second National AI Strategy (2025–2030), aiming to create 30,000 AI professionals. Nigeria and Zambia released draft national AI strategies. In 2025, 52 African states signed the Africa Declaration on Artificial Intelligence at the Global AI Summit on Africa in Kigali (Tech in Africa, 2026).

Globally, the EU's AI Act—the world's first comprehensive AI regulation—provides a risk-based framework that classifies AI systems into unacceptable, high, limited, and minimal risk categories. Health applications are classified as high risk and are subject to mandatory conformity assessments. The UNESCO Recommendation on the Ethics of Artificial Intelligence (adopted November 2021) is a global, nonbinding framework that urges states, industry, researchers, and civil society to ensure AI respects human rights, dignity, and the public interest by adopting human-centered design, human oversight, safety, privacy, fairness, nondiscrimination, transparency, accountability, and environmental and societal well-being. It recommends legal and policy measures (including prohibitions on rights-violating uses such as mass surveillance and social scoring), data governance, algorithmic impact assessments, documentation and explainability, mechanisms for redress and independent oversight, investment in education and capacity building, inclusive multistakeholder processes, support for research and open science, and international cooperation with monitoring and assistance to implement these principles—particularly to protect vulnerable groups and promote cultural diversity and equity.

ASEAN's Guide on AI Governance and Ethics sets out common regional principles. The 2024 Santiago Declaration for Latin America and the Caribbean aims to strengthen regional cooperation in AI governance. Canada's Artificial Intelligence and Data Act (AIDA), proposed alongside the Consumer Privacy Protection Act, establishes a framework for regulating high-impact AI systems. WHO's 2021 Ethics and Governance of Artificial Intelligence for Health guidance provides international normative reference points. In Africa, the challenge is to develop governance frameworks that ensure AI safety and fairness without stifling the innovation examined in Chapter 13—regulatory sandboxes, as proposed by the AU Continental AI Strategy, offer one mechanism for achieving this balance.

15.6 Health Data Standards and Interoperability Governance

Chapter 9 examines the governance of health data standards—establishing, mandating, and enforcing the technical and semantic standards that enable systems to exchange and meaningfully use shared data—from a technical perspective. This section addresses the governance and policy dimensions: how countries establish institutional authority for standards, create enforcement mechanisms, and balance standardization with the flexibility needed across diverse health system contexts.

Kenya's Health Data Standards and South Africa's National Health Normative Standards Framework for Interoperability (NHNSFI) exemplify national standards governance frameworks. Both establish technical standards aligned with international frameworks—HL7 FHIR, ICD, and SNOMED CT—while allowing flexibility for local contexts. India's ABDM mandates open standards and interoperability to prevent vendor lock-in, creating a federated architecture that keeps data at the source while enabling on-demand access. Indonesia's SATUSEHAT platform connects health facilities, providers, and systems to enable secure, patient-centered sharing of health information. It mandates integration for government-funded health facilities, making standards compliance a condition of public financing.

The EU's decade-long effort toward cross-border interoperability through the EHDS underscores both the importance and the difficulty of standards governance at the continental scale. Canada's Connected Care for Canadians Act mandates interoperability standards across provincial health systems. New Zealand's Health Information Standards Organization (HISO) offers a small-country model for national standards governance.

The African Medicines Regulatory Harmonization (AMRH) Initiative provides a continental platform for harmonizing digital health product regulation and standards across Africa. The AfCFTA's provisions on intellectual property and digital trade could create a more coherent continental framework. However, standards governance is only effective when paired with enforcement mechanisms—and enforcement capacity remains the weakest link in most African digital health governance structures.

15.7 Telemedicine and Digital Health Product Regulation

The COVID-19 pandemic dramatically accelerated telemedicine adoption across Africa, but regulatory frameworks have lagged. By 2024, only about 18 African countries had specific telemedicine regulations or guidelines, and many still relied on ad hoc arrangements established during the pandemic emergency (WHO, 2022). Major regulatory issues include cross-border provider licensing, platform standards and data security, reimbursement policies, liability concerns, and the scope of practice for different provider types.

In Latin America, Colombia's Law 1419 of 2010 on telemedicine is an early example of comprehensive legislation that mandates insurance coverage and sets technical standards. Uruguay has integrated telemedicine into its national health information system, enabling seamless referrals. The proliferation of digital health applications highlights the need for regulatory frameworks that ensure safety, efficacy, and quality. As of 2024, only 12 African countries had established certification processes for digital health products. The EU's Medical Device Regulation (MDR) and In Vitro Diagnostic Regulation (IVDR) provide detailed, risk-based frameworks for software as a medical device (SaMD).

Singapore's Health Sciences Authority has established a regulatory sandbox for AI-based medical devices, enabling testing in controlled clinical settings before full approval. Australia's Therapeutic Goods Administration (TGA) has issued specific guidance for software-based medical devices. The legal recognition of electronic signatures—crucial for digital prescriptions and health records—has been adopted in 28 African countries, with the Philippines and Singapore providing implementation models (UNCTAD, 2023; ASEAN, 2020).

15.8 Alignment with Continental and International Frameworks

National digital health governance does not operate in isolation. At the continental level, the AU's Digital Transformation Strategy for Africa (2020–2030) identifies health as a priority sector. The AU Continental AI Strategy (2024) and the Africa Declaration on Artificial Intelligence (2025) provide continental governance frameworks. Countries that integrate digital health into broader national digital transformation agendas benefit from shared infrastructure investments and coordinated regulatory development. Internationally, alignment with the WHO's Global Strategy on Digital Health and the SDGs provides coherence and access to technical assistance.

Table 15.1. Alignment of African Digital Health Governance with Continental and International Frameworks

Framework	Scope	Key Health Governance Provisions	Relevance to Africa
AU Digital Transformation (2020–2030)	Continental	Health as priority sector; data governance; regional integration	Direct mandate; aligns with Agenda 2063
AU Continental AI Strategy (2024)	Continental	Multi-tiered AI governance; healthcare as flagship sector; 2025–2030 roadmap	First continental AI governance framework; regulatory sandboxes proposed
EU GDPR / EHDS	Regional (EU)	Data protection; cross-border health data portability; secondary use regulation	Model for continental data governance; EHDS informs AfCFTA digital trade provisions
EU AI Act	Regional (EU)	Risk-based AI classification; health as high-risk; mandatory conformity assessments	Reference for Africa's AI governance; risk-based approach adaptable to African contexts
WHO Global Strategy on Digital Health	Global	Governance, evidence, implementation, enabling environment	Normative guidance; 2028–2033 strategy being developed with African input
ASEAN Digital Health Framework	Regional (Asia)	Interoperability standards; telemedicine regulation; cross-border data exchange	Lessons for RECs (ECOWAS, EAC, SADC) on regional harmonisation

Source: Author's Compilation

15.9 Monitoring and Evaluation

Strong M&E frameworks are essential for tracking governance effectiveness. The "Digital Health M&E Results Chain" presents a step-by-step model that shows how digital health investments translate into meaningful health improvements. It begins with inputs such as funding, human resources, infrastructure, and policy support, which enable key activities such as training, system deployment, and regulation. These activities generate immediate outputs, including deployed systems, trained staff, and enacted policies. In turn, these outputs contribute to improvements in access to services, data quality, and efficiency within the healthcare system. Ultimately, these outcomes have a broader impact on health and progress toward universal health coverage (UHC).

Figure 15.2. Digital Health M&E Results Chain Illustrating the Pathway From Inputs to Health Impact

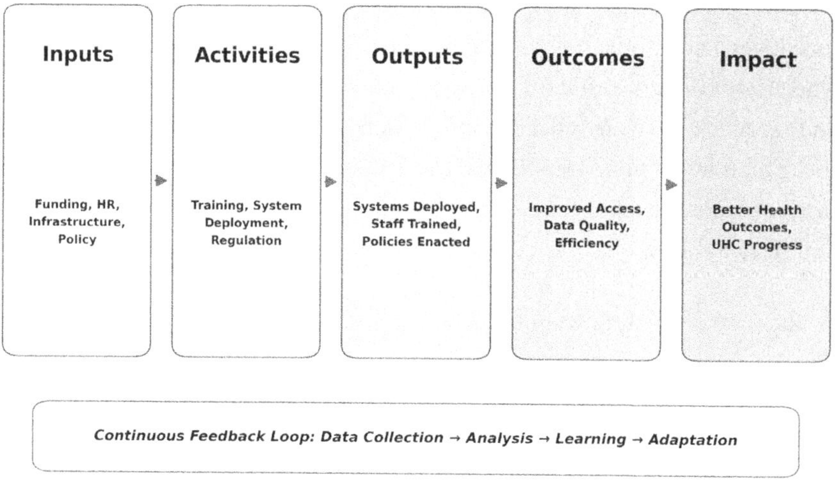

Source: Author's Elaboration

The monitoring and evaluation process is not linear but iterative, featuring a continuous feedback loop of data collection, analysis, learning, and adaptation. This loop ensures that insights from monitoring and evaluation inform refinement strategies and performance improvement at every stage of the results chain.

A 2021 WHO review found that fewer than half of African countries with strategies had functioning M&E frameworks with defined indicators, data collection mechanisms, and reporting cycles (WHO, 2022). The WHO Digital Health Atlas, the Global Digital Health Index (GDHI), and the PRISM framework have been adapted to African contexts. Chile's Salud Digital strategy includes quarterly progress reviews conducted by a dedicated M&E unit. Argentina's Federal Digital Health Strategy reports results through a public online dashboard—offering accountability models that African countries could adopt.

15.10 Change Management

Three core pillars are essential to successfully implementing digital health initiatives: People, Process, and Technology. Under the People pillar, the focus should be on leadership champions, training and capacity building, and incentives and motivation to drive adoption. The Process pillar emphasizes workflow redesign, standard operating procedures, and ongoing monitoring and feedback to ensure effective integration into routine practice. Meanwhile, the Technology pillar highlights the importance of user-centered design, interoperable systems, and continuous technical support to ensure usability and sustainability.

At the base of the framework is a strong foundation consisting of stakeholder buy-in, political will, institutional culture, and trust. This foundation supports all three pillars and is critical to long-term success. Effective digital health adoption requires a balanced approach that integrates human factors, organizational processes, and technological solutions, all grounded in a supportive enabling environment.

Even the most well-designed governance framework will fail without effective change management and sustained stakeholder support. In Morocco, digital health training includes modules on change management and professional development. Indonesia's SATUSEHAT program invested in 'digital health champions' at the community health center level.

Figure 15.3. A Three-Dimensional Change Management Framework for Digital Health Adoption

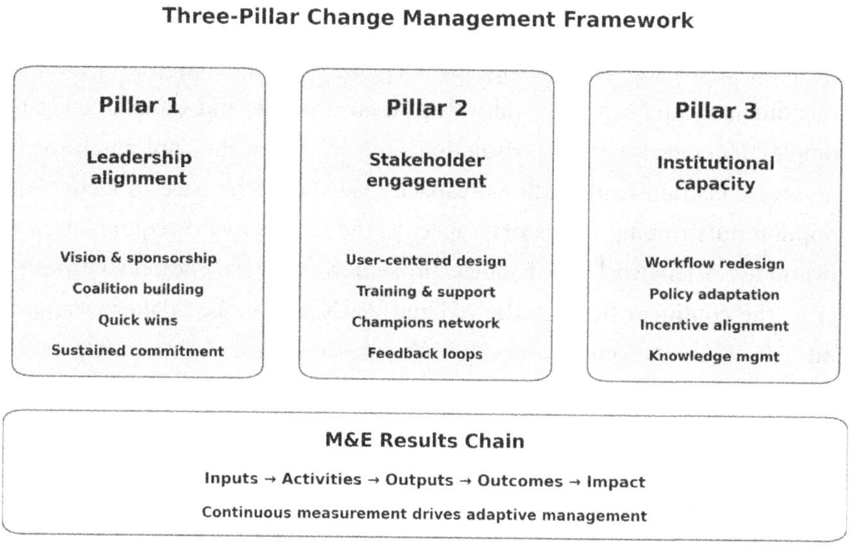

Source: Author's Elaboration

Rwanda's community health worker program links digital reporting to performance payments. In Uganda, community dialogues on digital health privacy have fostered trust. Jamaica's Digital Health Strategy incorporates public awareness campaigns and community feedback mechanisms. These experiences confirm that governance must address people, processes, and institutional culture alongside technical systems and legal frameworks.

15.11 Conclusion

This chapter has examined governance, policy, and standards—the most critical cross-cutting enabler in the Digital Health Technology Stack—as the institutional architecture that underpins strategy and enables the foundational layers to function. The evidence shows a continent making significant progress: 44 countries with data protection legislation, the AU Continental AI

Strategy adopted in 2024, 52 states signing the Africa Declaration on Artificial Intelligence in 2025, and rapid development of national AI strategies across 14 countries by 2025. Yet governance maturity remains uneven, enforcement capacity is limited, health-sector-specific regulations are underdeveloped, and cybersecurity governance is nascent.

The comparative analysis shows that governance challenges are universal—the EU took a decade to develop the EHDS, Australia required legislative amendments to reform My Health Record governance, and Canada navigates complex federal-provincial jurisdiction—but in Africa they are amplified by resource constraints, institutional capacity gaps, and the pace of technology adoption outstripping regulatory capacity. The path forward requires African governance frameworks to balance protection with innovation, harmonize across the continent through the AU and RECs, and embed data sovereignty and AI ethics as central—not peripheral—concerns. As the chapter on financing and sustainability (Chapter 17) will demonstrate, even the strongest governance frameworks cannot be sustained without predictable, long-term financing.

References

African Researchers Magazine. (2025). Data protection & AI governance in Africa: Key trends from 2024 & projections for 2025.

African Union Commission. (2020). Digital Transformation Strategy for Africa (2020–2030). AU.

African Union & Access Now. (2023). The state of data protection in Africa. Access Now.

ASEAN Secretariat. (2020). ASEAN digital integration framework. ASEAN.

AUDA-NEPAD. (2020). African Medicines Regulatory Harmonization Initiative: Strategic framework. AUDA-NEPAD.

Conduah, A. K., Ofoe, S., & Siaw-Marfo, D. (2025). Data privacy in healthcare: Global challenges and solutions. SAGE Digital Health.

European Commission. (2022). Proposal for a Regulation on the European Health Data Space. COM(2022) 197 final.

Future of Privacy Forum. (2024). The AU's Continental AI Strategy: Data protection and governance. FPF.

Ministry of Health, Kenya. (2020). National digital health strategy 2019–2024. Government of Kenya.

Ministry of Health, Rwanda. (2018). Health sector ICT strategic plan 2018–2024. Government of Rwanda.

Ministry of Public Health, Thailand. (2019). Thailand digital health strategic plan 2019–2023. MoPH Thailand.

PAHO. (2021). eHealth strategy for the Caribbean 2021–2025. PAHO.

Tech in Africa. (2026). Ethical AI: Navigating governance and compliance in Africa. Tech in Africa.

UNCTAD. (2023). Digital economy report 2023. UNCTAD.

WHO. (2021). Ethics and governance of artificial intelligence for health. WHO.

WHO. (2022). Global survey on digital health 2022. WHO.

WHO & ITU. (2012). National eHealth strategy toolkit. WHO.

Chapter 16 Regional Cooperation and Coordination of Digital Health

16.1 Overview

No single country—regardless of its resources or ambition—can address the full spectrum of digital health challenges alone. Regional collaboration enables resource pooling, harmonized standards, cross-border interoperability, collective problem-solving, and economies of scale needed to sustain investments in digital infrastructure and human capacity. This chapter examines continental and regional frameworks that shape digital health collaboration across Africa, analyzes the roles of the African Union, Regional Economic Communities, and pan-African health organizations, and explores cross-border health information exchange, regional interoperability, and training programs.

Drawing extensively on how other regions—the European Union, ASEAN, SAARC, PAHO, and the Americas—have fostered regional cooperation in digital health, the chapter identifies transferable models and governance architectures that Africa's regional institutions can adapt, while recognizing the African context's distinctive features: 55 AU Member States, enormous diversity, and the imperative to leapfrog rather than replicate incremental pathways.

16.2 African Union Digital Transformation Strategy

The African Union adopted the Digital Transformation Strategy for Africa (DTS) in February 2020, articulating a vision for an integrated, inclusive digital society across all sectors, including health. Health sector priorities under the DTS include establishing a continental interoperability framework, developing pan-African digital health platforms, harmonizing telemedicine and data protection regulations, enabling joint procurement of digital health technologies, and coordinating training programs. Implementation mechanisms include AU-led technical working groups, structured partnerships with Regional Economic Communities, and a monitoring framework aligned with Agenda 2063 (African Union, 2020).

Progress since adoption includes the African Digital Health Investment Framework, the AU Digital Health Technical Working Group, the Continental Interoperability Framework, and regional pilot projects. In 2024, the AU Executive Council endorsed the Continental AI Strategy, with healthcare as a flagship sector. In 2025, 52 states signed the Africa Declaration on Artificial Intelligence at the Global AI Summit in Kigali. However, challenges persist: limited dedicated funding, varying readiness across countries, and coordination among 55 AU Member States.

The AU's approach draws on and adapts models from other regional blocs. The European Union's Digital Decade program (2030) and the European Health Data Space (EHDS) provide the most mature model of supranational digital health governance, featuring binding regulatory instruments, dedicated funding (the EU4Health and Digital Europe programs), and institutional infrastructure. The 2025 PAHO Annual Report documented that 22 countries in the Americas joined the WHO's Global Digital Health Certification Network for cross-border interoperability, and that seven countries implemented the All-in-One Telehealth Platform—demonstrating the scale achievable through regional coordination supported by sustained institutional commitment (PAHO, 2026).

ASEAN's Digital Health Framework, adopted in 2021, shares similar objectives but uses a lighter governance approach, relying on voluntary harmonization. PAHO's 2025–2031 Subregional Cooperation Strategy for Central America, the Dominican Republic, and Mexico explicitly prioritizes digital transformation and interoperability of digital tools. Meanwhile, the EU–CELAC Summit in November 2025 promoted interregional cooperation to harmonize regulations between Europe and Latin America.

16.3 Regional Economic Communities and Digital Health

A comparative assessment of digital health maturity across African Regional Economic Communities (RECs) in 2024, using five key dimensions—policy frameworks, active programs, cross-border health information exchange (HIE), standards adoption, and training programs—finds that the East African Community (EAC) consistently leads across all indicators. EAC scores are particularly high in policy frameworks and active programs, reflecting strong institutional coordination, sustained investments, and relatively advanced implementation of digital health strategies. The Economic Community of West African States (ECOWAS) and the Southern African Development Community (SADC) follow at moderate levels, with ECOWAS performing better in policy and standards, while SADC shows more balanced but slightly lower scores across all dimensions.

In contrast, the Economic Community of Central African States (ECCAS) and the Arab Maghreb Union (AMU/UMA) lag significantly behind. ECCAS records the lowest scores across most categories—particularly in cross-border HIE and standards adoption—highlighting structural constraints such as weak institutional capacity, limited infrastructure, and fragmented governance. AMU/UMA performs somewhat better than ECCAS but still remains below continental averages, especially in training and interoperability. Notably, cross-border HIE and training programs are the weakest areas across nearly all RECs, underscoring ongoing challenges in interoperability, workforce capacity, and regional integration.

The EAC's eight partner states pursue integration through harmonized policies, shared infrastructure, and coordinated programs. Major projects include a cross-border HIE pilot linking Kenya, Uganda, and Tanzania, serving more than 50,000 patients—mainly migrant workers, cross-border traders, and refugees; regional telemedicine guidelines adopted by four partner states; and an annual joint digital health forum. The EAC's cross-border HIE experience parallels the EU's eHealth Digital Service Infrastructure (eHDSI), which enables the exchange of patient summaries and electronic prescriptions among member states—but the EU's project took more than ten years to develop. Notably, ASEAN's emerging digital health cooperation, formalized in its 2021 framework, is at an earlier stage than the EAC's, suggesting that Africa's regional pioneers may offer transferable lessons to Southeast Asian counterparts.

Figure 16.1. Digital Health Maturity Across Five Regional Economic Communities by Key Dimensions (2024)

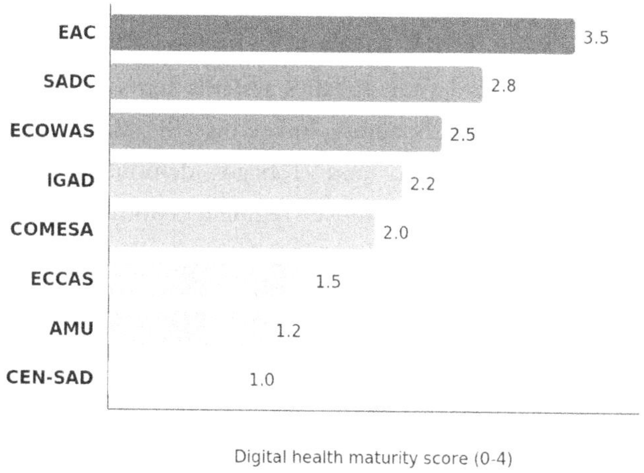

Source: REC Secretariats; WHO AFRO (2023); Development Partners' Reports

ECOWAS's 15 West African nations have prioritized digital health to strengthen regional health security. The digital yellow fever vaccination certificate pilot—tested in Benin, Burkina Faso, and Nigeria—achieved a 95% reduction in certificate forgery and demonstrated the viability of WHO-compatible digital health documentation standards for cross-border use. These standards feature offline capability, a mobile-first design, and simple interfaces for border officials. This initiative mirrors the EU's Digital COVID Certificate (DCC), which influenced the WHO's Global Digital Health Certification Network (GDHCN). PAHO's Digital Health Pass for the Americas pursued similar objectives. The 2025 revised ECOWAS Supplementary Data Protection Act, published for public comment, signals the community's growing focus on harmonized data governance.

SADC's 16 member states primarily pursue health cooperation through bilateral initiatives, including a regional malaria surveillance network that enables cross-border case tracking—achieving 40% faster outbreak detection—and shared telemedicine that connects smaller member states with South African specialist centers. South Africa's dominance creates both opportunities and challenges stemming from asymmetric power dynamics. ECCAS faces significant constraints due to political instability and limited infrastructure.

North African countries advance digital health through bilateral relationships and engagement with the OECD and the EU Neighborhood Policy. In the Caribbean, PAHO's 2025 initiative to improve the digital transformation of civil registration and vital statistics systems across 13 Caribbean countries—with interagency roadmapping involving The Bahamas, Guyana, Jamaica, Suriname, and Trinidad and Tobago—demonstrates how small island developing states can achieve regional coordination with multilateral institutional support.

16.4 Pan-African Health Organizations

The key Pan-African organizations are the Africa Centres for Disease Control and Prevention (Africa CDC), the continent's central technical authority for public health, which leads digital health initiatives in surveillance, health information systems, and pandemic preparedness (e.g., regional data platforms and digital surveillance architectures), and the World Health Organization (WHO AFRO), which leads digital health guidelines, interoperability frameworks, and country implementation support. Complementing these are technical, financial, and knowledge actors that enable implementation and scale.

Organizations such as Smart Africa, the African Telecommunications Union (ATU), and AfriNIC provide the digital infrastructure, standards, and connectivity backbone that digital health systems require. Development partners—including the World Bank, the International Telecommunication Union (ITU), and the African Development Bank (AfDB)—offer financing, technical assistance, and normative guidance. Research and civil society organizations, such as Research ICT Africa (RIA), contribute evidence, policy analysis, and advocacy.

16.4.1 Africa CDC and Digital Surveillance

Africa CDC has rapidly become the continent's leading institution for digital disease surveillance. Its Integrated Disease Surveillance and Response (IDSR) system links all 55 AU member states through five Regional Collaborating Centers. The COVID-19 continental dashboard provided unprecedented visibility into the pandemic's progress. The Africa Pathogen Genomics Initiative (Africa PGI) expanded sequencing capacity from fewer than 10 countries to more than 30 by 2024. Post-pandemic, the Africa CDC's cross-border surveillance supports malaria elimination, polio eradication, cholera response, and readiness for emerging pathogens.

Figure 16.2 Africa CDC Digital Disease Surveillance Architecture

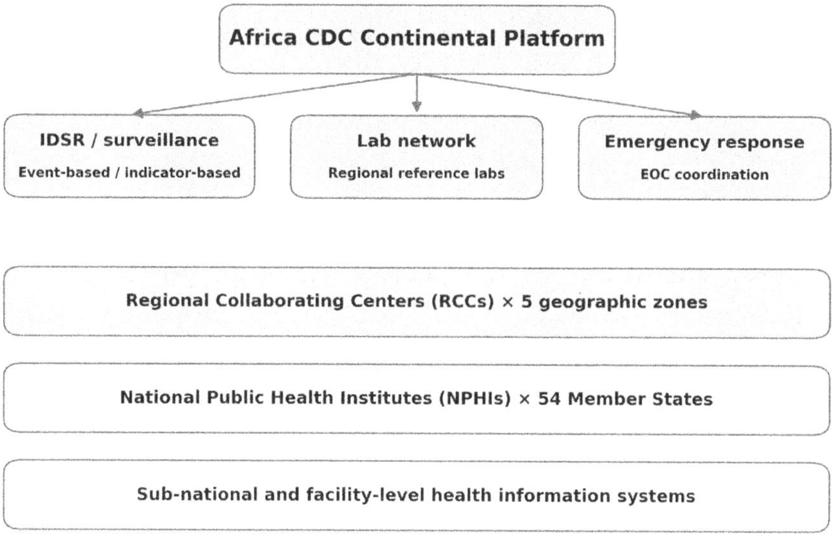

Source: Africa CDC (2021); Nkengasong & Mankoula (2020)

Africa CDC's launch of the Africa Health Security and Sovereignty Agenda underscored the institution's growing role in advancing African leadership in continental health data governance. Africa CDC's model draws on peer institutions yet differs from them. The European Center for Disease Prevention and Control (ECDC) collects data from 30 countries through TESSy. The ASEAN BioDiaspora Virtual Center oversees regional disease intelligence. In the Americas, PAHO's EIOS system for early detection of public health threats provides regional surveillance across 35 countries. Africa CDC's coordination mandate—covering 55 states with vastly different surveillance capacities—is arguably the most complex globally, making its achievements all the more notable.

16.4.2 WHO AFRO Digital Health Initiatives

WHO AFRO provides normative guidance, technical leadership, and coordination. The WHO Digital Health Atlas catalogs implementations. The WHO AFRO Digital Health Assessment Tool helps countries assess their readiness. Regional frameworks guide the deployment of telemedicine, mHealth, and clinical decision support. In 2025, WHO AFRO convened African regional consultations to shape the upcoming WHO Global Strategy on Digital Health (2028–2033), with a focus on governance, interoperability, AI, workforce, equity, and sustainable financing—ensuring that African priorities inform the global governance framework.

16.5 Regional Interoperability

A layered Pan-African Health Information Interoperability Framework presents interoperability as a structured stack of mutually reinforcing components, spanning from foundational infrastructure to high-level governance. At the base is the Infrastructure Layer, which encompasses essential enablers such as broadband connectivity, data centers, reliable power supply, and device access. This layer underpins all higher levels, underscoring that without robust digital infrastructure, interoperability cannot be effectively realized across health systems.

Above this sits the Technical Interoperability layer, which defines the standards and protocols that enable systems to communicate—such as HL7 FHIR, OpenHIE architectures, APIs, and cybersecurity protocols. Building on this is Semantic Interoperability, which ensures that exchanged data is consistently understood through shared terminology and coding systems such as ICD-10/11, SNOMED CT, and LOINC. The next level, Organizational Interoperability, focuses on aligning institutional processes, including shared workflows, data governance agreements, and trust frameworks across countries and institutions. At the top is the Governance & Policy Layer, which anchors the entire framework through continental and regional coordination, including African Union (AU) frameworks, REC-level harmonization, and national policy alignment.

Continental interoperability requires harmonized technical standards across governance, organizational, semantic, technical, and infrastructure layers. The OpenHIE reference architecture has gained significant traction and is being adopted by Rwanda, Kenya, Tanzania, Uganda, Mozambique, and Sierra Leone. HL7 FHIR's mobile-friendly, RESTful design makes it particularly suitable for African environments. Semantic interoperability depends on ICD-10/11, SNOMED CT, and LOINC, though costs, linguistic challenges, and training needs remain barriers.

Figure 16.3 Pan-African Health Information Interoperability Framework

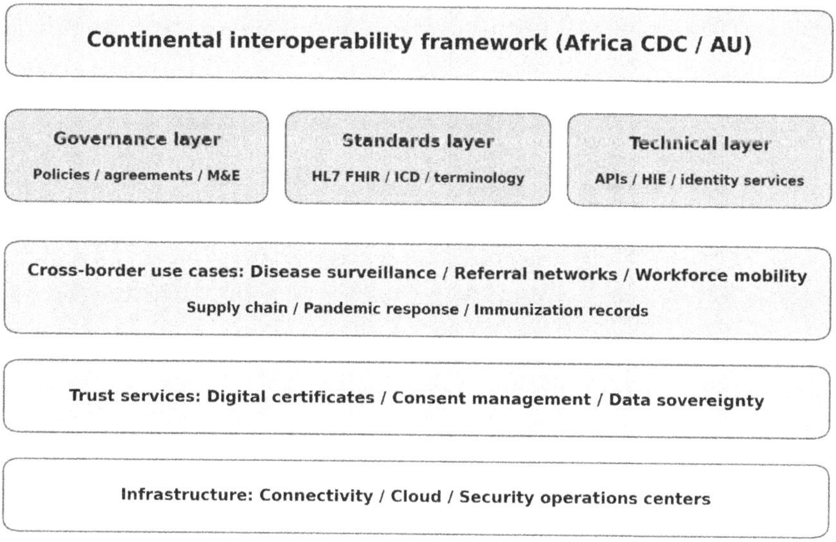

Source: Adapted from OpenHIE (2022); Moodley et al. (2012)

In the Americas, PAHO developed the offline-capable 'Vacuna Offline' immunization application in collaboration with Peru's Ministry of Health. It is built on WHO SMART Guidelines interoperability standards—achieving a 30% reduction in data entry time and demonstrating how offline-first, standards-compliant tools can serve cross-border indigenous communities in the Amazon-Andean region (PAHO, 2025). This model is directly relevant to Africa's cross-border populations in similarly remote, connectivity-challenged settings. Australia's National Healthcare Interoperability Plan and Canada's pan-Canadian interoperability mandates provide mature frameworks for standards governance in federated systems. New Zealand's HISO offers a small-country standards governance model.

Operational pilots demonstrate the feasibility of interoperability in Africa: the EAC HIE reduced duplicate tests by 60%; the ECOWAS vaccination system cut fraud by 95%; the SADC malaria network detected outbreaks 40% faster; and the West African TB laboratory network improved drug-resistance monitoring. Scaling from pilot to routine operations requires formal data governance agreements, harmonized data protection laws, and sustainable financing.

Figure 16.4 Documented Impact of Cross-border Health Information Exchange Pilots in Africa

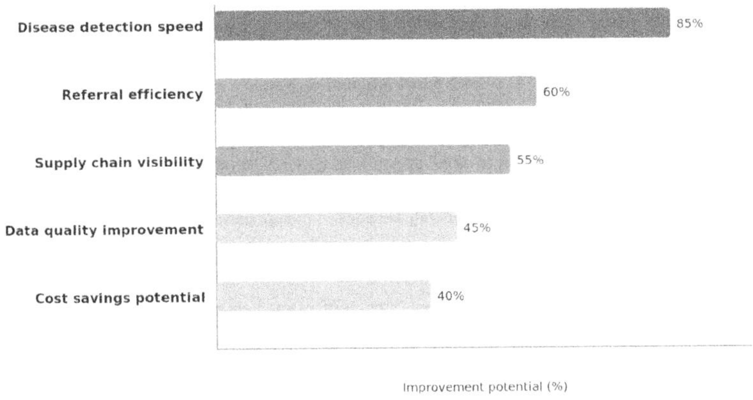

Source: EAC (2021); ECOWAS (2020); SADC (2020)

16.6 Cross-Border Health Information Exchange

Millions of Africans regularly cross national borders. The AfCFTA is expected to further accelerate cross-border mobility. Without access to their home-country health records, mobile populations face duplicate testing, medication errors, and fragmented care. The EAC HIE pilot demonstrated measurable impact: a 60% reduction in duplicate laboratory tests, a 40% decrease in medication errors, and a significant improvement in patient satisfaction. Africa hosts over 30 million refugees and displaced persons, whose medical records often become inaccessible during displacement (Kiberu et al., 2019).

The EU's eHDSI provides a mature reference—since 2019, it has enabled cross-border exchange of patient summaries and electronic prescriptions—but required more than a decade of development. The EAC's more pragmatic approach, focused on specific border populations and critical use cases rather than full interoperability, offers a model better suited to African realities, where perfect interoperability should not stand in the way of practical, high-impact data exchange. In the Americas, PAHO's 2025–2031 Subregional Cooperation Strategy for Central America explicitly addresses access to health services for migrant populations through intergovernmental agreements and interoperable digital tools—directly paralleling Africa's challenge of serving mobile populations across porous borders.

COVID-19 highlighted both the value and the limitations of cross-border disease surveillance: Africa CDC's continental platform enabled regional outbreak detection about 40% faster than pre-pandemic systems, but gaps in data completeness and standardization reduced accuracy. Post-pandemic, surveillance capabilities support malaria elimination, polio eradication, and readiness for emerging pathogens. The New Public Health Order initiative, endorsed by AU Heads of State in 2022, commits AU Member States to establishing digitally enabled surveillance with cross-border data sharing as a foundational requirement.

16.7 Regional Training and Capacity Building

Regional training programs leverage economies of scale and build pan-African professional networks. The DHIS2 Academy has trained more than 15,000 professionals through regional academies in Dar es Salaam, Dakar, and Cape Town. The African Field Epidemiology Network (AFENET) has trained over 5,000 professionals in surveillance and health information systems across 19 countries. HELINA facilitates curriculum development and research collaboration. The EAC Digital Health Community of Practice connects more than 200 professionals

Figure 16.5 Regional Digital Health Training Programs: Cumulative Participants (2024)

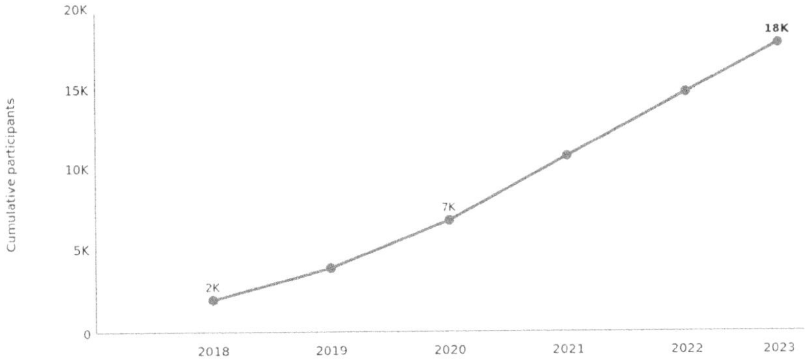

Source: HISP (2023); AFENET (2022); HELINA (2022); EAC (2021)

Compared with other regions, the EU invests significantly through the European Health Workforce Network and Horizon Europe. India's ABDM workforce component aims to train 500,000 health IT professionals by 2030. PAHO's Virtual Campus for Public Health provides online training across the Americas, and in 2025, PAHO's Digital Literacy Program trained more than 70,000 health-sector staff—the fastest regional-scale digital-literacy rollout in the Global South. The Caribbean Public Health Agency (CARPHA)'s model consolidates training resources across 24 Caribbean nations, achieving scale no single country could afford—a model highly relevant to Africa's RECs.

Africa's estimated shortfall of more than 50,000 health informatics professionals calls for expanding training through online courses, regional centers of excellence, and public-private partnerships, as discussed in Chapter 11.

16.8 Global Comparison: Regional Collaboration Models

A global comparative assessment of regional health collaboration in 2024, evaluating six dimensions—cross-border health information exchange (HIE), harmonized regulations, regional surveillance, shared standards, joint training, and coordinated procurement—reveals a clear performance hierarchy, with the European Union (EU) consistently leading across all indicators. The EU's high scores reflect decades of institutional integration, robust legal frameworks, and investments in cross-border digital health infrastructure, including the European Health Data Space.

Africa shows uneven but growing progress, with relatively stronger performance in regional surveillance and joint training, reflecting gains from continental initiatives and REC-level coordination. However, Africa lags significantly in harmonized regulations and coordinated procurement, indicating ongoing fragmentation of legal frameworks and limited pooled procurement mechanisms. Asia (ASEAN/SAARC) and Latin America & the Caribbean occupy middle positions, with moderate achievements in surveillance and training but weaker integration of standards and cross-border systems.

The European Union leads comprehensively through binding regulatory instruments (EHDS, AI Act, NIS2), dedicated funding (EU4Health: EUR 5.3 billion for 2021–2027; Digital Europe program), and mature institutional infrastructure (ECDC, European Health and Digital Executive Agency). Cross-border patient data exchange via the eHDSI, standardized digital health documentation via the Digital COVID Certificate, and interregional cooperation via the EU–CELAC Summit demonstrate the depth of EU digital health regionalism. The 2025 PAHO–EU–CELAC partnership for regulatory harmonization between Europe and Latin America illustrates emerging interregional cooperation models.

Figure 16.6 Regional Health Collaboration Maturity: Global Comparison Across Key Dimensions (2024)

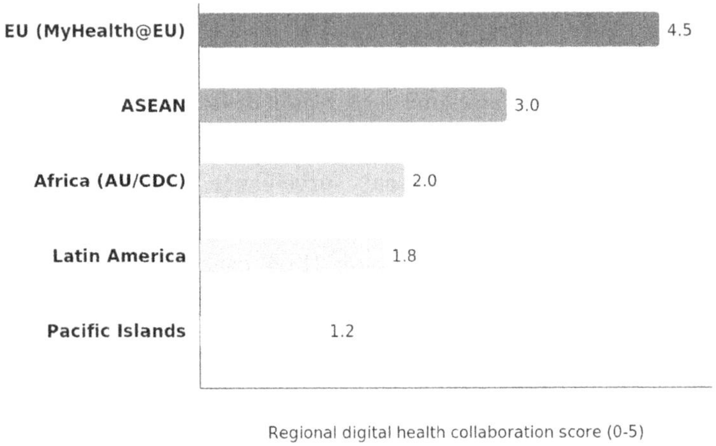

Source: WHO; ITU; Regional Organisation Assessments

PAHO and the Americas demonstrate strengths in regional surveillance through the EIOS system, in regional procurement through the Revolving Funds (procuring over USD 900 million in vaccines, technologies, and health supplies in the 2024–2025 biennium), in joint training through the Virtual Campus, in digital innovation through the Vacuna Offline application, and in subregional cooperation strategies for Central America and the Caribbean. PAHO's 2025 Annual Report documented 22 countries joining the Global Digital Health Certification Network and seven implementing the All-in-One Telehealth Platform, demonstrating how sustained institutional commitment translates into regional-scale digital health adoption.

ASEAN promotes consensus-based, voluntary harmonization through its Digital Health Framework (2021), the ASEAN BioDiaspora Virtual Center for disease intelligence, and emerging cross-border telemedicine guidelines. ASEAN's governance model—delivering results without binding regulation—

offers lessons for African RECs operating within similar consensus-based institutional frameworks.

Africa's distinctive strengths include strong institutional structures (AU, RECs, Africa CDC, WHO AFRO), crisis-driven coordination capacity (the COVID-19 continental response), leadership in open-source platforms (DHIS2, OpenMRS, OpenHIE) that inherently facilitate cross-border interoperability, and vibrant professional networks. The most urgent gaps are in cross-border data governance frameworks, harmonized regulatory environments, sustained financing for regional initiatives, and scaling interoperability pilots from proof of concept to routine operations.

AU and WHO AFRO consultations indicate that mobilizing sustainable financing is the top priority, underscoring the central role of long-term, predictable funding in scaling up digital health systems and cross-border initiatives. This is followed by strengthening continental data governance and enhancing African Union (AU) coordination, reflecting the need for coherent policy frameworks, trusted data-sharing mechanisms, and stronger supranational leadership to drive harmonization across countries and Regional Economic Communities (RECs).

Figure 16.8. Priority Actions for Strengthening Regional Digital Health Collaboration in Africa (2024)

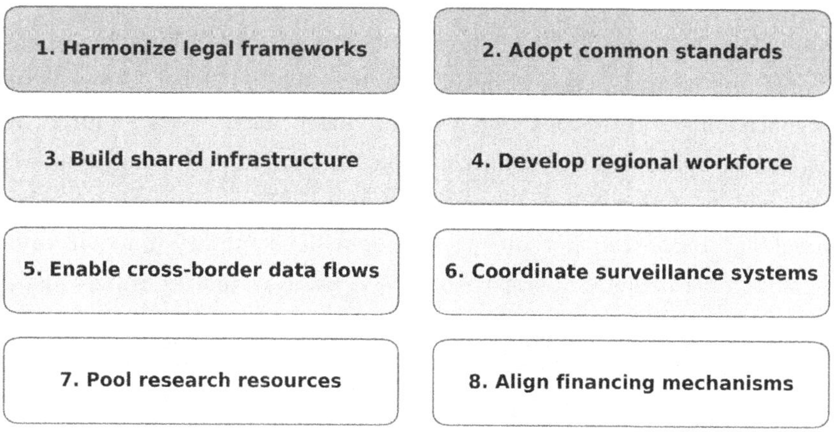

Source: AU and WHO AFRO Consultations

Mid-tier priorities, such as increasing REC-level investment and expanding cross-border health information exchange, underscore the importance of both regional financial commitments and the operationalization of interoperability frameworks. The relatively lower—though still significant—priority assigned to scaling training programs suggests that, while human capacity development is essential, stakeholders view governance, financing, and system integration as more immediate constraints.

16.9 Conclusion

This chapter has explored regional cooperation and coordination as a vital element spanning all enablers and foundational layers of the Digital Health Technology Stack. Africa's regional structure—the AU, eight RECs, Africa CDC, and WHO AFRO—provides institutional support unmatched in ambition and complexity. The EAC's cross-border HIE serving over 50,000 patients, ECOWAS's digital vaccination certificates achieving a 95% reduction in fraud, Africa CDC's continental surveillance linking 55 member states, and the Africa Pathogen Genomics Initiative expanding sequencing capacity from 10 to more than 30 countries demonstrate that African regional digital health collaboration is delivering tangible results.

The comparative analysis shows that regional health collaboration is essential yet time-consuming: the EU's cross-border health data exchange took more than a decade to develop, supported by sustained political backing and binding regulations. PAHO's 2025 accomplishments—training more than 70,000 professionals, connecting 22 countries to the Global Digital Health Certification Network, deploying telehealth platforms in seven countries, and advancing digital CRVS transformation in the Caribbean—demonstrate what sustained institutional commitment can achieve. Africa's pragmatic, use-case-driven approach—centered on specific populations and key functions rather than full interoperability—offers a feasible pathway that prioritizes impact while gradually building more integrated regional digital health ecosystems.

References

Africa CDC. (2021). Framework for integrated disease surveillance and response. Africa CDC.

African Field Epidemiology Network. (2022). Annual report 2022. AFENET.

African Union. (2020). Digital Transformation Strategy for Africa (2020–2030). AU Commission.

African Union Commission. (2021). African digital health investment framework. AUC.

EAC. (2021). EAC health sector strategic plan 2020–2025. EAC Secretariat.

ECOWAS. (2020). Regional health intervention plan 2020–2025. ECOWAS.

HELINA. (2022). Health informatics in Africa: Advances and challenges. HELINA.

HISP. (2023). Health information systems programme: Global impact report 2023. University of Oslo.

Kiberu, V. M., et al. (2019). Barriers and opportunities for sustainable e-health in Uganda. Afr J Prim Health Care, 11(1), e1–e10.

Moodley, D., et al. (2012). Open architectures for national HIS in developing countries. MEDINFO 2012. IOS Press.

Nkengasong, J. N., & Mankoula, W. (2020). Looming threat of COVID-19 in Africa. The Lancet, 395, 841–842.

OpenHIE. (2022). OpenHIE architecture specification version 2.0. OpenHIE.

PAHO. (2025). Digital innovation for vaccination in cross-border indigenous communities. PAHO.

PAHO. (2025). 2025–2031 subregional cooperation strategy for Central America. PAHO.

PAHO. (2026). 2025 Annual Report: Driving innovation, delivering impact. PAHO.

SADC. (2020). Regional indicative strategic development plan 2020–2030. SADC Secretariat.

WHO AFRO. (2019). Framework for digital health services in the African Region. WHO AFRO.

WHO AFRO. (2023). Digital health in the African Region: Progress report 2023. WHO AFRO.

WHO AFRO. (2025). Shaping the next global strategy on digital health (2028–2033): African Region consultation. WHO AFRO.

Chapter 17 Financing and Sustainability

17.1. Overview

This chapter addresses financing and sustainability—the final cross-cutting enabler in the Digital Health Technology Stack (Figure 4.1)—and examines one of the most critical and persistent challenges in Africa's digital health transformation. It estimates the cost of a comprehensive digital health transformation, maps the current and rapidly shifting funding landscape, examines how health financing mechanisms can integrate digital tools, assesses return on investment, explores innovative financing models, and analyzes the often underestimated total cost of ownership.

The chapter is written at a moment of profound disruption in global health financing. The restructuring of PEPFAR, the dissolution of USAID, and the introduction of bilateral health agreements with bundled data-sharing requirements have created a USD 12 billion shortfall in Africa's healthcare financing and have fundamentally altered the relationship between external funding and health system sovereignty. Drawing on practices from India, Brazil, Thailand, Colombia, the EU, Chile, Australia, and the Caribbean, the chapter provides a practical guide to building domestically anchored, diversified, and sustainable financing for digital health.

17.2 The Cost of Digital Health Transformation

The Broadband Commission estimated in 2020 that achieving meaningful digital health coverage across low- and middle-income countries would require annual investments of about USD 2 per capita, or roughly USD 2.6 billion per year for sub-Saharan Africa alone (Broadband Commission, 2020). PATH Digital Square estimated that a comprehensive transformation program for a typical African country of 30 million people would require USD 200–400 million in initial capital and USD 50–100 million in annual recurring costs over ten years. At the continental level, total investment needs are estimated at USD 15–25 billion over the decade to 2030, with annual recurring costs of USD 5–8 billion (PATH Digital Square, 2022; AfDB, 2022).

Figure 17.1. Estimated Cost Components of Digital Health Transformation in Africa, Initial Capital and Recurring Costs

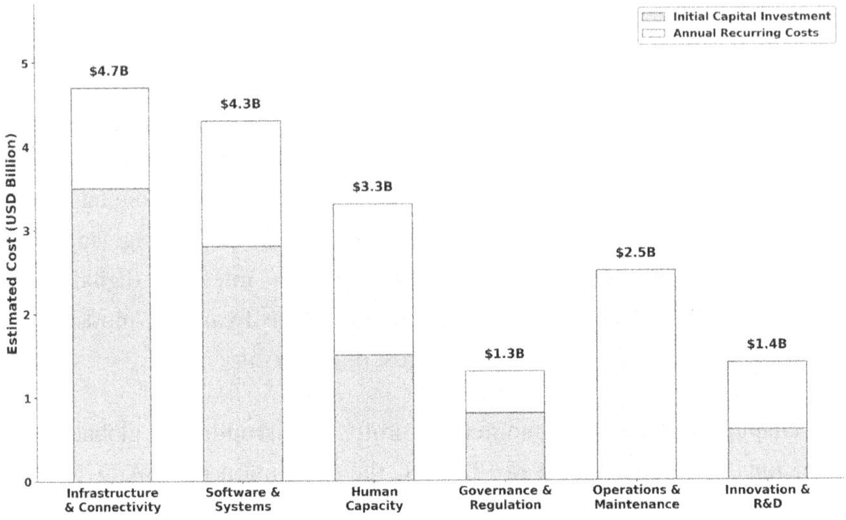

Source: PATH Digital Square (2022); Author's Elaboration

India's ABDM allocated approximately USD 200 million for the initial phase (2021–2023), and state-level costs brought the total investment to over USD 1 billion for 1.4 billion people (National Health Authority India, 2022). Brazil's RNDS investment is estimated at approximately USD 500 million, co-financed by the federal budget and World Bank lending (World Bank, 2021). Australia's National Digital Health Strategy is supported by the Australian Digital Health Agency's annual budget of approximately AUD 350 million. These comparators underscore that although Africa's investment needs are substantial, they represent only 2–5 percent of projected health expenditure—a fraction that can yield returns many times the investment.

17.3 The Funding Landscape in Crisis and Transition

Comparing the current funding mix (2023) with a target financing structure for 2030 shows that digital health financing in Africa is heavily donor-dependent, with development partners and donors contributing the largest share (42%), followed by government budgets (25%) and the private sector

(18%). Philanthropic foundations account for about 10%, while other sources contribute a small 5%. This distribution highlights a financing model that is externally driven, with limited domestic resource mobilization and relatively modest private-sector participation.

Figure 17.2. Evolution of Digital Health Financing Sources in Africa: Current Mix versus Target

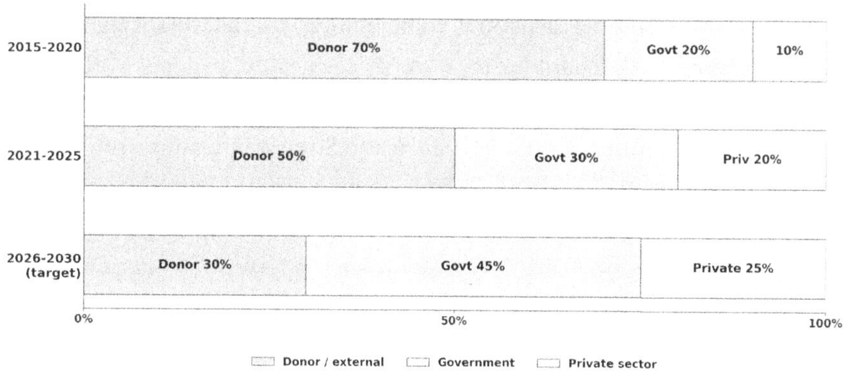

Source: Nutley & Reynolds (2023); WHO AFRO (2023); Author's Update

A strategic shift toward a more sustainable and diversified financing model by 2030 requires that government funding become the largest contributor (35% to 45%), reflecting increased domestic ownership and fiscal commitment. In this scenario, the private sector expands to 25%, signaling a growing role for investment, innovation, and public–private partnerships. Meanwhile, reliance on development partners is expected to decline to 18%, indicating reduced dependence on external aid. A notable addition is innovative financing (10%), such as blended finance and impact investment, while philanthropic contributions slightly decrease to 7%. Overall, the scenario calls for a transition from a donor-driven model to a more balanced, domestically anchored, and market-enabled financing ecosystem, which is critical to the long-term sustainability of digital health systems in Africa.

17.3.1 The 2025 Financing Fracture

The year 2025 marked a structural rupture in Africa's health financing landscape. The restructuring of PEPFAR and the dissolution of USAID created an estimated USD 12 billion shortfall in Africa's healthcare financing (CGD, 2025). The US cut bilateral HIV/AIDS funding by 86% in early 2025, halting programs that supported 21 million people on antiretroviral therapy. In South Africa, over 8,000 healthcare workers lost their jobs, clinics closed, and essential HIV services were significantly reduced (ScienceOpen, 2025). Africa's spiraling debt—countries are expected to service USD 81 billion by 2025—further erodes fiscal space (Africa CDC, 2025).

This crisis has exposed a structural vulnerability: external financing and out-of-pocket payments account for most of Africa's health financing, with foreign aid constituting roughly 70% of HIV financing. The 26 bilateral health MOUs signed under the America First Global Health Strategy are not merely funding agreements but digital governance agreements, bundled with specimen- and data-sharing sub-agreements that raise fundamental questions about data sovereignty (ICTworks, 2026). Kenya's court intervention suspending its agreement over data privacy concerns shows that organized legal challenges can work—but such leverage depends on the strength of domestic data protection frameworks and judicial independence.

17.3.2 Government Budgets

Government health expenditure remains the primary determinant of digital health investment capacity. Only three countries—Rwanda, Botswana, and Cabo Verde—have consistently met the Abuja Declaration's 15% target, while more than 30 remain below 10% (Africa CDC, 2025). Digital health typically receives less than 1% of health budgets. Rwanda allocates 2–3% of its health budget to health IT, and South Africa's NHI includes ring-fenced technology funding. The African Leadership Meeting (ALM) initiative, co-led by the Finance and Health Ministries, is translating political commitments into budgetary reforms and fiscal accountability (Health Policy Watch, 2026).

17.3.3 Development Partners, Private Sector, and Philanthropy

Development partners currently account for about 40–45% of digital health financing in Africa, creating significant sustainability risks because project-based, time-limited funding fosters parallel systems. The Global Fund's co-financing requirements—mandating progressive domestic contributions—

offer a model for managed transitions. Private-sector investment (about 18%) has grown through venture capital (USD 4 billion+ cumulative since 2019, as detailed in Chapter 13), telecommunications partnerships (Safaricom, MTN), and corporate investment. Philanthropic funding (about 10%) is anchored by the Gates Foundation (over USD 500 million in African digital health over the past decade), complemented by the Rockefeller Foundation, Skoll Foundation, and Mastercard Foundation.

17.4 Health Financing Mechanisms and Digital Integration

Sustainable health financing in Africa increasingly depends on the convergence of multiple financing mechanisms and robust digital public infrastructure, enabling inclusivity, efficiency, and system-wide coordination. A comprehensive framework for health financing mechanisms in Africa and their integration with digital systems can be organized around six key financing models, each supported by a common digital enabling layer. At the core are National Health Insurance (NHI) schemes, which leverage digital tools for enrollment, claims processing, and fraud detection (e.g., Ghana, Rwanda, and Kenya).

Alongside these are mobile money and digital payment systems, which facilitate out-of-pocket payments and microtransactions through platforms such as M-Pesa and MTN MoMo, significantly expanding financial access. Performance-based financing (PBF), in which digital systems support verification, results tracking, and automated disbursement of funds, as seen in Rwanda and Cameroon, is another approach. Together, these mechanisms illustrate how digitalization enhances efficiency, transparency, and accountability in health financing.

The second set of mechanisms includes tax-based financing, where digital tools improve revenue collection and transparency (e.g., Kenya's digital health levy); community-based health financing, which uses digital platforms for savings groups, micro-insurance, and crowdfunding (e.g., M-TIBA, Jamii Africa); and blended finance and impact investment, involving instruments such as social impact bonds and development finance co-investment (e.g., IFC

Health initiatives). Underpinning all these models is a digital enabling layer comprising interoperable payment systems, digital identity, data analytics, and regulatory frameworks. This foundation enables diverse financing streams to be integrated, tracked, and scaled effectively.

Figure 17.3. Six Principal Health Financing Mechanisms and Their Integration with Digital Health Tools

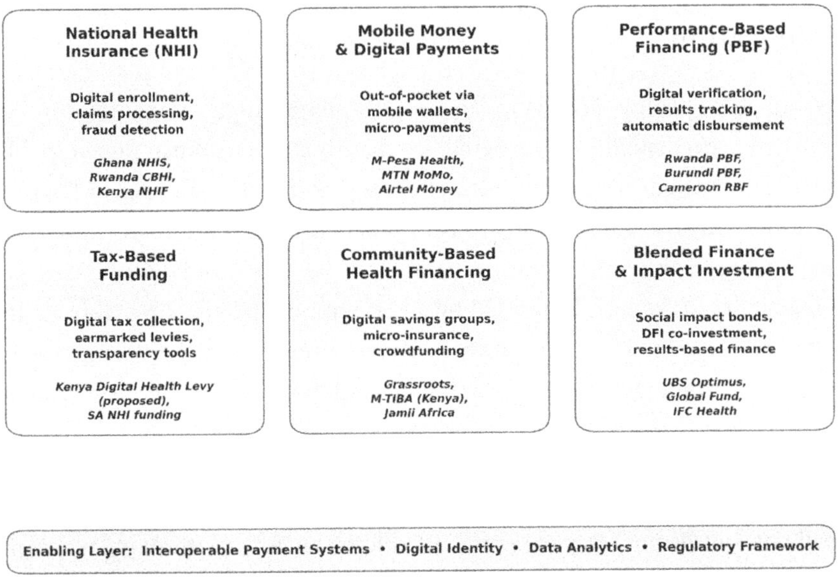

Source: Author's Elaboration

National health insurance schemes are powerful vehicles for digital integration. Ghana's NHIS has progressively digitized enrollment, claims processing, and fraud detection. Biometric registration has expanded coverage, and digital claims processing has reduced turnaround from months to weeks (NHIA Ghana, 2023). Rwanda's Community-Based Health Insurance (CBHI), which covers over 80% of the population, uses digital tools for enrollment, mobile money for premium payments, and real-time utilization reporting. Kenya's Social Health Authority has beem implementing a platform that integrates registration, accreditation, claims management, and analytics.

Thailand's Universal Coverage Scheme provides an instructive model, using a comprehensive digital platform to serve 47 million beneficiaries and maintaining administrative costs at approximately 1.5% of total expenditure (NHSO Thailand, 2022). Colombia's health insurance regimes use mobile enrollment to expand coverage among informal sector workers. Australia's Medicare digital infrastructure enables real-time claims processing across the universal health system.

In Africa, mobile money is transformative: M-TIBA in Kenya has processed over USD 60 million in health transactions, connecting 5 million users to accredited facilities (CarePay, 2023). Tanzania's Jamii Africa provides mobile micro-insurance for informal sector workers. Performance-based financing in Rwanda links digital reporting to payments, while Cameroon's Result-Based Financing program reduced payment delays from 6 months to 6 weeks through digital verification (World Bank, 2022).

17.5 Return on Investment

The McKinsey Global Institute estimated that digitalizing healthcare in sub-Saharan Africa could generate USD 40–60 billion annually by 2030 through improved efficiency, reduced waste, expanded access, and better outcomes. All digital health interventions generate positive returns above break-even, though the magnitude varies. Digital payment systems deliver the highest potential returns, ranging from 6x to 15x, reflecting their strong impact on efficiency, reduced leakage, improved revenue collection, and financial inclusion. Similarly, digital disease surveillance (5x–12x) and mHealth for maternal and child health (4x–9x) demonstrate substantial returns, driven by improved early detection, prevention outcomes, and reduced treatment costs. Supply chain digitization (4x–8x) also performs strongly by reducing stockouts, waste, and logistics inefficiencies.

DHIS2 generates 3–5 times its cost through improved data quality. Telemedicine in South Africa and Mozambique yields 30–50% cost savings compared with traditional referrals. mHealth reminders reduce missed appointments by 25–40% and increase vaccination coverage by 10–20 percentage points (Watterson et al., 2015).

Figure 17.4. Estimated return on investment for selected digital health interventions in Africa over a five-year horizon

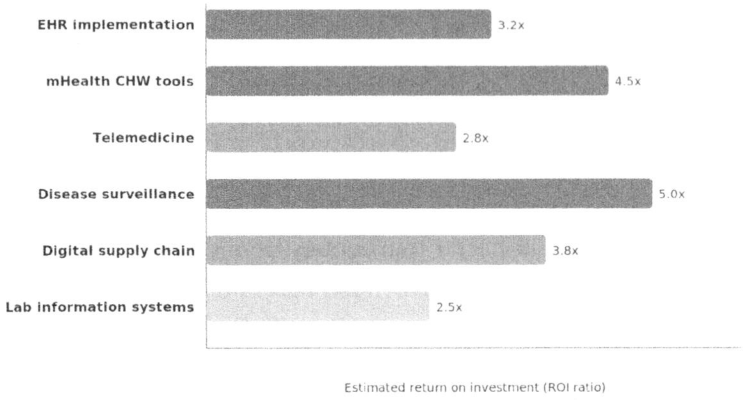

Source: McKinsey (2020); Braa & Sahay (2017); Mars (2013); author's compilation

Electronic health records (EHRs) also show moderate returns (2x–5x), reflecting longer implementation timelines and higher upfront costs, despite their long-term system benefits. Overall, surveys highlight that investments in foundational digital health infrastructure and platforms yield significant economic and health returns, particularly when they improve system efficiency, scale service delivery, and reduce costs. It also suggests that prioritizing high-impact areas such as payments, surveillance, and supply chains can accelerate financial sustainability and improve health outcomes across African health systems.

India's e-Sanjeevani telemedicine platform facilitated over 100 million teleconsultations (2020–2023), with estimated savings of approximately USD 3 per consultation from avoided travel costs—totaling over USD 300 million. Uruguay's national telemedicine network returned approximately 7 times its initial investment over 8 years. Australia's COVID-19-era telehealth expansion, which was permanently retained, demonstrated significant cost savings for rural specialist access. However, evidence of Africa-specific ROI remains limited, and investment in rigorous economic evaluation is needed to build the domestic investment case.

17.6 Innovative Financing Models

The financing spectrum for digital health in Africa spans the transition from highly concessional funding to fully commercial investment models. On the left side of the spectrum are grants and philanthropy, including foundation support, bilateral aid, and multilateral funding—typically used for early-stage pilots, public goods, and high-risk interventions. This is followed by concessional loans, such as Development Finance Institution (DFI) lending and soft loans, which provide affordable capital to scale foundational infrastructure. Further along, social impact bonds introduce results-based financing mechanisms in which returns are linked to measurable outcomes, while blended finance combines public and private capital—often with first-loss guarantees—to de-risk investments and attract private participation.

Figure 17.5. The Financing Spectrum for Digital Health: From Concessional Grants to Commercial Capital

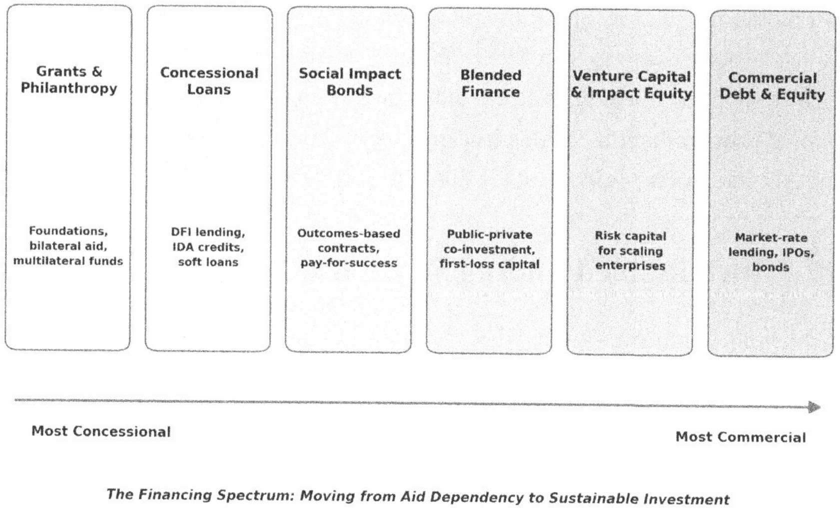

Source: Author's Elaboration

On the right side of the spectrum are more market-driven instruments, including venture capital and impact equity, which provide risk capital to scale digital health enterprises, and commercial debt and equity, which represent fully market-based financing, such as bonds, IPOs, and private lending. The spectrum reflects a strategic shift from aid dependency toward sustainable, investment-driven financing models, with instruments playing complementary roles at different stages of maturity. This underscores the importance of layering financing mechanisms—from concessional to commercial—to build scalable, resilient digital health ecosystems across Africa.

Impact bonds, blended finance, crowdfunding, and diaspora bonds are innovative instruments that complement traditional sources. India's Utkrisht Impact Bond uses digital tools to track maternal health outcomes in real time. The Global Innovation Fund's investment in mPharma combined grant funding with growth equity. Crowdfunding platforms such as M-Changa Kenya and Thundafund South Africa provide seed capital for innovation. Diaspora bonds—Ethiopia (2008, 2011) and Nigeria (2017)—demonstrate the feasibility of tapping diaspora savings.

Africa CDC is piloting innovative health financing options as the traditional aid model restructures (Health Policy Watch, 2025). PAHO's Revolving Funds, which procured more than USD 900 million in vaccines, technologies, and health supplies during the 2024–2025 biennium, demonstrate that regional pooled procurement mechanisms can achieve scale and affordability—a model the AU and RECs could adapt for digital health technologies.

17.7 Sustainable Funding Strategies

Achieving sustainable digital health financing in Africa requires a holistic, multi-source strategy that integrates public, private, and innovative financing approaches within a robust governance and accountability framework. Sustainability also requires a deliberate shift from donor dependence to domestically anchored financing. A strategic framework for sustainable digital health funding in Africa can be structured around four complementary financing pillars, supported by a strong foundational layer.

- The first pillar, **domestic resource mobilizatio**n, emphasizes strengthening national ownership through mechanisms such as government budget allocations, earmarked levies on health technologies, and revenues from national health insurance schemes.

- The second pillar, **external resource optimization**, focuses on improving the effectiveness of donor funding through strategic alignment, South–South cooperation, and a gradual transition from aid dependence to investment-oriented models. Together, these two pillars underscore the importance of balancing domestic financing with smarter use of external support to ensure sustainability.

- The third pillar, **private sector engagement**, underscores the role of market-driven approaches, including public–private partnerships (PPPs), enterprise licensing revenues, and the attraction of venture capital to scale digital health solutions.

- The fourth pillar, **innovative financing instruments**, introduces mechanisms such as impact bonds, blended finance facilities, and crowdfunding or diaspora bonds to diversify funding sources.

Underpinning all four pillars is a foundational layer comprising investment case development, total cost of ownership (TCO) planning, monitoring and evaluation (M&E) for value, financial governance, and accountability.

Domestic resource mobilization is the cornerstone: governments must increase the share of health budgets allocated to digital health from less than 1% to 3–5%. Kenya's proposed Digital Health Levy is expected to add a surcharge to mobile money health transactions. Earmarked technology levies —similar to telecommunications universal service levies—could provide dedicated, predictable revenue. The Lusaka Agenda (2023) emphasizes greater domestic investment, pooled funding mechanisms, and accountability frameworks.

The EU's Digital Europe Program, which allocates EUR 7.5 billion to digital transformation, including health, offers a model of supranational co-financing on a matched-funding basis. Africa's RECs and the AU could explore similar mechanisms using the AfDB, regional development funds, and instruments such as the Africa50 infrastructure fund.

Figure 17.6. A Four-pillar Framework for Sustainable Digital Health Funding Strategies

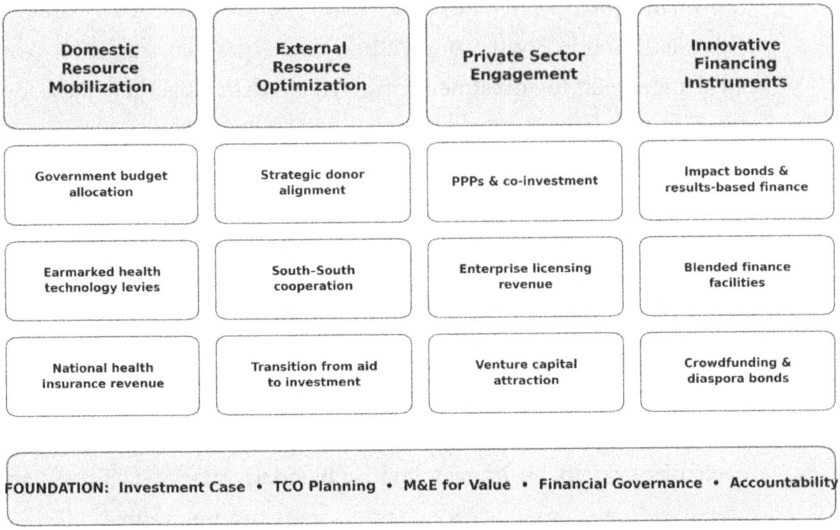

Source: Author's Elaboration

External resource optimization means shifting from dependency to strategic partnership—using external funding to catalyze domestic and private resources, with explicit transition strategies. Canada's approach through the IDRC, which co-finances digital health research partnerships on a matched basis with domestic institutions, demonstrates partnership-based financing. New Zealand's approach of treating digital health as core health infrastructure within its unified health system budget provides a model for embedding digital health financing within routine health expenditure.

17.8 Total Cost of Ownership

Digital health investment requires comprehensive Total Cost of Ownership (TCO) planning, realistic budgeting, and long-term financing strategies to ensure sustainability and prevent system failures caused by underfunded downstream costs. An iceberg metaphor can illustrate the TCO of digital health systems, highlighting the gap between visible upfront costs and the much higher, often underestimated hidden costs. The small portion above the waterline represents visible costs (20–30%), typically including hardware procurement, software licenses, and system installation. These are the most apparent and commonly budgeted expenditures, often forming the basis for initial project planning and funding proposals.

Figure 17.7. The Digital Health TCO Iceberg

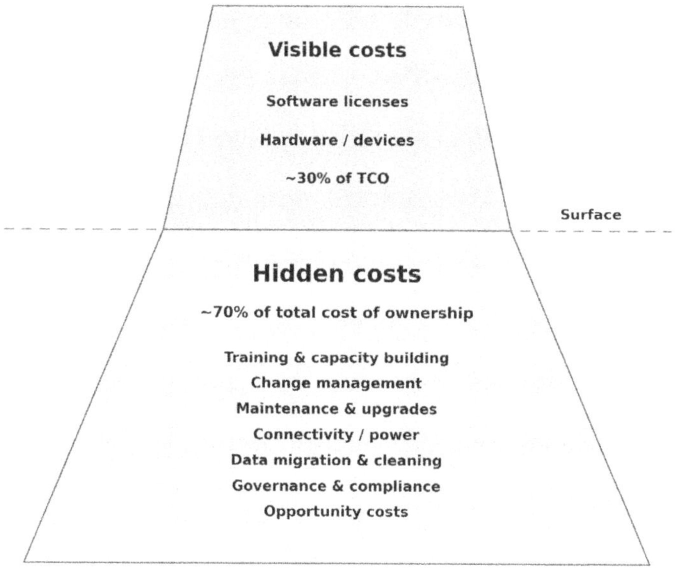

Source: Author's Elaboration

However, the much larger submerged portion represents hidden costs (70–80%), which constitute the majority of long-term investment requirements. These include training and capacity building, change management, system integration and interoperability, data migration and cleaning, ongoing maintenance and updates, technical support, infrastructure dependencies such as electricity and connectivity, and opportunity costs.

Successful digital health implementation depends less on initial capital expenditure and more on sustained operational and system-wide investments.

A WHO costing study in East Africa found that operational costs typically exceeded initial implementation costs within 3–5 years (WHO, 2020).

Table 17.1. Illustrative Five-Year Total Cost of Ownership for an EHR System sSrving 50 Health Facilities

Cost Category	Year 1 (USD)	Years 2–5 Annual	5-Year Total
Hardware & devices	500,000	50,000	700,000
Software	300,000	75,000	600,000
Installation	150,000	0	150,000
Training & capacity	200,000	80,000	520,000
Change management	100,000	40,000	260,000
Data migration	120,000	30,000	240,000
Maintenance & support	50,000	120,000	530,000
Connectivity & electricity	80,000	80,000	400,000
Staff time & opportunity	150,000	100,000	550,000
TOTAL	1,650,000	575,000	3,950,000

Source: Author's Estimates Based on WHO (2020) and PATH (2022)

Chile requires all digital health project proposals to include five-year TCO projections for approval (Ministry of Health Chile, 2022). The UK's NHS requires Total Economic Impact assessments for major digital investments. Australia's Digital Health Agency requires lifecycle cost analyses for all national platform investments. These models should be adopted by African health ministries to prevent the pattern of system abandonment that has plagued too many digital health projects on the continent.

17.9 Conclusion

This chapter has examined financing and sustainability—the most critical cross-cutting enabler in the Digital Health Technology Stack—at a moment of unprecedented disruption in global health financing. The restructuring of PEPFAR, the dissolution of USAID, and the introduction of bilateral billion shortfall, exposing the structural vulnerability of donor-dependent health financing. Africa's spiraling debt, with countries servicing USD 81 billion in 2025, further constrains fiscal space.

Yet the crisis has also accelerated overdue conversations about health financing sovereignty. The African Leadership Meeting, the Lusaka Agenda, and Africa CDC's New Public Health Order all position domestic resource mobilization and health financing self-reliance as strategic imperatives. Evidence from India (ABDM phased investment), Brazil (World Bank co-financing), Thailand (lean UHC administration), Colombia (mobile-enabled insurance), Chile (mandatory TCO budgeting), the EU (Digital Europe matched funding), PAHO (Revolving Funds and regional procurement), and Australia (statutory agency financing) shows that sustainable digital health financing is achievable when embedded in deliberate policy architectures.

Africa's digital health transformation requires estimated investments of USD 15–25 billion over the decade to 2030—substantial but representing only 2–5% of projected health expenditure and yielding returns of 2–15 times the investment. The path forward requires domestic resource mobilization as the cornerstone, diversified funding sources, lifecycle cost planning, innovative financing instruments, and alignment of financing with the national strategies (Chapter 14), governance frameworks (Chapter 15), regional cooperation (Chapter 16), and the other enablers examined throughout this book.

References

AfDB. (2022). Digital Moonshot for Africa. African Development Bank.

Africa CDC. (2025). Africa's health financing in a new era. Africa CDC.

African Union Commission. (2020). Digital Transformation Strategy for Africa. AU.

Basinga, P., et al. (2011). Effect on maternal and child health services in Rwanda. The Lancet, 377, 1421–1428.

Braa, J., & Sahay, S. (2017). The DHIS2 open source platform. In Global Health Informatics. MIT Press.

Broadband Commission. (2020). Digital health: A call for government leadership. ITU/UNESCO.

CarePay. (2023). M-TIBA health wallet impact report 2023. CarePay.

CGD. (2025). A new era for global health: Can African countries agree on a new compact? Center for Global Development.

European Commission. (2023). Digital Europe Programme: Work programme 2023–2024. EC.

Gates Foundation. (2023). Digital health portfolio: Africa overview. Gates Foundation.

Health Policy Watch. (2025). Africa CDC to pilot new health financing options. Health Policy Watch.

Health Policy Watch. (2026). As the aid model collapses, Africa rewrites its health future. Health Policy Watch.

ICTworks. (2026). African digital health data is a condition of global health funding. ICTworks.

Mars, M. (2013). Telemedicine in Africa. Progress in Cardiovascular Diseases, 56(3), 326–335.

McKinsey Global Institute. (2020). How digital health could catalyze growth in SSA. McKinsey.

Ministry of Health Chile. (2022). Digital health investment guidelines: TCO requirements. MoH Chile.

Ministry of Health, Rwanda. (2022). Health sector performance report 2021–2022. MoH Rwanda.

National Health Authority India. (2022). ABDM financial framework. NHA India.

NHIA Ghana. (2023). Annual report 2022–2023. NHIA Ghana.

NHSO Thailand. (2022). Universal Coverage Scheme: Digital platform review. NHSO Thailand.

Nutley, T., & Reynolds, H. W. (2023). Improving use of health data. BMC Health Services Research.

PATH Digital Square. (2022). Costing digital health transformation. PATH.

ScienceOpen. (2025). Impact of US cuts on South African healthcare. ScienceOpen.

Watterson, J. L., et al. (2015). Using mHealth for ANC and immunization. BioMed Research International.

WHO. (2020). HIS costing study: East Africa findings. WHO.

WHO. (2021). Global strategy on digital health 2020–2025. WHO.

WHO AFRO. (2023). Health Financing in the African Region. WHO AFRO.

World Bank. (2021). Brazil digital health project completion report. World Bank.

World Bank. (2022). Cameroon RBF digital platform evaluation. World Bank.

PART 4

Strategic Pathways for Transforming Digital Health in Africa

Chapter 18 Priorities and Path Forward

18.1 Overview

This final chapter synthesizes the analysis presented throughout this book into an actionable framework for Africa's digital health transformation. It identifies priority investment areas grounded in the five foundation layers and seven cross-cutting enablers of the Digital Health Technology Stack, organizes these investments into a phased roadmap spanning short-, medium-, and long-term horizons, clarifies the roles of stakeholders at the national and regional levels, establishes how progress can be measured using readiness and maturity assessment tools, and concludes with a call to action that articulates both the urgency and achievability of the continent's digital health ambitions.

The chapter is written at a moment of profound transition: the 2025 disruption in global health financing has made the case for domestically anchored, strategically sequenced digital health investment more urgent than ever. Yet Africa enters this period with formidable assets: near-universal coverage of digital health strategies; continental leadership through the AU and Africa CDC; a maturing healthTech ecosystem that has attracted more than USD 4 billion in cumulative investment; leadership in open-source platforms through DHIS2 and OpenMRS; and a young, digitally native population of 1.4 billion. The question is no longer whether Africa can achieve digital health transformation, but whether it will invest with the discipline, coherence, and sustained commitment the evidence demands in the post-COVID-19 era.

18.2 Priority Investment Areas

The Digital Health Technology Stack, introduced in Chapter 4 and explored throughout Chapters 7–17, provides the integrating framework for identifying and sequencing priority investments. The stack model rests on a fundamental insight: digital health applications—the tools that clinicians, patients, and public health officials interact with directly—depend on layers of infrastructure, identity, interoperability, and analytics beneath them, as well as enablers of strategy, governance, workforce, research, ecosystem, cooperation, and financing that cut across all layers. A weakness at any level cascades across the entire stack, undermining investments elsewhere.

This means Africa's digital health transformation cannot be achieved through application-layer investments alone. A telemedicine platform requires reliable connectivity (Layer 1), authenticated user identities (Layer 2), access to patient records from other systems (Layer 3), and analytical capabilities for clinical decision support (Layer 4). It also requires a supportive strategy, governance and regulation, a workforce capable of using it, evidence that it works in local contexts, an ecosystem that can maintain and improve it, regional cooperation, and sustainable financing to keep it running. Countries that invest in applications without building the foundations and enablers create fragile, project-dependent implementations that collapse when donor funding ends or key technical staff depart.

18.2.1 Foundation Layer Priorities

Layer 1: Infrastructure and Connectivity. The physical infrastructure layer—telecommunications networks, data centers, cloud platforms, end-user devices, and electricity—is the bedrock of all digital health systems. Mobile network coverage reaches about 84% of Africa's population, yet meaningful broadband connectivity remains limited in rural areas, where health needs are often greatest.

Priority investments include expanding mobile broadband to health facilities (targeting 80% coverage by 2030), deploying solar power at off-grid health posts, investing in cloud infrastructure and in national or regional data centers, and leveraging satellite connectivity for remote areas.

Without reliable infrastructure, every investment in the layers above is compromised.

The infrastructure challenge is not unique to Africa—Australia and Canada face similar rural connectivity gaps—but it is more acute. India's BharatNet program, which aims to connect 250,000 village councils with optical fiber, shows how government-led infrastructure investment can provide the connectivity foundation digital health requires. African countries should explore similar dedicated connectivity programs for health facilities and other anchor institutions, such as schools and libraries, potentially leveraging universal service fund obligations imposed on telecommunications operators.

Layer 2: Digital Identity and Registries. Effective digital health systems must uniquely identify patients, health workers, and health facilities. Without a reliable identity infrastructure, data cannot be linked across encounters and institutions, undermining the value of digitalization. Kenya's Master Patient Index covers 28 million citizens, and India's Ayushman Bharat Health Account (ABHA) covers over 770 million. Rwanda's community-based health insurance uses a unique identification system integrated with the national EMR platform. **Priority investments include deploying a unique national patient identifier system, establishing registries for health workers and facilities, and building an authentication infrastructure to enable secure access to health records.**

The identity layer is a critical early investment that unlocks downstream value across clinical care, public health surveillance, and health financing. Countries that delay building identity infrastructure cannot link patient records, track disease outbreaks to individual cases, or verify insurance enrollment—problems that become more expensive to fix as digital systems proliferate without shared identifiers. Estonia's national e-ID system, which authenticates nearly all residents for access to health and government services, demonstrates the transformative value of investing early in identity infrastructure.

Layer 3: Interoperability and Data Exchange. The interoperability layer enables different health information systems to communicate, exchange, and meaningfully use shared data through health information exchange platforms, application programming interfaces, messaging standards such as HL7 FHIR, and terminology services such as ICD-11, SNOMED CT, and LOINC. DHIS2 is deployed in 47 African countries, but primarily supports aggregate-level data reporting; individual-level data exchange—critical for care coordination—requires additional interoperability infrastructure. **Priority investments include establishing national health information exchanges based on the OpenHIE architecture, mandating HL7 FHIR for all new system acquisitions, and building semantic interoperability to enable meaningful data exchange.**

Without interoperability, digital health systems become silos—generating data that cannot be shared across facilities, programs, or jurisdictions. The result is duplication, fragmentation, and an inability to build comprehensive patient records and population-level analytics that justify investment in digital health. Rwanda's national HIE, which connects OpenMRS implementations across 45 district hospitals to laboratory, pharmacy, and insurance systems, demonstrates what an integrated architecture can achieve. The EU's decade-long effort to achieve cross-border interoperability through the European Health Data Space underscores that this is both essential and difficult—but the cost of not investing early is far higher than the cost of investing.

Layer 4: Data Management and Analytics. This layer transforms raw health data into actionable insights using data warehouses, business intelligence tools, machine learning platforms, and analytical pipelines. South Africa's Health Data Research Network enables local researchers to generate evidence from de-identified health data. Brazil's e-SUS platform aggregates data from more than 5,400 municipalities to power national dashboards. **Priority investments include building data warehouses and analytical pipelines, deploying dashboards for real-time decision-making, and developing AI and machine learning capabilities validated on African datasets—recognizing that AI tools trained on non-African data may yield biased results when applied to African populations.**

The analytics layer is where data generates value—informing clinical decisions, guiding resource allocation, detecting outbreaks, and evaluating program effectiveness. Countries that invest in data collection without investing in analytics create data graveyards: vast repositories of information that go unused. India's CoWIN platform, originally developed for COVID-19 vaccination, produced datasets that informed real-time policy decisions on vaccine distribution and coverage gaps, demonstrating how analytics infrastructure can transform public health response.

Layer 5: Applications and Services. The application layer is the most visible component of the digital health technology stack—where clinicians, patients, administrators, and public health officials interact with digital tools. It encompasses electronic medical records, telemedicine platforms, mobile health applications, clinical decision support systems, laboratory information systems, supply chain management software, and digital learning platforms. Priority investments include scaling EHRs (targeting 50% facility coverage by 2027 and 80% by 2030), deploying national telemedicine platforms that connect primary care with specialists, implementing mHealth for maternal and child health, strengthening digital disease surveillance, and establishing electronic immunization registries.

Electronic health records should be deployed through a phased national program, starting with district-level hospitals and progressively extending to primary health centers. Countries should adopt open-source platforms such as OpenMRS or commercially viable cloud-based SaaS solutions, mandate HL7 FHIR interoperability for all new EHR procurements, integrate EHRs with the national health information exchange and the unique patient identifier system, and provide sustained training and help desk support at every deployment site. India's phased EHR deployment under the ABDM, Rwanda's OpenMRS implementation across 45 district hospitals, and Brazil's progressive e-SUS deployment across 5,400 municipalities each demonstrate that national-scale EHR coverage is achievable when supported by clear standards, phased timelines, and sustained investment in both technology and the workforce to operate it.

Telemedicine platforms should be developed as national networks linking primary health centers—especially in rural and underserved areas—to specialist centers, supporting both synchronous video consultations and store-and-forward modalities for dermatology, radiology, and pathology. Countries must establish comprehensive regulatory frameworks that address provider licensing across geographic boundaries, reimbursement parity with in-person consultations, prescribing and referral protocols, liability allocation, and data protection. The platforms should integrate with EHRs and health information exchanges rather than operate as stand-alone systems. Rwanda's partnership with Babyl (serving over two million subscribers), South Africa's national telemedicine program, India's e-Sanjeevani (over 100 million teleconsultations), and the Philippines' Telehealth Act of 2023 each offer models that African countries can adapt to their regulatory and infrastructure contexts.

Mobile health (mHealth) for maternal and child health is the most evidence-supported, high-impact quick win available to African countries. Countries should build or scale trusted national or subnational digital channels—using SMS, voice, WhatsApp, or apps in local languages—for antenatal care reminders, immunization scheduling, danger-sign messaging, breastfeeding support, and community health worker-linked follow-up. These tools must be linked to real services, including facilities, teleconsultation, transport and referral mechanisms, and immunization programs, and be designed for inclusion by supporting low-bandwidth tools, basic phones, offline workflows, and multilingual content. Rwanda's RapidSMS, Tanzania's Wazazi Nipendeni, and PAHO's experience across Latin America demonstrate that mHealth for MCH is most effective when integrated into primary healthcare strengthening rather than as a standalone innovation project.

Digital disease surveillance systems should be strengthened through a phased approach: in the near term, fully digitize routine surveillance within the Integrated Disease Surveillance and Response (IDSR) framework; in the medium term, integrate laboratory, genomic, and cross-border intelligence functions through Africa CDC platforms; and over time, add AI-assisted signal detection and broader environmental surveillance, including wastewater monitoring. Countries should expand event-based surveillance using community reports, hotline data, and media monitoring; adopt common data standards so national systems can connect to regional platforms; invest in the surveillance workforce—epidemiologists, informaticians, and data analysts—not only in software; and ensure that surveillance systems are linked to actual response mechanisms, because early warning without field investigation and action has limited value. Nigeria's SORMAS, Africa CDC's continental IDSR platform, and WHO's Epidemic Intelligence from Open Sources (EIOS) initiative each demonstrate components of an effective digital surveillance architecture.

Electronic immunization registries (EIRs) should be built as person-based systems using unique identifiers for each child, linked where possible to civil registration or broader digital health identity systems, and integrated into routine immunization workflows at the facility and outreach levels, with offline capability for low-connectivity settings. Registries should include core operational functions: due-dose forecasting, defaulter tracing, reminders and recalls, coverage dashboards, certificate generation, and integration with DHIS2, supply chain systems, and maternal and child health records. Africa CDC reported that DTP3 coverage in Africa was 76% in 2024, unchanged from 2023, with approximately 7.8 million children missing DTP1—underscoring the urgent need for individual-level tracking and follow-up through EIRs. Tanzania's EIR, integrated with DHIS2, covers over 90% of districts; Rwanda's system provides real-time vaccination data; and PAHO's experience across Latin America (where EIR coverage exceeds 70% in many countries) provides a maturity benchmark. Countries should phase rollouts, starting with high-priority districts, and budget for devices, maintenance, connectivity, training, and supportive supervision.

Application layer investments must be guided by the principle that applications depend on all lower layers to be effective. A telemedicine application deployed without reliable connectivity will frustrate users. An EHR system deployed without interoperability standards will become another data silo. An AI diagnostic tool deployed without local validation will yield unreliable results. The insight is clear: invest in foundations first, then deploy applications that leverage them—rather than deploying applications in isolation and retrofitting the foundations later.

18.2.2 Cross-Cutting Enabler Priorities

The seven enablers examined in Chapters 11–17 determine whether foundation-layer investments succeed or fail. Each enabler spans all five foundation layers, and a weakness in any one can undermine investments across the entire stack. Countries that build excellent infrastructure but lack governance will see their systems compromised by data breaches. Countries that develop strong governance but neglect workforce development will have standards that no one can implement. Countries that produce innovative applications but fail to finance their maintenance will watch those applications decay within years.

Digital health skills and workforce are perhaps the most critical enablers. Africa faces a health informatics workforce deficit of an order of magnitude—approximately 1 professional per 100,000 population, compared with 10–15 in high-income countries—amounting to an estimated deficit of over 50,000 professionals across the continent.

Priority investments include embedding digital competencies in pre-service health worker education (the Ethiopian model, with 30+ universities producing 2,000+ graduates annually), establishing regional training hubs (the CARPHA Caribbean model of pooled resources), generating workforce demand through policy mandates (the Indian ABDM model), and developing professional certification frameworks (the Australian CHIA model).

Research and development must build Africa's capacity in implementation science, AI validation using representative datasets, genomics research, and health technology assessment. Sub-Saharan Africa accounts for fewer than 5% of global digital health publications, despite bearing a disproportionate disease burden.

Priority investments include strengthening academic research institutions, building AI validation infrastructure, expanding genomics capacity through initiatives such as H3Africa and the Africa Pathogen Genomics Initiative, and establishing institutionalized health technology assessment units within ministries of health.

Specifically, countries should embed implementation science in every major digital health deployment to generate the evidence needed to understand how, why, and under what conditions interventions work across diverse African settings. AI tools developed for African healthcare must be validated on local datasets before deployment—the risk of algorithmic bias from tools trained on non-African populations is well documented and can lead to harmful clinical outcomes. Genomics research should be expanded through continental initiatives such as H3Africa and the Africa Pathogen Genomics Initiative, as well as through emerging partnerships with Latin American genomics programs (LatinCells, Project JAGUAR) that face analogous challenges in population representation. Health technology assessment should become routine, with dedicated HTA units informing procurement decisions—following Thailand's HITAP model, which has become a globally recognized center for health technology assessment led by low- and middle-income countries and informs coverage decisions under universal health coverage.

The healthTech ecosystem comprises startups, social enterprises, and innovation hubs that develop and maintain digital health products. Africa's ecosystem has attracted more than USD 4 billion in cumulative investment and hosts more than 120 health-focused technology hubs.

Priority investments include regulatory sandboxes that enable innovation while managing risk, government procurement from local innovators (the anchor-buyer model), open data and digital public goods that lower barriers to entry, and structured public–private partnerships that channel private-sector innovation toward public health priorities.

The healthTech ecosystem challenge is not merely about supporting startups but about connecting innovation to health system demand. Governments should act as anchor buyers, committing to procure digital health solutions from local enterprises to create the market demand that enables companies to achieve the scale needed for financial sustainability. Kenya's Access to Government Procurement Opportunities program, Brazil's SUS procurement framework, and Australia's Digital Health Agency conformance testing requirements each demonstrate how procurement policy can catalyze domestic innovation. Open data initiatives—making non-sensitive health data, including aggregated epidemiological data, facility registries, drug pricing information, and health workforce data—available enable innovators to develop solutions that address real health system needs. The Digital Public Goods Alliance's registry of recognized DPGs, including DHIS2, OpenMRS, and OpenCRVS, provides shared foundations that reduce barriers to entry and prevent vendor lock-in.

Digital health strategy must be treated as a living document—costed, funded, governed, and iteratively refined—rather than a static policy instrument. As of 2024, the vast majority of African countries have some form of digital health strategy, but only a fraction have complete implementation plans, adequate financing, and functioning monitoring and evaluation frameworks. Countries should develop costed implementation plans with identified funding sources and multi-year budget commitments, and review and update strategies annually based on implementation evidence.

The most effective strategies globally—Rwanda's, India's ABDM, Australia's National Digital Health Strategy 2023–2028, and Brazil's ESD28—share key features: they are linked to investment plans with identified funding; they include implementation timelines with milestones and accountability mechanisms; they are regularly reviewed and revised using performance data; and they are aligned with broader national development agendas. African countries should adopt these practices, treating strategy documents not as endpoints but as the starting point for a continuous cycle of planning, implementation, monitoring, and adaptation. The WHO's upcoming Global Strategy on Digital Health 2028–2033, being developed with input from African regions, provides an opportunity for countries to align their next-generation strategies with global governance frameworks.

Governance, policy, and standards encompass data protection legislation, cybersecurity frameworks, AI ethics guidelines, telemedicine regulation, digital health product certification, and institutional oversight. As of 2026, over 40 African countries have enacted data protection legislation; the AU Continental AI Strategy has been endorsed; and 52 states have signed the Africa Declaration on Artificial Intelligence. However, health-sector-specific regulations, enforcement capacity, and cybersecurity governance remain underdeveloped. The 2025 bilateral data-sharing agreements underscore the urgency of robust, enforceable data governance frameworks to protect African health data sovereignty.

In practice, this means every African country should enact comprehensive data protection legislation with health-sector-specific provisions and establish a functioning data protection authority with the capacity to enforce compliance. Countries should develop national cybersecurity strategies that set mandatory requirements for health-sector entities, including incident reporting and regular security audits. Building on the AU Continental AI Strategy's multi-tiered approach, countries should establish a risk-based classification of AI health applications, require local validation before deployment, and create regulatory sandboxes for testing innovative tools. Standards governance must be accompanied by enforcement mechanisms: mandating HL7 FHIR for new system acquisitions, requiring interoperability certification for government procurement, and establishing penalties for non-compliance. Singapore's AI medical device sandbox, the EU's risk-based AI Act, and Kenya's 2024 sector-specific data protection directives for healthcare each offer adaptable models.

Financing and sustainability determine whether other investments can be sustained. The 2025 disruption—with a USD 12 billion shortfall from PEPFAR/USAID restructuring and African countries servicing USD 81 billion in debt—has exposed the structural vulnerability of donor-dependent financing.

Priority interventions include increasing government health budget allocations for digital health from less than 1% to 3–5%, developing innovative financing instruments (earmarked levies, blended finance, diaspora bonds), implementing mandatory lifecycle cost planning (the Chilean model of five-year TCO projections), and building regional co-financing mechanisms modeled after the EU's Digital Europe Program and PAHO's Revolving Funds.

The financing transition must be both structural and cultural. Structurally, countries must create dedicated digital health budget lines within health budgets—rather than relying on ad hoc allocations or ICT ministry funding—and treat digital health infrastructure as essential health infrastructure, comparable to hospitals and laboratories. Every digital health investment must include five-year total cost-of-ownership projections, in line with Chile's mandatory requirement, because upfront costs represent only 20–30% of total system costs. Failure to budget for training, maintenance, support, and connectivity is the single most common cause of digital health project failure. Culturally, the shift from viewing digital health as a donor-funded project to a domestically financed public good is the most important mindset change required. The African Leadership Meeting, the Lusaka Agenda, and Africa CDC's New Public Health Order articulate this shift at the continental level—individual countries must translate it into budget reality.

Regional cooperation enables resource pooling, harmonized standards, cross-border interoperability, and economies of scale that no single country can achieve alone. The EAC's cross-border HIE serving 50,000+ patients, ECOWAS's digital vaccination certificates, which have reduced fraud by 95%, and Africa CDC's continental surveillance, which connects 55 AU Member States, demonstrate the potential of regional collaboration. Priority investments include shared health informatics training hubs anchored by regional universities, harmonized data protection regulations within RECs, continental interoperability frameworks, and joint procurement arrangements.

Regional cooperation is not optional—it is essential to achieving the scale, harmonized standards, and economies of scale that no individual African country can achieve alone. The CARPHA model in the Caribbean, which pools training resources across 24 small island developing states, demonstrates how countries too small to sustain comprehensive health informatics programs independently can achieve quality and scale through regional cooperation. PAHO's 2025 Digital Literacy Program trained more than 70,000 health sector personnel across the Americas through regional coordination. The EU's Digital Europe Program allocated EUR 7.5 billion for digital transformation, including health, on a co-financing basis. RECs should emulate these models by establishing shared training hubs (a Francophone West African hub at UCAD in Senegal, an East African hub at MUHAS in Tanzania, and a Southern African hub at UCT), harmonizing data protection regulations within their blocs, and developing regional procurement frameworks for digital health technologies that provide the buying power individual countries lack.

18.3 Phased Implementation Roadmap

Digital health transformation cannot be achieved across all dimensions at once. Evidence from every successful national program—India's ABDM, Brazil's RNDS, Estonia's X-Road, and Thailand's Universal Coverage digitization—demonstrates that phased, incremental approaches succeed where comprehensive, simultaneous transformation fails. Phasing enables organizational learning, builds capacity progressively, generates early wins that demonstrate value and sustain political momentum, and prevents the catastrophic failures that result from attempting too much too quickly.

The following roadmap organizes Africa's digital health transformation across seven dimensions over three time horizons. The short-term phase focuses on foundations and quick wins: establishing governance structures, deploying foundational systems, building basic workforce capacity, and securing initial financing commitments.

Figure 18.1. Phased Implementation Roadmap

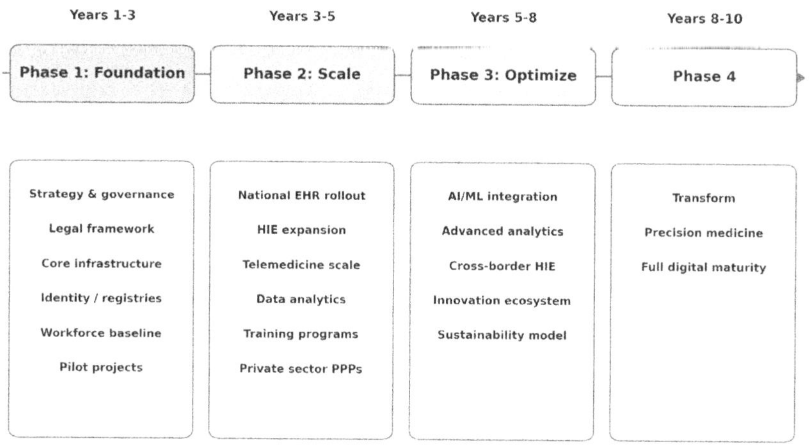

Source: Author's Elaboration

The medium-term phase) focuses on scaling and integration: expanding EHRs to 50% of facilities, establishing national HIE platforms, enforcing interoperability standards, and transitioning from donor-funded to domestically financed operations. The long-term phase aims for genuine transformation: achieving 80% EHR coverage, deploying AI-assisted diagnostics, establishing continental digital health platforms, and securing full domestic financing for digital health operations.

In Phase 1, the focus should be on establishing foundational digital health building blocks to deliver immediate impact and prepare the system for scaling. Key interventions include introducing unique patient identifiers, implementing digital literacy programs for health workers, and expanding mobile health (mHealth) services, particularly for maternal and child health. This phase also emphasizes strengthening digital disease surveillance systems and developing a telemedicine policy framework to ensure that early gains are practical and policy-supported. Overall, Phase 1 prioritizes low-cost, high-impact initiatives that improve access, data visibility, and workforce readiness.

Phase 2 shifts toward system integration and the institutionalization of digital health infrastructure. During this period, countries need to expand electronic health record systems to the district level, supported by the development of health information exchange (HIE) platforms. A critical focus is on enforcing interoperability standards to ensure different systems can communicate effectively. The phase also includes regional data exchange pilots, reflecting the growing importance of cross-border health data flows within Africa's broader Digital Single Market agenda. Additionally, support for the innovation ecosystem must be revamped to foster local solutions and private-sector participation, marking a transition from isolated pilots to coordinated national systems.

In Phase 3 the roadmap envisions a fully digital, data-driven, and intelligent health system. This includes deploying AI-assisted diagnostics and clinical decision-support tools, as well as achieving nationwide EHR coverage. At the continental level, the focus must expand to integrated digital health platforms and cross-country interoperability, aligning with Africa-wide digital integration efforts. The phase also highlights the need for sustainable domestic financing mechanisms to ensure long-term viability and reduce dependence on donors. At this stage, advanced capabilities such as predictive analytics and precision medicine become feasible, signaling a shift toward high-value, personalized, and efficient healthcare delivery.

The phased implementation plan should closely track progress across seven core dimensions—infrastructure, governance, human capital, data systems, innovation, financing, and regional integration—across three time horizons (short-, medium-, and long-term). In the short term, the emphasis should be on establishing foundational capabilities and policy frameworks. Infrastructure efforts should focus on mapping facility connectivity, expanding mobile broadband, and piloting solar power solutions to address energy gaps. Governance priorities should include establishing digital health units, enacting data protection laws, and developing telemedicine and AI ethics frameworks. At the same time, early investments in human capital development, with a focus on digital literacy for frontline health workers and pre-service training, are essential. Data systems should begin with unique patient identifiers. Countries need to strengthen DHIS2 and deploy surveillance and immunization platforms. In this phase, innovation is catalyzed through regulatory sandboxes and startup support, while financing efforts prioritize developing investment cases and aligning with donors. Regionally, coordination must begin with REC-led collaboration and cross-border surveillance pilots.

In the medium term, there should be a shift from pilots and fragmented initiatives to systematic scale-up and institutionalization. Infrastructure is expected to expand to achieve 50% broadband connectivity across health facilities, supported by cloud infrastructure and large-scale device procurement. Governance structures are expected to mature through the establishment of national digital health agencies, enforcement of interoperability standards, and the introduction of monitoring and evaluation (M&E) frameworks. Human capital development deepens through university-level programs, regional training hubs, and professional certification systems, ensuring a more specialized workforce. Data systems are expected to evolve significantly, with electronic health records reaching 50% of facilities, supported by national health information exchanges and enforced interoperability. Innovation ecosystems are expected to expand, with governments acting as anchor buyers, fostering public-private partnerships (PPPs) and regional innovation hubs. Financing becomes more structured, with 3–5% of national health budgets allocated to digital health, alongside blended finance models and gradual donor transition strategies. At the regional level, collaboration advances toward operational cross-border HIEs, continental frameworks, and joint procurement mechanisms.

Table 18.1. Phased implementation matrix across seven dimensions and three horizons.

Dimension	Short-Term (Yr 1–2)	Medium-Term (Yr 3–5)	Long-Term (Yr 5–10)
Infrastructure	Facility connectivity mapping; mobile broadband leveraging;	50% facility broadband; cloud infrastructure; device procurement at	80% broadband; national/ regional data centres; IoT-enabled facilities
Governance	Digital health unit; data protection law; telemedicine regulation;	National digital health agency; interoperability enforcement; M&E	Mature governance; cross-border harmonisation; AI regulation
Human Capital	Digital literacy for frontline workers; pre-service curricula;	University programmes; regional training hubs; professional certification	PhD programmes; competitive careers; self-sustaining workforce
Data Systems	Unique patient IDs; DHIS2 strengthening; e-immunisation;	EHR at 50% of facilities; national HIE; interoperability enforced	80% EHR coverage; AI-assisted diagnostics; real-time analytics
Innovation	Regulatory sandboxes; startup support; open	Government as anchor buyer; PPPs; regional	Vibrant domestic healthtech; African
Financing	Investment case development; initial budget commitments;	3–5% health budget to digital; blended finance; donor transition	Full domestic financing; sustainable recurrent funding
Regional	REC coordination; cross-border surveillance pilots;	Operational cross-border HIE; continental framework; joint	Pan-African platform; seamless cross-border care; continental

Source: Author's synthesis from Chapters 7–17

Over the long term, the implementation plan envisions a fully mature, integrated, and self-sustaining digital health ecosystem across Africa. Infrastructure targets include 80% broadband coverage, complemented by national and regional data centers and the deployment of IoT-enabled health facilities. Governance systems become highly advanced, marked by cross-border regulatory harmonization, mature institutional arrangements, and comprehensive AI regulation frameworks. Human capital reaches a sustainable stage, with PhD-level training programs, competitive career pathways, and a self-replenishing workforce. Data systems achieve 80% EHR coverage, enhanced by AI-assisted diagnostics and real-time analytics, enabling predictive and precision healthcare. Innovation ecosystems mature into vibrant domestic health technology industries, with African solutions scaling globally. Financing transitions fully to domestic, sustainable funding models, reducing reliance on external donors. Finally, regional integration culminates in a pan-African digital health platform that enables seamless cross-border care and is supported by continental governance mechanisms, closely aligning with the broader vision of Africa's Digital Single Market.

The phasing must be adaptive rather than rigid. Countries at different starting points will enter the framework at different stages—Rwanda and Kenya may already be in medium-term implementation for some dimensions, while still in short-term for others. The assessment tools described in Section 18.5 enable each country to locate itself on the maturity continuum and to develop a contextually appropriate implementation sequence. The key principle is not that every country follows the same timeline, but that every country invests in foundations before applications and enablers alongside layers.

18.4 Stakeholder Roles

Digital health transformation is not the responsibility of any single actor. It requires coordinated action across government, the private sector, development partners, civil society, and academic institutions, each playing distinct yet complementary roles. The governance structures described in Chapter 15—dedicated digital health units, multi-stakeholder steering committees, and cross-sector coordination mechanisms—provide the institutional framework for this coordination.

Governments bear primary responsibility for strategy, governance, financing, and accountability. They must establish dedicated digital health units or agencies with clear mandates, authority, and resources—as Kenya has done with its Division of Digital Health and Australia with its statutory Australian Digital Health Agency. Governments must develop and enforce data standards, data protection, and cybersecurity regulations. They must allocate 3–5% of health budgets to digital health, moving from the current average of less than 1%. They must procure from local innovators, creating market demand that enables domestic enterprises to grow. And they must embed digital health in health worker training curricula at all levels.

India's ABDM, led by the National Health Authority and backed by the Prime Minister's direct endorsement, underscores the importance of high-level political ownership. Brazil's phased digitalization of the SUS demonstrates how governments can sequence investments across a federated system. Thailand's embedding of digital health within the national economic transformation agenda ensures sustained political attention. For African governments, the key insight is that digital health is not an ICT project—it is a health system transformation that requires leadership from the health ministry, cross-ministerial coordination, and sustained political commitment from the highest levels.

The private sector drives innovation, develops context-appropriate solutions, and builds sustainable business models. Africa's healthTech ecosystem—with over 120 health-focused technology hubs, enterprises such as mPharma, Helium Health, Vezeeta, and LifeBank, and cumulative investment exceeding USD 4 billion—represents a formidable asset. Governments should engage the private sector as partners, not merely as vendors, through regulatory sandboxes that enable innovation while managing risk, anchor buyer commitments that create predictable demand, public-private partnerships that align commercial incentives with public health objectives, and co-investment platforms that aggregate resources.

The private sector also includes telecommunications companies (Safaricom, MTN, Orange, Airtel), global technology firms (Microsoft, Google, AWS), and pharmaceutical companies—each bringing infrastructure, expertise, and investment capacity to accelerate digital health transformation. The key governance challenge is ensuring that private-sector engagement serves public health priorities, that data sovereignty is protected, and that commercial incentives align with equity and access—concerns examined in detail in Chapters 13 and 15.

Development partners must shift from project-based funding to strategic partnerships. They provide over 40% of digital health financing in Africa and have been instrumental in catalyzing digital health initiatives—but the dominance of external financing creates sustainability risks. Donor funding is typically project-based and time-limited, leading to parallel systems that may not be maintained. The 2025 financing disruption has made this transition urgent rather than optional.

Development partners should align investments with national strategies rather than donor preferences, use external funding to catalyze domestic and private resources rather than to substitute for them, plan explicit transition strategies that shift financial responsibility to domestic sources, and coordinate to avoid fragmentation that leads to incompatible systems. The Global Fund's co-financing requirements, Canada's IDRC matched-funding approach, and the Digital Investment Principles provide frameworks for this reformed partnership model.

Civil society and communities provide accountability, advocate for equity, and build the trust essential to digital health adoption. Community engagement is not a nice-to-have—it is a prerequisite for sustainable digital health. In Uganda, community dialogues on digital health privacy have built trust in electronic health records. In Jamaica, the Digital Health Strategy includes public awareness campaigns and community feedback mechanisms. In New Zealand, the Te Mana Raraunga Māori Data Sovereignty Network has asserted indigenous rights to community-derived health data.

Civil society organizations can serve as watchdogs, ensuring that digital health governance protects patient rights; as advocates, ensuring that marginalized populations are not excluded from digital health benefits; and as intermediaries, translating community needs into design requirements for digital health systems. Countries that deploy digital health technologies without building community trust risk adoption failure—a lesson reinforced by resistance and circumvention that have undermined digital health projects across the continent.

Academic and research institutions generate evidence, train the workforce, and develop innovations that sustain transformation. Africa's university system must expand health informatics programs to close the 50,000+ professional deficit documented in Chapter 11. Ethiopia's model, with 30+ universities producing 2,000+ health informatics graduates annually, demonstrates what is achievable through political commitment and systematic scaling at the university level.

Research institutions must embed implementation science in digital health deployments, build AI validation capacity using African datasets, and develop health technology assessment capacity to inform investment decisions—priorities examined in Chapter 12. The partnership between universities and the healthTech ecosystem—exemplified by UCT's d-school, Makerere's AI Lab, and Strathmore's @iLabAfrica—creates a virtuous cycle in which academic research generates innovations that enterprises scale, and enterprise experience generates research questions that academics investigate.

18.5 Regional Bodies Roles

No single African country—regardless of its resources or ambition—can address the full spectrum of digital health challenges independently. Regional collaboration enables resource pooling, harmonized standards, cross-border interoperability, collective problem-solving, and the economies of scale necessary to sustain investments in digital infrastructure and human capacity. Chapter 16 examined Africa's regional architecture in detail; this section highlights the specific roles that each institution must play in the decade ahead.

The African Union provides continental strategic direction through the Digital Transformation Strategy (2020–2030), the Continental AI Strategy (2024), and the Africa Declaration on Artificial Intelligence (2025). The AU has established the institutional framework—the Digital Health Technical Working Group, the Continental Interoperability Framework, and the African

Digital Health Investment Framework—but must now translate these frameworks into operational mechanisms with dedicated financing.

Specifically, the AU should develop a continental co-financing mechanism for digital health—modeled on the EU's Digital Europe Program, which allocates EUR 7.5 billion, or on PAHO's Revolving Funds, which procured more than USD 900 million in health supplies during the 2024–2025 biennium. Such a mechanism could mobilize and pool resources from bilateral and multilateral sources, multilateral development banks, including the African Development Bank, regional development funds, and instruments such as the Africa50 infrastructure fund to co-finance national digital health infrastructure on a matched-funding basis, thereby incentivizing domestic investment and providing catalytic external support.

Africa CDC has emerged as the continent's preeminent institution for digital disease surveillance, with the Integrated Disease Surveillance and Response system connecting all 55 AU Member States; the Africa Pathogen Genomics Initiative expanding sequencing capacity from fewer than 10 to more than 30 countries; and the 2025 Health Security and Sovereignty Agenda asserting African leadership in health data governance. Africa CDC's role should expand beyond surveillance to serve as a continental center of excellence for digital health governance, standards harmonization, and workforce development—comparable to the ECDC's role in Europe and complementary to WHO AFRO's normative function.

The 2025 bilateral health MOU negotiations have underscored Africa CDC's unique role as the institutional voice for African health data sovereignty. Africa CDC's declaration that health sovereignty 'does not mean isolation but signals a new model of partnership articulates a principle that should guide the continent's digital health governance: African countries must retain control over their health data while remaining connected to global health networks. Africa CDC should develop continental guidelines for health data-sharing agreements that protect sovereignty while enabling essential cross-border collaboration for pandemic preparedness and health security.

Regional Economic Communities are the building blocks of African integration and the operational vehicles for cross-border digital health collaboration. The EAC's cross-border HIE serving 50,000+ patients, ECOWAS's digital vaccination certificates, which have achieved a 95% reduction in fraud, and SADC's malaria surveillance network, which has achieved 40% faster outbreak detection, demonstrate what RECs can accomplish. Looking ahead, RECs should establish shared health informatics training hubs serving clusters of countries with similar linguistic and health system characteristics—a Francophone West African hub anchored by UCAD in Senegal, an East African hub at MUHAS in Tanzania, and a Southern African hub at UCT.

RECs should also harmonize data protection regulations across their blocs, develop regional procurement frameworks for digital health technologies, and pilot cross-border telemedicine services that connect smaller member states to specialist centers in larger ones. PAHO's 2025–2031 Subregional Cooperation Strategy for Central America—which addresses digital transformation, interoperability, and access to migrant health care—provides a model for REC-level digital health coordination that explicitly links digital tools to health service access for mobile populations.

WHO AFRO provides normative guidance, technical leadership, and coordination through the Digital Health Atlas, assessment tools, and regional frameworks. WHO AFRO should strengthen its role as the knowledge broker linking national implementations to global evidence and standards, and develop a continental benchmarking dashboard that tracks digital health maturity across all member states and enables peer learning.

18.6 Measuring Progress: Readiness and Maturity Assessment

Digital health maturity models provide structured frameworks for assessing the sophistication, reach, and effectiveness of a country's digital health ecosystem. They serve as diagnostic tools and strategic roadmaps, enabling governments, development partners, and the private sector to assess current capabilities, benchmark performance against peers, and prioritize investments to maximize impact. In the African context—where resources are scarce, and health needs are acute—maturity models are indispensable for ensuring that investments are targeted, sequenced, and sustainable.

Figure 18.2. Digital Health Maturity Progression from Nascent to Leading

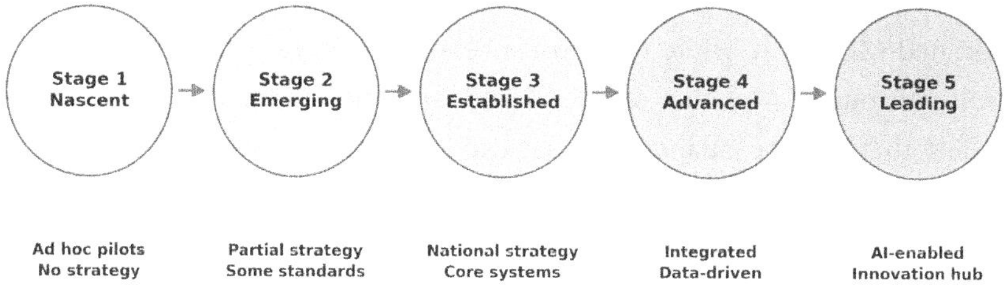

Source: Adapted from WHO (2022); Author's Elaboration

Most maturity models follow a five-stage progression.

- At the nascent stage, digital health efforts are ad hoc, donor-driven, and fragmented, with no national strategy or standards in place.
- At the early stage, countries have begun developing strategies and piloting systems, but interoperability remains limited.
- The established stage features a national strategy, allocated budgets, core operational systems, and a cadre of trained professionals.
- Advanced countries have achieved widespread interoperability, data-driven decision-making, and robust innovation ecosystems.
- The leading stage—aspirational for most—features AI-enabled health systems, real-time analytics, and a vibrant digital health economy.

Several validated tools support digital health assessment. The WHO Global Digital Health Monitor (GDHM) scores countries on a composite index covering leadership and governance, strategy, legislation, workforce, standards, infrastructure, and services. The Global Digital Health Index, developed by HealthEnabled, assesses readiness across seven categories closely aligned with the technology stack discussed in this book. The Performance of Routine Information System Management (PRISM) framework has been adapted for digital health in Tanzania, Uganda, and Ghana. The WHO Digital Health Atlas catalogs implementations and enables cross-country comparisons.

Chile's Salud Digital strategy includes quarterly progress reviews with a dedicated M&E unit, while Argentina's Federal Digital Health Strategy reports results through a public online dashboard—both offering accountability models that can be adapted by African countries. Brazil's RNDS employs staged rollouts, managing complexity through incremental maturation. Estonia's X-Road evolved from basic data exchange to a comprehensive digital public infrastructure over two decades.

The distribution of digital health maturity across African regions, based on the WHO Global Digital Health Monitor, shows that East Africa has a relatively balanced profile, with most countries in the Emerging stage (45%), followed by Established (25%), Nascent (20%), and Advanced (10%), indicating steady progress toward system integration. West Africa presents a mixed picture, with a high share in both Nascent (35%) and Emerging (40%) stages, alongside 20% in the Established stage and only 5% in the Advanced stage, suggesting ongoing expansion of foundational systems but limited advancement toward fully mature ecosystems. In contrast, Southern Africa demonstrates stronger maturity, with lower Nascent levels (15%) and higher proportions in Established (30%) and Advanced (20%), reflecting relatively robust infrastructure and institutional capacity.

Central Africa remains the least mature region, with a majority of countries in the Nascent stage (55%) and minimal representation in the Established (8%) and Advanced (2%) stages, underscoring persistent structural and institutional challenges. By contrast, North Africa exhibits one of the most advanced profiles, with only 10% in the Nascent stage and substantial shares in the Established (35%) and Advanced (25%) stages, indicating stronger policy frameworks, infrastructure, and system integration.

Figure 18.3. Benchmarking Countries in African Regions

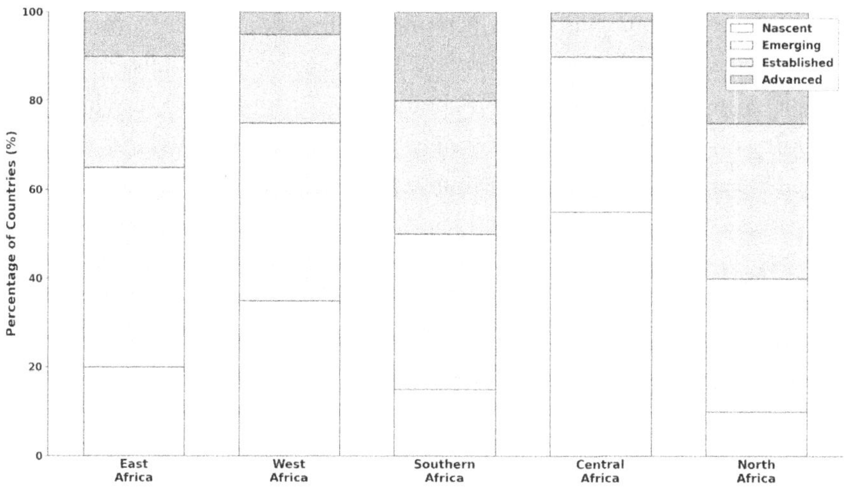

Source: WHO GDHM (2023); GDHI (2023); Country Reports

Overall, significant regional disparities persist across the continent, with Southern and North Africa leading in maturity, East and West Africa progressing through transitional phases, and Central Africa lagging, underscoring the need for targeted investments and coordinated policy interventions.

Country journeys offer transferable lessons: Rwanda achieved government-led transformation through centralized governance and alignment with universal health coverage; Kenya leveraged its innovation ecosystem and multi-stakeholder governance; Ethiopia built foundations at scale through pre-service health informatics training at 30+ universities; Nigeria harnessed private-sector innovation amid governance complexity. These trajectories show that rapid advancement in maturity is achievable—but only with sustained political commitment, adequate investment, and disciplined execution of phased strategies.

The critical lesson is that assessment should drive action through a practical five-step framework: countries need to conduct a comprehensive baseline assessment using validated tools; translate findings into a quantified gap analysis that identifies the most critical weaknesses; develop and update their digital health strategies, along with costed implementation plans that include measurable targets, identified funding, and clear accountability; implement phased interventions with built-in monitoring; and establish learning loops that enable evidence-based course correction. The assessment phase should be completed within six months and should actively involve all stakeholders—including the private sector, civil society, and development partners—to foster ownership and ensure the strategy reflects diverse perspectives.

18.7 Path Forward

Africa enters this decade of transformation with competitive advantages unmatched by any other region. The world's youngest and fastest-growing population—with a median age of 19 years—creates both demand for digital health services and the workforce capacity to deliver them. Mobile-first innovation has already produced globally significant solutions: M-Pesa transformed financial inclusion; DHIS2 became the world's most widely used health information system; and Zipline pioneered drone-delivered medical supplies. The continent's leapfrog potential enables the adoption of emerging technologies—cloud computing, AI, and genomics—without replicating the legacy-system constraints that burden high-income health systems. A disease burden that includes HIV, TB, malaria, and emerging infectious diseases, along with a rising non-communicable disease profile, creates urgent demand that drives innovation. Growing political momentum through the AU, Africa CDC, and RECs provides the institutional scaffolding for continental coordination.

The evidence presented across eighteen chapters leads to seven commitments that Africa's digital health stakeholders must make:

1. **Invest in foundations before applications.** Infrastructure, identity, interoperability, and analytics must be prioritized as the layers on which all applications depend. Countries that invest in these foundational layers build sustainable digital health ecosystems; those that invest only in applications create fragile, project-dependent implementations that collapse when donor funding ends. The sequencing principle is clear: connectivity before

telemedicine, identifiers before records, standards before exchange, and analytics before AI.

This does not mean delaying application deployment—it means deploying applications on solid foundations. Kenya's simultaneous investment in its Master Patient Index, national HIE, and KenyaEMR shows that foundations and applications can advance in parallel when guided by an integrated architecture. The mistake is deploying applications in isolation, without the underlying layers to sustain performance.

2. Finance for sustainability, not for projects. The shift from donor-dependent, project-based financing to domestically anchored, lifecycle-costed investment is the single most important structural reform the digital health sector in Africa must undertake. The 2025 financing disruption—with a USD 12 billion shortfall from PEPFAR/USAID restructuring—has demonstrated, with devastating clarity, the vulnerability of external dependence.

Africa requires a balanced financing mix, with heavy upfront investment in infrastructure and sustained support for systems, skills, and governance. Infrastructure accounts for approximately $12.5 billion in total investment requirements, far exceeding those of all other pillars. This reflects the high cost of expanding broadband connectivity, data centers, cloud infrastructure, and reliable power systems. Notably, infrastructure financing is relatively balanced across the three sources, with strong contributions from both governments and the private sector. Data systems and standards follow at around $4.5 billion, driven by the need for interoperable health information systems, electronic health records, and national health information exchanges. Innovation ecosystems ($4.0 billion) and human capacity development ($3.5 billion) also require substantial investment, highlighting the importance of building local digital health innovation, workforce skills, and institutional capabilities.

Figure 18.4. Estimated Investment Need by Strategic Pillar (2024-2030)

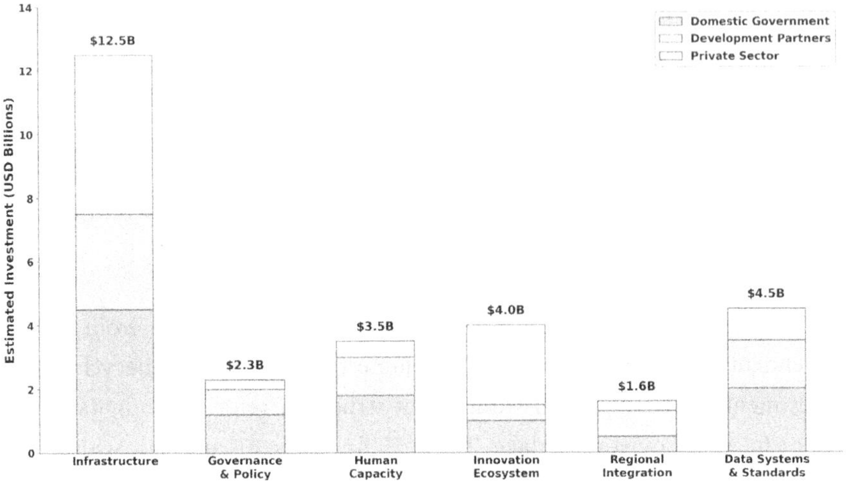

Source: Author's Elaboration

Governance and regulatory frameworks ($2.3 billion) and regional integration ($1.6 billion) are comparatively smaller but remain critical areas of investment. Governance investments focus on policy development, regulatory strengthening, and institutional coordination, while regional integration supports cross-border data sharing, interoperability frameworks, and continental alignment through initiatives such as the African Digital Single Market. Across most pillars, domestic governments must provide the largest share of funding, particularly for governance and human capacity, while development partners play a significant complementary role, especially in capacity building and regional initiatives. The private sector needs to play a key role in infrastructure and innovation investment, where commercial incentives and public–private partnerships are strongest.

Governments must increase digital health budget allocations from less than 1% to 3–5% of health budgets. Every digital health investment must include five-year total cost-of-ownership projections—consistent with Chile's mandatory requirement. Innovative financing instruments—earmarked technology levies, blended finance, and diaspora bonds—must complement traditional budget allocations. Regional co-financing mechanisms modeled on the EU's Digital Europe Program and PAHO's Revolving Funds should pool resources across countries. The African Leadership Meeting, the Lusaka Agenda, and Africa CDC's New Public Health Order all position domestic resource mobilization as a strategic imperative. It is time to translate these commitments into budget lines.

3. **Build the workforce the stack demands.** The estimated 50,000+ professional deficit in health informatics is the single most significant barrier to sustainable digital health transformation. Without the people to design, implement, manage, and improve digital health systems, every other investment is at risk. The deficit cannot be closed by conventional training pipelines alone—it requires creative approaches that integrate pre-service training, regional training hubs, online and blended learning, professional certification, and demand-generating policy mandates.

Concretely, countries should take five workforce actions.

- First, create or update national digital health competency frameworks for various cadres—doctors, nurses, community health workers, health information officers, managers, and educators.
- Second, embed those competencies in pre-service curricula at medical, nursing, public health, and allied health training institutions, rather than adding them only after graduation.
- Third, integrate digital health training into continuing professional development and licensing renewal to keep skills current as systems evolve.
- Fourth, ensure that every rollout of an EHR, telemedicine, or surveillance system includes facility-level coaching, super-users, and help desks—not only classroom training.
- Fifth, develop professional certification frameworks and career pathways to retain talent in the public sector, recognizing that without competitive salaries and clear career progression, trained professionals will leave for the private sector or abroad.

4. **Govern for trust.** Data protection, cybersecurity, AI ethics, and data sovereignty must be embedded as central—not peripheral—governance priorities. Digital health systems that are not trusted will not be used. Systems that are not secure will be compromised. Unvalidated AI tools will produce biased results. Data-sharing agreements that are not governed will erode sovereignty. The governance architecture described in Chapter 15 provides the framework; the political will to enforce it must come from the highest levels.

The 2025 bilateral data-sharing agreements between the US and African countries—bundled with health funding and requiring pathogen specimen sharing within five days—have made data governance an urgent strategic issue rather than an abstract policy concern. Kenya's court intervention suspending its agreement on data privacy grounds shows that strong domestic governance frameworks provide leverage. Africa CDC's Health Security and Sovereignty Agenda offers continental guidance. Every country must ensure that its data protection framework is robust enough to govern health data amid growing international pressure.

5. **Innovate locally, collaborate regionally, connect globally.** Africa's healthTech ecosystem, leadership in open-source platforms, and infrastructure for cross-border collaboration position the continent to develop solutions that serve African populations and contribute to global digital health. The healthTech enterprises examined in Chapter 13—mPharma, Helium Health, Vezeeta, LifeBank, Access Afya, and Zipline—demonstrate that African innovation can achieve significant scale and impact.

Regional collaboration through the AU, RECs, and Africa CDC enables the pooling of resources, harmonization of standards, and economies of scale that no single country can achieve alone. The EAC's cross-border HIE, ECOWAS's digital vaccination certificates, and SADC's surveillance network demonstrate what is achievable. Global connections—through the WHO's Global Strategy on Digital Health 2028–2033, the I-DAIR collaborative, and South–South partnerships with India, Brazil, and the Caribbean—ensure that Africa both contributes to and benefits from global knowledge flows.

6. **Measure what matters.** Readiness and maturity assessments must move from periodic exercises to institutionalized governance tools. Assessment without action is academic; action without measurement is blind. Countries should conduct comprehensive baseline assessments using validated tools (GDHM, GDHI), establish national digital health dashboards with publicly accessible indicators, implement quarterly progress reviews with defined accountability mechanisms, and build learning loops to enable evidence-based course correction.

Chile's quarterly M&E reviews, Argentina's public online dashboards, and India's ABDM real-time monitoring provide models. The WHO's Digital Health Atlas and the Global Digital Health Index provide internationally comparable frameworks. Africa should develop a continental benchmarking mechanism—managed by WHO AFRO or Africa CDC—that tracks maturity across all member states and enables peer learning, healthy competition, and collective accountability.

7. **Act with urgency.** The convergence of health system challenges, demographic pressures, technological opportunities, and financing disruption creates a window of action that will not remain open indefinitely. Africa's population is projected to double by 2050, reaching 2.5 billion. The burden of communicable diseases persists, while non-communicable diseases are rising rapidly. Climate change is expanding the geographic range of vector-borne diseases. The 2025 financing disruption has exposed the fragility of externally dependent health systems. The technologies needed for transformation—mobile platforms, cloud computing, AI, genomics—are available, affordable, and increasingly proven in African contexts.

Africa's digital health transformation is not a luxury—it is a prerequisite for universal health coverage, health security, and the health outcomes that 1.4 billion people deserve. Every year of delay increases the cost of transformation, widens the gap between Africa and other regions, and prolongs preventable suffering that digitally enabled health systems can reduce. The foundations described in this book are achievable. The enablers are identifiable. The roadmap is clear. What remains is sustained commitment —from governments, the private sector, development partners, civil society, and the health professionals who will build and operate these systems—to invest with discipline, execute with coherence, and persist with the patience that systemic transformation demands.

18.8 Conclusion

This book has presented a comprehensive analysis of digital health in Africa: its foundations, enablers, challenges, and extraordinary potential. The Digital Health Technology Stack—five foundational layers and six cross-cutting enablers—provides a unifying analytical framework that situates individual interventions within their broader architectural context and reveals the interdependencies that determine success or failure.

The chapters preceding this one documented the scale of the challenge and the grounds for measured optimism. Africa has achieved near-universal coverage of digital health strategies, deployed DHIS2 in 47 countries, built a healthTech ecosystem that has attracted billions in investment, established continental governance through the AU and Africa CDC, expanded genomics capacity from 10 to 30+ countries, trained thousands of health informatics professionals through regional academies, and demonstrated the capacity for rapid, crisis-driven innovation during COVID-19. The continent possesses competitive advantages—a young population, a mobile-first innovation culture, leapfrog potential, and growing political momentum—that no other region can match.

Yet the gaps between strategy and implementation, between pilot and scale, and between aspiration and sustained investment remain Africa's central challenge. The evidence is unequivocal: deploying technology without parallel investment in governance, workforce, research, ecosystem support, regional cooperation, and sustainable financing produces systems that cannot be maintained, data that cannot be used, and innovations that cannot be sustained. The Digital Health Technology Stack is only as strong as its weakest layer.

The path forward is clear, though demanding. Invest in foundations. Finance for sustainability. Build the workforce. Govern with trust. Innovate locally, collaborate regionally, and connect globally. Measure what matters. Act with urgency. Africa's 1.4 billion people—and the generations that follow—depend on this path.

References

African Union Commission. (2015). Agenda 2063: The Africa We Want. AUC.

African Union Commission. (2020). Digital Transformation Strategy for Africa (2020–2030). AUC.

HealthEnabled. (2020). Global Digital Health Index: Methodology. HealthEnabled.

Ministry of Health, Kenya. (2021). National Digital Health Strategic Framework 2021–2025. GoK.

National Health Authority India. (2022). ABDM implementation progress report. NHA India.

PAHO. (2022). Information Systems for Health (IS4H): Regional framework. PAHO.

PATH Digital Square. (2022). Costing digital health transformation. PATH.

WHO. (2022). Global Digital Health Monitor: Country assessments. WHO.

WHO. (2023). Global strategy on digital health 2020–2025: Implementation review. WHO.

Index

E

G

S

T

V

List of Abbreviations

A4AI	The Alliance for Affordable Internet
ABDM	Ayushman Bharat Digital Mission
ABHA	Ayushman Bharat Health Account
ACHEST	African Center for Global Health and Social Transformation
ADHA	Australian Digital Health Agency
AfDB	African Development Bank
AFENET	The African Field Epidemiology Network
AFIDEP	African Institute for Development Policy
AFRO	WHO Regional Office for Africa
AHDO	Africa Health Data Observatory
AHIMA	American Health Information Management Association
AI	Artificial Intelligence
AIDA	Artificial Intelligence and Data Act
AIHW	The Australian Institute of Health and Welfare
AIMS	African Institute for Mathematical Sciences
ALM	The African Leadership Meeting
AMRH	African Medicines Regulatory Harmonization
AMU/UMA	Arab Maghreb Union
ANVISA	The Brazilian Health Regulatory Agency
AR	Augmented Reality
ASHA	Accredited Social Health Activist
ATU	African Telecommunications Union
AU	African Union
B2B	Business-to-Business

B2C	Business-to-Consumer
B2G	Business-to-Government
CARPHA	The Caribbean Public Health Agency
CBHI	Community-Based Health Insurance
CCSS	Caja Costarricense de Seguro Social (Costa Rica Social Security Fund)
CDA	Clinical Document Architecture
CDC	Centers for Disease Control and Prevention
CDISAH	Classification of Digital Interventions, Services and Applications in Health
CDSS	Clinical Decision Support Systems
CFIR	The Consolidated Framework for Implementation Research
CHAP	Climate Health Analytics Platform
CHT	Community Health Toolkit
CHW	Community Health Worker
CIHI	Canadian Institute for Health Information
CME	Continuing Medical Education
COSECSA	College of Surgeons of East, Central and Southern Africa
COVID-19	Coronavirus Disease 2019
CPD	Continuing Professional Development
CRTC	Canadian Radio-television and Telecommunications Commission
CSIRO	Commonwealth Scientific and Industrial Research Organization
DCC	Digital COVID Certificate
DFI	Development Finance Institution
DHIS2	District Health Information Software
DHTA	Digital Health Technology Assessment
DPGA	The Digital Public Goods Alliance
DPI	India has built a Digital Public Infrastructure

DS4H	Data Science for Health
DTS	Digital Transformation Strategy
EAC	East African Community
ECCAS	In contrast, the Economic Community of Central African States
ECDC	The European Center for Disease Prevention and Control
ECOWAS	Economic Community of West African States
EDCTP	The European and Developing Countries Clinical Trials Partnership
EHDS	European Health Data Space
EHIS	Estonian Health Information System
EHR	Electronic Health Record
EIOS	Epidemic Intelligence from Open Sources
ELSI	Research into ethical, legal, and social implications
EMR	Electronic Medical Record
ENAHPA	Ethiopian North American Health Professionals Association
ETL	Data warehouses ensure data quality through extract-transform-load
EU	European Union
FHIR	Fast Healthcare Interoperability Resources
GAVI	Global Alliance for Vaccines and Immunization
GCI	The latest International Telecommunication Union Global Cybersecurity Index
GDHCN	Global Digital Health Certification Network
GDHI	The WHO Digital Health Atlas, the Global Digital Health Index
GDHM	The WHO Global Digital Health Monitor
GDP	Gross Domestic Product
GDPR	General Data Protection Regulation
GIS	Geographic Information System
GSMA	Global System for Mobile Communications Association

GWAS	Genome-Wide Association Studies
HAQAA	Harmonization of African Higher Education Quality Assurance and Accreditation
HCEN	Historia Clinica Electronica Nacional
HDC	Health Data Center
HELINA	The Health and Biomedical Informatics Association of Sub-Saharan Africa
HIE	Health Information Exchange
HIE-CM	Health Information Exchange and Consent Manager
HIKM	Health Informatics Knowledge Management
HIM	Building on this, the health information management
HIS	Health Information System
HISO	Health Information Standards Organization
HISP	Health Information Systems Programme
HITAP	Health Intervention and Technology Assessment Program
HIV/AIDS	Human Immunodeficiency Virus / Acquired Immunodeficiency Syndrome
HMIS	National Informatics Center, provides a Hospital Management Information System
HPRS	Health Patient Registration System
HRIS	Human resource information systems
HTA	Health Technology Assessment
HTHA	The HealthTech Hub Africa
I-DAIR	The International Digital Health and AI Research Collaborative
ICD	International Classification of Diseases
ICD-10	The use of the International Classification of Diseases
ICT	Information and Communication Technology
ICU	Intensive Care Unit
IDI	Integrated Data Infrastructure
IDRC	International Development Research Center

IDSR	Integrated Disease Surveillance and Response
IHE	FHIR and Integrating the Healthcare Enterprise
IHI	Individual Healthcare Identifier
IMIA	The International Medical Informatics Association
IoT	Internet of Things
IP	Intellectual Property
IS4H	Information Systems for Health
IT	Information Technology
ITU	World Bank, the International Telecommunication Union
IVDR	In Vitro Diagnostic Regulation
JKUAT	Jomo Kenyata University of Agriculture and Technology
KNUST	Kwame Nkrumah University of Science and Technology
LEO	Low Earth Orbit
LGPD	Lei Geral de Proteção de Dados (Brazil General Data Protection Law)
LOINC	Logical Observation Identifiers, Names and Codes
LTE	Long-Term Evolution (4G standard)
MAST	Model for Assessment of Telemedicine
MDR	Medical Device Regulation
MFL	Master Facility List
MHRA	Medicines and Healthcare products Regulatory Agency
ML	Machine Learning
MOTECH	Mobile Technology for Community Health
MPI	Master Patient Index
MUHAS	MSc programs, including Muhimbili University of Health and Allied Sciences
NBN	National Broadband Network
NEHR	National Electronic Health Record

NGO	Non-Governmental Organization
NHA	National Health Authority (India)
NHI	National Health Index
NHMRC	National Health and Medical Research Council
NHNSFI	National Health Normative Standards Framework for Interoperability
NIMC	National Identity Management Commission
NIN	National Identification Number
NIS2	Network and Information Security
NITDA	National Information Technology Development Agency
NPRS	Namibia National Population Registry
OECD	Organisation for Economic Co-operation and Development
OOP	Out-of-Pocket (health payments)
PAHO	In the Caribbean, the Pan American Health Organization
PAVM	Information Exchange framework, the Partnership for African Vaccine Manufacturing
PBF	Performance-based financing
PEPFAR	Emergency Plan for AIDS and Relief
PHC	Primary Health Care
PHDC	Provincial Health Data Center
PIDA	Program for Infrastructure Development in Africa
PIPEDA	Personal Information Protection and Electronic Documents Act
PMIR	The Patient Master Identity Registry
POPIA	Protection of Personal Information Act
PPP	Public-Private Partnership
PRISM	The Performance of Routine Information System Management
RE-AIM	The Reach, Effectiveness, Adoption, Implementation, Maintenance
RIA	Research ICT Africa

RNDS	Rede Nacional de Dados em Saude
ROI	Return on Investment
SADC	Southern African Development Community
SARA	Service Availability and Readiness Assessment
SDG	Sustainable Development Goal
SMS	These technologies range from simple short message service
SUS	Unified Health System
TCO	Digital health investment requires comprehensive Total Cost of Ownership
TGA	Therapeutic Goods Administration
TI	Transparency International
UCSF	University of California, San Francisco
UHC	Universal Health Coverage
UPI	Unified Patient Identifier
USAID	United States Agency for International Development
USD	United States Dollar
VR	Virtual and Augmented Reality for Medical Training Virtual reality
WACS	West African College of Surgeons
WHO	World Health Organization

Made in the USA
Monee, IL
05 November 2026

67914385R00262